THE INVULNERABLE CHILD

THE INVULNERABLE CHILD

Edited by

E. James Anthony, MD
and
Bertram J. Cohler, PhD

The Guilford Press
New York   London

© 1987 The Guilford Press
A Division of Guilford Publications, Inc.
200 Park Avenue South, New York, N.Y. 10003

Printed in the United States of America

Library of Congress Cataloging-in-Publication Data

The Invulnerable child.

(The Guilford psychiatry series)
Includes bibliographies and indexes.
1. Children—Mental health—Forecasting.
2. Resilience (Personality trait)   3. Adjustment
(Psychology)   4. Mental illness—Social aspects.
I. Anthony, E. James (Elwyn James), 1916-   .
II. Cohler, Bertram J.   III. Series. [DNLM: 1. Adaptation, Psychological—in infancy & childhood.   2. Ego—in infancy & childhood.   3. Parent-Child Relations.
4. Personality Disorders—in infancy & childhood.
5. Probability.   WS 350.8.P3 I62]
RJ499.I68   1987   618.92′89   86-27120
ISBN 0-89862-227-1

To Beatrice and Irving Edison, my good companions and cherished friends for so many years who have loved me and helped me to build a little world of research and scholarship, a part of which is represented in this book. Our lives have been blended together in the common purpose of understanding the children better.

—E. James Anthony

To the families who have shown me how to be strong in the face of crisis, and who have so generously shared their experiences with me and with my collaborators in good times and in times of adversity.

—Bertram J. Cohler

Contributors

E. James Anthony, MD, Director of Psychotherapy, Chestnut Lodge, Rockville, Maryland

William Beardslee, MD, Department of Psychiatry, Harvard Medical School, Boston, Massachusetts

Bertram J. Cohler, PhD, Department of Behavioral Sciences, University of Chicago, Chicago, Illinois

Robert E. Cole, PhD, Department of Psychiatry, University of Rochester, Rochester, New York

Felton Earls, MD, Department of Psychiatry, Washington University School of Medicine, St. Louis, Missouri

Byron Egeland, PhD, Department of Educational Psychology, University of Minnesota, Minneapolis, Minnesota

Ellen A. Farber, PhD, Department of Psychology, State University of New York, Buffalo, New York

J. Kirk Felsman, EdD, Department of Psychiatry, Dartmouth Medical School, Hanover, New Hampshire

Lawrence Fisher, PhD, Veterans Administration Medical Center, Fresno, California, and the University of California at San Francisco, San Francisco, California

William Garrison, MD, Department of Psychiatry, Washington University School of Medicine, St. Louis, Missouri

Judith Goldman, ACSW, Erikson Institute, Chicago, Illinois

Cynthia L. Janes, MD, Department of Psychiatry, Washington University School of Medicine, St. Louis, Missouri

Ronald F. Kokes, PhD, Veterans Administration Medical Center, Fresno, California, and the University of California at San Francisco, San Francisco, California

Alice E. Moriarty, formerly Senior Psychologist, The Menninger Foundation, Topeka, Kansas

Lois Barclay Murphy, formerly of the Menninger Foundation, Topeka, Kansas

Judith S. Musick, PhD, Ounce of Prevention Fund, Chicago, Illinois

Edwin C. Peck, Jr., MD, PhD, Private Practice, Irvine, California

Patricia M. Perkins, MD, Department of Psychiatry, University of Rochester, Rochester, New York

Arnold J. Sameroff, MD, Department of Psychiatry and Human Behavior, Brown University Program in Medicine, Providence, Rhode Island

Ronald Seifer, MD, Department of Psychiatry and Human Behavior, Brown University Program in Medicine, Providence, Rhode Island

Katherine Klehr Spencer, PhD, formerly of the Department of Psychology, Northwestern University, Evanston, Illinois

Frances M. Stott, PhD, Erikson Institute, Chicago, Illinois

George E. Vaillant, MD, Department of Psychiatry, Dartmouth Medical School, Hanover, New Hampshire

David G. Weeks, MD, Department of Psychiatry, Washington University School of Medicine, St. Louis, Missouri

Julien Worland, MD, Department of Psychiatry, Washington University School of Medicine, St. Louis, Missouri

Lyman C. Wynne, MD, Department of Psychiatry, University of Rochester, Rochester, New York

Preface

There are several points about this book that should help to guide the reader through the theoretical and practical entanglements of a relatively new field of inquiry. First of all, the editors would like to emphasize that it is made up of *original* papers written specifically for this publication and devoted, one and all, to the central issues of resilience and competence. There is therefore a unity of aim and purpose but not in content and design that adds to the richness of the general offering. Second, having explored the field thoroughly, the editors were struck by the sparseness of the literature dealing with this important topic and sympathized with the comment of Garmezy and Nuechterlein that "only an occasional article brings some life into this empty scene." This may reflect the state of the art but what could account for this developmental lag? One would have thought that the picture of children triumphing over despairing, degrading, depressing, depriving, and deficient circumstances would have caught the immediate attention of both clinicians and researchers, but the survivors and thrivers appeared to pass almost unnoticed amidst the holocaust of disadvantage and the tragedies of those who succumbed to it. The clinical eye, since Hypocratic times, has been trained to detect even the most miniscule aspects of disease, while at the same time paying little heed to the health and well-being of those who would scarcely bring themselves to the attention of clinicians. And if by chance they make their appearance in the clinic, there are no professional schedules to record them. Whereas mental illness has generated a plethora of nosologies, health continues to be looked at as something outside the scope of clinical work. One can say somewhat simply that the mentally sound child or adult works well, plays well, feels well, loves well, copes well, and hopes well, but how would one set about pinning down the label. In more turgid terms, as put forward in the midtown-Manhattan project, the healthy ones are those who have resources that are "eugenically fortifying and immunizing against the potentially shattering impact of extreme exogenous adversity." There was no mention of what these resources might be, but clearly some stabilizing and organizing forces (whether internal or external), must help to counteract the powerful environmental pathogens.

Third, the reader should bear in mind that the age of this new field of risk is relatively young, being hardly more than 25 years old and that it is only in the last 15 years that the concept of invulnerability has taken its place alongside the clinical focus on vulnerability. In this short period of time, there has been a shift away from the disease entities toward good psychosocial capacities such as competence, coping, creativity, and confidence.

When the editors set us to put this book together, they were aware of the new knowledge that was scattered disconnectedly through the literature of the data being churned out independently in different locations and of the incipient theoretical constructions that were being grounded out but not too coherently. They did not seem to feel that the field was ready for a coordinated and comprehensive systematization. At present, it would appear that the major value of this publication is as a stimulus to the clinician, the researcher, and the theoretician. Each chapter was designed to add something to the total picture with beginning and ending overviews intended to offer the uninformed reader a helpful frame of reference. Among the experts involved are developmentalists, child clinicians, infant psychologists, risk researchers, psychophysiologists, and psychoanalysts. It is a pleasure to have among the collaborators two of the pioneers in this field, Lois Barclay Murphy and Alice Moriarty. What they had to say 10 years ago in their monumental, *Vulnerability, Coping and Growth* (1976), is still pertinent to our understanding of the field.

> Along the continuum of vulnerability, children may be distributed in different numbers: few if any are so robust, so completely lacking in small as well as moderate or major handicaps as to be totally free from some zone of vulnerability. Most children have a checkerboard fo strengths and weaknesses, or an Achilles heel, or a cluster of tendencies that interact in such a way as to produce one or another pattern of vulnerability as well as strength. Given an infant of greater or lesser initial adequacy decreases in vulnerability depend on outcomes of interaction between this child and its environment and the extent to which these outcomes compensate for early deficiences or allow for progress in mastery. Increases in vulnerability are seen when the interaction between the child and the environment results in new limitations or difficulties, new threats to homeostasis and to integration, new obstacles to learning, increased difficulties in mastering anxiety, or negative expectancies.

Those of us working in the field today are especially aware of this "continuum of vulnerability," this "checkerboard of strengths and weaknesses," this "interaction between the child and its environment" and the "compensations" that development continuously brings with it. With such an approach, one can set about the task of preventive interventions with more assurance than ever before, so that in time, the promise of primary prevention, almost an alchemist's dream a few decades ago, may be within the range of fulfillment. The concept of continuum also serves to remind us of the importance of individual differences even in the same family of children and within the same twinship.

We have preferred to use the term "invulnerability" rather than resilience in the title of this book because it seemed to us to make the point of psychological invincibility much more strikingly than the term resilience. We would however, agree with Murphy and Moriarty (1976) when they say:

> in our use of "vulnerability" there is no completely invulnerable child—we are concerned with the degree and locus of vulnerability in relation to the intensity and quality of stress. When the child's most vulnerable area is confronted by severe stress for that area, *some degree* of breakdown (somatic or psychological "disintegrative reaction") is likely to occur even though the child does not become delinquent or mentally ill. (p. 248)

To this we would add that the child is also relatively invulnerable when the stress is meaningless within the frame of the child's phase of development, which psychoanalysts refer to as "nonspecific trauma."

Most of the contributions to this book have a longitudinal perspective, allowing for the data to be examined prospectively, retrospectively, or cross-sectionally, thus illuminating the process of development under conditions of risk. Scrutinizing this "epigenetic landscape," as Piaget and Waddington have referred to it, brings into closer view the vicissitudes of resilience during the course of the life history with robustness giving place to vulnerability and *vice versa*, and the two together create a rich and varied tapestry of strength and weakness. Here, in this book, our major concern is with the elements of strength.

As with all undertakings of this nature, we have acknowledgments to make: to our publishers who have helped us so much behind the scenes; to all of our contributors who have waited patiently for the outcome and have generously rewritten sections on request; and to Professor Norman Garmezy who recently shared a podium in Sweden discussing vulnerability with one of the editors (EJA) and, as always, generously shared his thinking in this area. Finally, one of us (EJA) whose resilience was taxed by fate a few years ago, owes a large debt of gratitude to his wife, Virginia Q. Anthony (Ginger), whose loving vitality (as in many instances of risk) harnassed the forces of his recuperation.

E. James Anthony, MD
Bertram Cohler, PhD

Contents

Introduction I

1

Risk, Vulnerability, and Resilience: An Overview

E. JAMES ANTHONY
Chestnut Lodge Hospital

The limits of thought in any age are set not so much from the outside, by the fullness or poverty of experience that meets the mind, as from within, by the power of conception and the wealth of formulative notions with which the mind meets experience (Langer, 1942). Most new discoveries, as Langer points out, are "suddenly-seen things" that were always there. What the new idea does is to illuminate presences that simply had no form before the light fell on them and lit up the entire intellectual landscape. As one examines the history of science, one can see such ideas at work in different minds from the same era. At such times, it would seem as if scientific opinion was highly receptive and resonant to these ideational seeds germinating in certain prepared minds. They are not theories, but rudiments of potential theories; yet they raise crucial questions that coalesce the thoughtful activities of a field. Such ideas might be termed "generative," since they precede the formation of theory, ask the important questions, and are conducive to necessary research. Being striking in themselves, they also tend to captivate the popular mind and so accumulate a mythology that adds distortion and misconception to the aura of novelty. Despite this, their vitality is such that increasing numbers of researchers are drawn toward their investigation.

A Generative Group of Ideas

The generative ideas presented here are those concerned with risk, vulnerability, and resilience, together with neighboring concepts that have grown along side them and contributed to their elucidation.

In discussing "risk," one has first to remember that in addition to being a scientific abstraction, this potent idea also relates to the terrible actualities of life that equally encompass the worlds of researcher and rescuer and therefore are likely to contaminate their appraisal. Where risk is concerned, no man is an island. Each individual is someone in particular who is constantly subjected to an individually perceived barrage of hazards. Furthermore, because risks are also internally represented, the actualities, bad enough in themselves, undergo transmogrification and may become grotesquely alarming. The processes involved in risk are therefore both external and internal, both objective and subjective, and both consciously and unconsciously determined. These elaborations add further dimensions to traumatic exposures and amplify the experience by degrees that are difficult at the present time to evaluate precisely. Depending, therefore, on what the individual mind does with it, the selfsame risk may be apprehended by one individual as a trivial event and by another as a personal disaster.

The notion of "vulnerability" first came to prominence when individual and group differences at various stages of life were being investigated, and there were growing concerns with individuality and identity. As in much research, it took time and effort to establish the truism that people are different and react differently to seemingly similar events, and that the differences are located in the apperceptive mechanisms, the biological makeup, and the psychosocial setting. For example, in animal research, a high degree of variance was found with respect to the lethal effects of certain poisons on laboratory rats. When they were grouped together, their vulnerability significantly decreased, and when they were placed in isolation, their vulnerability increased. It was also found that the hypervulnerable reaction could be transmitted across generations by selective breeding. It would appear, then, that as with many complex behaviors in the biopsychosocial field, the expression of vulnerability is a function of transactions between the different areas of the field.

Now, at the opposite end to this heightened susceptibility, "resilience" was discovered to be similarly detectable in both animal and human subjects. For instance, when laboratory rats were placed in various types of extreme environments, a certain small percentage not only survived the ordeal but seemingly thrived on it, as evidenced in greater maze-running resourcefulness and enhanced exploratory behavior.

The resilience of human subjects emerged in epidemiological studies on susceptibility to coronary heart disease, where time sampling showed that the patterns of illness created by different susceptibilities were likely to continue for as long as 20 years or more, with the vulnerable subjects maintaining their higher illness rates and the resilient ones remaining comparatively healthy (Hinkle, 1972). Linked to this dispositional tendency was a responsiveness to significant changes in social and interpersonal relations. These findings were followed by the surprising observation that a small number of individuals could live through major changes in relationships, deprivations, and dislocations, and yet exhibit little if any overt evidence of illness. The phenomenon was associated with two factors: no history of any pre-existing susceptibilities, and the presence of certain personality characteristics that "insulated" the individual from detrimental life experiences (Hinkle, 1974).

> The healthiest members of our samples often showed little psychological reaction to events and situations which caused profound reactions in other members of the group. The loss of a husband or wife, the separation from one's family, the isolation from one's friends, community or country, the frustration of apparent important desires, or the failure to obtain apparently important goals produced no profound or lasting reaction. (Hinkle, 1974, pp. 40–41)

The investigators were so intrigued by this apparent "psychoimmunity" to the effects of deprivation and change that they took a closer look at the psychological concomitants and came up with what I call here the "Meursault phenomenon," from the name of the leading character in *The Stranger* by Camus (1954). Hinkle (1974) referred to an "almost sociopathic flavor" typifying these "invulnerables," reminiscent of some form of narcissistic disorder.

> Many of these people displayed a distinct awareness of their own limitations and their physiological needs. They behaved as if their own wellbeing were one of their primary concerns. They avoided situations that would make demands on them if they felt they could not, or did not want to meet these demands. An employed man or woman might refuse a promotion because he did not want the increased responsibility, refuse a transfer because it was "too much trouble," or refuse to work overtime because it might be too tiring—despite the fact that each of these changes might have increased his income, increased his prestige, or increased his opportunity to go ahead in his occupation. As family members, such people might refuse to take the responsibility for an aged or ill parent or sibling, giving as an explanation a statement implying that it would be "too much for me." If such a person learned that family members or relatives in a foreign country were in need, or were being oppressed, he might give little evidence of concern about this, and he might explain, if asked, that he saw no reason to worry about it since there was nothing he could do about it. If it was the lot and life of such a person to be poorer, or to live alone, he seemed to feel no need to be unhappy about this or to rebel against it. (p. 41)

In turning to Meursault (Camus, 1954), we first encounter him as he reacts to his mother's death, and our first clue to his nature is that he does *not* react. In fact, he feels no emotion stronger than annoyance. His mother's death is an imposition upon him, since he must trouble himself to appear grieved, to accept condolences, and to pretend that their relationship was meaningful to him. He preserves a flat level of affect. After the burial, he begins a desultory love affair, but again feels nothing. When he is offered a better job, he refuses. His job means nothing more than onerous routine. Indeed, the idea of "better" or "worse" among his activities and relationships is quite foreign to him. Anything is as good as any other thing. In fact, there is a strategic and utter selfishness based solely on the convenience and comfort of the self—a rational egotism. Meursault is a passive, detached observer of life who will not involve himself or engage himself in the world around him. This detachment, this defensive distancing, insulates him from all disturbing psychosocial impingements from the environment. As will become clear later, this represents only one form of invulnerability, but the mechanisms involved are a contribution to our understanding of psychoimmunization.

Neighboring Concepts

One of the surprises constantly encountered in psychiatric research (as in many other areas of research) is the way in which language determines the shape and direction of investigations. Researchers may begin their exploratory operations in the same research area, but they then proceed to look at the phenomena confronting them differently; what is more, they label them differently. As a result, parallel processes of inquiry are established, each with its own lexicon, and the language differences give rise to the illusion that one is dealing with quite different study areas. Eventually some inquisitive researcher calls attention to the overlapping concepts and the basic similarities of the research fields.

Stress investigators coming from varied theoretical and empirical backgrounds may currently be converging on a central group of factors related to both stress-induced illness and resilience. What makes it difficult to encompass this development within a single conceptual framework is the fact that different researchers have tended to confine their work to particular amounts of stress. For example, some have focused on acute life-threatening stresses leading to posttraumatic stress disorders; others have confined themselves to subacute life-changing stresses (with changes for better or for worse) resulting in different forms of psychosomatic illnesses; and, more recently, a few have examined chronic life-irritating stresses that constitute the wear and tear of everyday life in pressuring modern environments. It may turn out that those at one extreme of the spectrum are vulnerable to any degree or kind of stress—reacting typically with exquisite awareness to the slightest threats from the outside (Cohen & Lazarus, 1973), feeling themselves to be at the mercy of external controlling forces (Rotter, 1966), competing constantly and excessively against everyone and everything (Friedman & Rosenman, 1974), and eventually collapsing into helpless and hopeless positions (Schmale, 1972). In contrast, there may be others who respond to stress by maintaining a confident control over the environment, by remaining hopeful and helpful in distressing situations, and by taking responsibility for what occurs to them. In some studies, the internal locus of control expectancy has been equated with competence, coping ability, and *relative invulnerability* to debilitating effects of stressful events (Campbell, Converse, & Rodgers, 1976). With respect to sensitivity, laboratory research on physiological and psychological responses to threatening stimuli has demonstrated that certain individuals tend to repress their awareness of such stimuli and that this repression is associated with better recovery or "bouncing back" (Cohen & Lazarus, 1973). However, further study could reveal that this "ostrich-type" behavior, while working to advantage in some circumstances, could prove deleterious and dysfunctional when survival is at stake and flight reactions are imperative.

So far, only a very limited notion of "invulnerability" has emerged from stress theory. Some investigators have argued that early experience with certain types of events may "inoculate" the individual against later stressful events (Bornstein, Clayton, Halikas, Maurice, & Robins, 1973) and perhaps increase resilience. There have also been suggestions, based on reasonably good empirical data, that a strong support system in the social environment may add to psychoimmunization (Caplan & Killilea, 1976), in that highly stressful events combined with high social support have been found to be significantly less pathogenic than highly stressful events in combination with low social support. However, it is still not clear at the present time how such family, neighborhood, and friendship networks function in the life stress process; what are needed are objective measures regarding such structures and the degree of the individual's participation in them.

During recent years, stress research has passed through a series of constructs manifesting increasing sophistication. Earlier, there was a "victimization" hypothesis (drawn from studies of extreme situations such as combat and concentration camps); this was followed by the suggestion of psychophysiological strain as an intermediating adverse change, and then by the notion of a preceding disorder in the individual that conduces to stress, which in turn exacerbates the original disorder. It is only recently that a "vulnerability" hypothesis has taken shape, possibly influenced by risk research, that takes into account the dispositional characteristics of the individual and the "holding" and "facilitating" qualities of the milieu (Dohrenwend & Dohrenwend, 1981).

In a stress–vulnerability model (Gore, 1981), interactions are considered in terms of life changes, objectively and subjectively appraised, and in terms of the buffering provided by measurable social supports that help to mitigate the strain on the individual and release his coping behavior. However, in this model, the main focus is on the transactional activities set in motion by the supportive network, and not on the individual's resistance.

The methodologies of stress and risk research have also gone different ways. First, risk research has been more prospective and stress research more retrospective in design; second, the former has engaged in broad-range assessment procedures, whereas the latter has confined itself in general to pinpointing proximal events; and finally, risk research has for the past decade occupied itself more thoroughly than stress research with notions of resilience and invulnerability. In brief, stress has tended to be investigated in the laboratory and risk in the field. This has resulted in stress research's being more controlled, more precise, more quantitative, more event-conscious than life-conscious, more restricted in its general clinical application, and more atheoretical. Kellam (1974) has recalled the distinction put forward by Berlin (1953) between people who are temperamentally "hedgehogs" and constantly on the lookout for connections and unifying theories, and people who are "foxes" and content to examine in detail the individual aspects of life without searching for interrelationships, theoretical frameworks, or comprehensive theories. The general trend would suggest that stress researchers are inclined to be "foxes"—strictly empirical in their approach, parsimonious in the use of theory, and stuck with relatively simple atheoretical inventories of life events that are thought to be stressful. Kellam is of the opinion that it is high time for them to move on to a second stage that would explore the conceptual framework of stressful life events more broadly. Risk researchers are more inclined to be "hedgehogs." The elaborate scientific stronghold that they have constructed in the past decades is almost confusing in its patterned interrelations, its colorful clinical illustrations, and its profusion of "grounded" theory. And, like hedgehogs, they can be prickly in defense of their more clinically diffuse investigations.

For reasons that are not quite clear, the stress concept has not appealed to clinicians with a psychodynamic orientation as much as the trauma concept has, although psychiatrists have found the nosological concept of stress disorders, particularly the posttraumatic variety, highly pertinent to their work. The notion of trauma was crucial to Freud's earlier thinking, at first as a recent etiological agent but subsequently as a remoter causal one reaching back into early childhood. As Freud's understanding of intrapsychic conflict grew, he began to relinquish the traumatic hypothesis, in which he had invested so much, until it almost faded out of the picture altogether. Its usefulness persisted in the notion of a traumatic neurosis with a limited time span and a fairly characteristic clinical picture that ran parallel, at least for a while, to the ongoing developmental conflict and interacted with it.

In the psychoanalytic concept of trauma, the basic function of the mental apparatus is the re-establishment of stability after a disturbance by external stimuli through combinations of discharge and "binding." When the homeostasis is affected, a state of emergency exists, and one is then concerned with the capacity to master the situation. This capacity was thought to depend on both constitutional and acquired experiential factors: "There are stimuli of such overwhelming intensity that they have a traumatic effect on anyone; other stimuli are harmless for most persons but traumatic for certain types with a readiness to become overwhelmed traumatically. Such 'weakness' may have a constitutional root" (Fenichel, 1945, p. 117). One view of the ego is that it develops for the purpose of avoiding traumatic states by discharging and binding; by organizing; by anticipating in play, fantasy, or thought; and, in recurrently disturbing situations, by building up reserves of counterenergy to deal with overwhelming excitations.

The human organism also has more primitive ways of protecting itself: It can interpose a buffer (*Reizschutz*) that prevents new stimulation from getting through and can thus afford to lie fallow (Freud, 1922). Engel and Schmale's (1972) "conservation–withdrawal" thesis serves the same purpose throughout the phylogenetic series. The repetitive dreaming and visual imagery of the posttraumatic phase also represent a regression to a primitive mode of mastery; by experiencing again and again what once had to be endured, the individual can slowly re-establish control.

The neurotic conflicts that lie behind the trauma or precede it historically are factors in determining the "breaking point" of the individual: The more intense the prior conflicts, the more likely it is for an experience to become traumatic. In this sense, the trauma may be looked upon as having a screening function for the earlier infantile neuroses. Following a traumatic exposure, hypervulnerable individuals move not toward a spontaneous recovery, but toward the development of lasting defects of the personality, such as an impoverishment of ego functions, a diminished interest in the external world, and a readiness to withdraw from contact with reality, all summarized in the picture of a general restriction of the personality. Within this theoretical context, resilience may ensue if infantile threats and anxieties are minimal and complications of a narcissistic nature have not developed; a pseudoresilience may result if a strong counterphobic attitude develops and becomes associated with a false confidence in the "noncastrating" nature of the environment.

The Historical Role of Adversity

From time immemorial, adversity has been regarded negatively as an integral part of the human condition to be suffered and endured, but positively as a testing ground for the heroism of man. "Sweet are the uses of adversity," wrote Shakespeare in *As You Like it*; on one side it is "ugly and venomous," like a toad, but it also is "a precious jewel." There is almost contempt for the easy life. "Plenty and peace breeds cowards; hardness ever of hardness is Mother," he stated in *Cymbeline*. Francis Bacon (who, according to Freud, wrote under the pseudonym of Shakespeare) had much the same attitude. "He knows not his own strength that hath not met adversity," Bacon noted; in his essay "Adversity," he saw it as outshining prosperity in that it "best discovers virtue," and its virtue is fortitude, of which stuff heroes are made. Oliver Goldsmith considered that the greatest object in the universe was "a good man struggling with adversity." In this century, Arnold Toynbee, the historian, came out with a challenge-and-response theory to throw light on the vicissitudes through which human societies pass (Toynbee, 1972). He described three kinds of responses: a disintegrating one, characteristic of the most vulnerable societies; a transient disintegration followed by reintegration, as the social group first succumbs to the adversity and then overcomes it; and, finally, the apparent ability to thrive on adversity and come out stronger, more cohesive, and more creative as a result of exposure to it. Elsewhere (Anthony, 1970), I have made use of the Toynbee model to explain the clinical outcome in families who lived under the duress of psychosis. I have also noted that Koos (1946), in his study of a family's inadversity, found the same basic responses: Some became totally and permanently disorganized; some went downhill but recovered, at times reaching the original baseline and at times remaining below the original level of functioning. However, there has been a small percentage in all studies of societies, families, and individuals where the outcome has been better than the initial status.

In another work (Anthony, 1974a), in attempting to clarify the concepts of risk, vulnerability, and resilience, I have used the analogy of three dolls made of glass, plastic, and steel and exposed to the same risk, the blow of a hammer. The first doll breaks down completely, the second shows a dent that it carries permanently, and the third doll gives out a fine metallic sound. Of course, the "outcome" for the three dolls would be different if their "environments" were to buffer the blows from the hammer by interposing some type of "umbrella" between the external attack and the recipient. Furthermore, there is another element in the analogy that is untrue to life: The risks to which children are exposed are as variable in their severity and nature as the vulnerabilities and resiliences with which the children confront them. These considerations make the prediction of outcome extremely difficult. What Freud referred to as "too searching a destiny" represents an accumulation of adversity that may eventually tax the toughest constitution or the most propitious environmental setting. But there are "favorites of fortune," born to the role or endlessly lucky in life. The oft-quoted remark by Freud (1925) undoubtedly has a face validity: "A man who has been the indisputable favorite of his mother keeps for life the feeling of a conqueror, that confidence of success that often induces real success" (p. 26). It is this sense of confidence that seems to be the hallmark of many invulnerables.

The Dynamics of Vulnerability and Invulnerability

Anxiety, for Freud, had two aspects. There is anxiety that results as a reaction to a traumatic situation and that is paralyzing, overwhelming, and productive of a "fright-neurosis"; on the other hand, there is anxiety that protects against such a powerful experience by signaling and thus preparing the subject beforehand for the disturbing encounter (Freud, 1922). In order to enable us to appreciate the situation of risk, Freud has asked us to visualize the situation of one of our cells attempting to deal with the encircling danger—that is, the living vesicle with its receptive cortical layer. "This little fragment of living substance is suspended in the middle of an external world charged with the most powerful energies; and it would be killed by the stimulation emanating from these if it were not provided with a protective shield against stimuli" (Freud, 1922, p. 27). In other words, it acquires a skin that functions as a resistant membrane or special envelope. Because of this shield, the strong stimuli from the outer world are able to penetrate the living organism, but with only a small fraction of their actual intensity. As Freud pointed out, "protection against stimuli is an almost more important function for the living organism than reception of stimuli" (p. 27). The organism can thus sample the external excitations because the barrier imposes a threshold that blocks the possibility of an "overdose." The two surface layers function synergistically: The other layer is protective and the inner layer receptive.

If one extends this idea in two ways—from cell to human individual, and from physical to psychological experience—the barrier hypothesis continues to stand us in good stead. If the shield is breached in some limited area, the organism falls back on a second line of defense. "Cathectic energy is summoned from all sides to provide sufficiently high cathexes of energy in the environs of the breach. And 'anticathexis' on a grand scale is set up, for whose benefit all the other psychical systems are impoverished, so that the remaining psychical functions are extensively paralyzed or reduced (Freud, 1922, p. 30). In this way, the invading energy is "bound." The metapsychological notion of "anticathexis" was therefore put forward by Freud as an additional way that the individual has for dealing with too much excitation.

The primary and secondary buffering systems have been inherent in the thinking of developmentalists for a long time, since not only the helplessness but the vulnerability of the newborn human infant was very apparent, and it was argued without much scientific basis that "something" must be interposed between this extremely immature organism and the external excitatory impingements to protect from such overwhelming stressors. William James (1890) concluded that the baby is relatively immune from such booming and buzzing because the brain is plunged in a deep sleep and consciousness is practically nonexistent, so that it takes a strong message from the sense organs to break this slumber (pp. 7–8). This speculative notion of a sleepy, largely inactive cortex has gained some support from more recent studies that have allowed cerebral functioning to be directly visualized.

The third component of the buffering system is generally more efficient through its specificity. It derives from caretakers who regard it as an essential part of their job to provide the infant with as optimal a milieu as possible (Anthony, 1958). In normal practice, its functioning can best be described as "good enough," depending on the psychophysiological well-being of the caretaker. The human element allows it to work within a generally acceptable range of empathy. To the degree that the mother feels the comforts and discomforts of her baby as if they were her own, this makes it possible for her to grade her interventions in accordance with this subjective criterion. It is customary to label the mothering as "good" or "bad," depending on the level of comfort maintained for the baby. When ministrations are inept or neglectful on the one side, verging on or amounting to abuse, or so excessive on the other side as to seriously interfere with the child's capacity to assume protectiveness for himself; the mothering is considered "bad."

This brings us to consider the fourth component of the buffering system, which evolves along with the child's ego activities.

The Ego and Its Mechanism of Resilience

Whereas there is no selection in the first two buffering systems, and only a modicum of selectivity relating to maternal empathy, the ego's autonomous buffering has the potential to become a highly calibrated and sensitive perceptual instrument. Even when the ego is handicapped by disorders of the sensory apparatus, it is surprising how it is possible for it to compensate for such deficiencies.

Redl (1969) introduced the concept of "ego resilience," which comprises two aspects: (1) the capacity to withstand pathogenic pressures, and (2) its ability to recover rapidly from a temporary collapse even without outside help and to bounce back to normal or even supernormal levels of functioning. What had surprised Redl in his clinical work was not that individuals broke down, but rather that their egos held up "under conditions that seemed insupportable to health" (p. 98) and where the traumatic weight of adverse circumstances would have made it humanly excusable to succumb. Another factor that puzzled him in the face of this "astounding degree of ego resilience" (p. 97) was why the psychiatric literature continued to focus so exclusively on vulnerability and clinical failure, and yet had little or nothing to say either practically or theoretically on the occurrence of unexpected health. A look at the ego from this novel viewpoint seemed warranted.

"A catalogue of ego functions," said Hartmann (1950), "would be rather long" (p. 114); rather than cover the area encyclopedically, one could follow Freud and center one's attention on the ego's relation to reality and the outside world. As it organizes and controls motility and perception, the ego "serves as a protective barrier against excessive external and, in a somewhat different sense, internal stimuli" (Hartmann, 1950, p. 115). The protection against inner dangers involves a more complex set of inhibiting and defensive functions, which run the gamut of internal "flight" responses that may begin to operate even before the ego as a definite system has evolved. At this time, such functions as the postponement of discharge are more passively effected, but are incorporated more actively later on by the ego in its more subtle and age-appropriate deployment of defenses; these functions come into being negatively, under the pressure of conflict, or positively, as a habitual mode of maintaining a "conflict-free sphere" through the use of "neutralization" and a wide range of autonomous ego functions. In this way, Hartmann attempted to relate primordial forms of buffering activity to later characteristics of the developed ego and to hypothesize a genetic correlation between individual differences in primary delaying reactions to the eventual choice of defense mechanisms. He intended this as an appeal to analysts who had opportunities for conducting longitudinal developmental studies on children to verify or refute this hypothesis.

Bergman and Escalona (1949) used the concept of a "thin" protective shield against stimuli in accounting for the unusual sensitivities of children who may be in some phase of schizophrenic development. Their assumption was that this "thinness" may lead to precocious ego development, thus setting ego functioning at risk. Even when these children subsequently achieve a comparatively high degree of secondary autonomy, their psychological resistance is impaired and may contribute to the vulnerability of defense and neutralization, as well as of other ego functions, that antedates the development of schizophrenia. Bergman and Escalona were here presupposing that both vulnerabilities and invulnerabilities of defense and ego resilience have a hereditary core. In this, their thinking was similar to that of Freud (1937).

There is much more to the ego than defensiveness and passivity. When confronted with challenge, the ego does more than retreat or safeguard itself; it attempts to master the stimulus and bend it to its needs. In this sense, it copes interactively with the environment, overcoming impediments and transforming situations rather than permitting itself to be transformed by them. "Coping" is now regarded as a broader concept than "defense" and employs many more ego skills than are required for purely defensive purposes. The distinctions between the two may appear to be more semantic than real, but as the definitions have been refined, "coping" has come to imply something over and beyond intrapsychic defensive maneuvering, with its close tie to the operations of instinct and affect. However, it would by no means be accurate to define "defense" as something pathological and internally directed, as contrasted with "coping" with its normal concerns and outer directedness. Defined in this way, "coping" would include the mastering of both objective and subjective anxiety and a heightening of frustration tolerance. It was said that while defenses need to be analyzed, coping can be taught and learned, which also means that parent figures can serve as appropriate models. It is as if the ego has two strategies at its command: one that operates less consciously but more stereotypically, and another that is both more conscious and more competent and creative in its activities. The main differences, therefore, appear to lie between habitual and spontaneous behavior, between the fixed and the flexible, and between the internally determined and the externally responsive. On first inspection, the resilient are more inclined to use the less rigidly applied defenses and a wider range of coping mechansims. Kroeber (1963) has made the useful suggestion that defensive and coping responses are clinical and nonclinical facets of a broad range of ego functions (see Table 1-1).

Kroeber's analysis of the ego's coping functions is weighted on the side of health. He speaks approvingly of the "new ego psychology" that is trying to reorient itself from "a preoccupation with pathology" and is making it its major concern to conceptualize "nonneurotic, adaptive functioning" (1963, p. 181). As epitomized by Rapaport (1960), it is assumed that "the inborn ego apparatuses enter conflicts as independent factors and that their function is not primarily dependent on

Table 1-1. Defensive and Coping Ego Functions

Ego function	Defensive response	Coping response
Discrimination	Isolation	Objectivation
Detachment	Intellectualization	Intellectual activity
Symbolization	Rationalization	Logical analysis
Attention	Denial	Focused activity
Sensitivity	Projection	Empathy
Postponement	Procrastination	Heightened frustration tolerance
Remembering	Wishful regression	Regression in service of ego
Impulse diversion	Displacement	Sublimation
Impulse transformation	Reaction formation	Substitute activity
Impulse control	Repression	Suppression
	Where defense is, let coping be.	

Note. After Kroeber (1963).

drives" (p. 54–55). According to Kroeber (1963), in the new ego model, the ego mechanisms can take on either defensive or coping functions. Coping mechanisms differ from defense mechanisms in being flexible, purposive, selected, and oriented toward present reality and future planning; in involving largely conscious, "secondary-process" thinking; and in operating in accordance with individual needs and ordered, tempered, open impulse satisfactions. The autonomy of ego functioning depends on the relative use of coping over defense mechanisms, with the latter indicating the more clinical proclivity. For instance, the ego function of the selective awareness can be distorted by the defense of denial, with a refusal to face up to painful sights, thoughts, and feelings; on the other side, it may be enhanced by the capacity to concentrate on the task at hand and deal with it as effectively as possible.

Whether all these complex operations can be represented within a single equation is a moot point, even though depicted as an "informal statement of relationship" (Kroeber, 1963, p. 197):

$$\text{Mental health} = f \left(\frac{\text{sum } C \ E, \ Dr}{\text{sum } D} \right)$$

where sum C represents the sum of ratings of coping mechanisms; sum D, the sum of ratings of defense mechanisms; E, the total of general ego mechanisms (themselves sums of their coping and defensive parts); and Dr, an estimate of drive. In terms of robustness and resilience, such a conception of mental health would imply that high energy availability, coupled with channeling and control through adequate coping mechanisms, would lead to *the greatest potential for creative and productive use.*

Another look at coping comes from the studies of Murphy and Moriarty (1976). They point out that the term "coping" should not be used as the healthy antonym to "defense," since an extensive literature exists on healthy and universal defense structures. According to them, normal children use defense mechanisms and autonomous ego functions in a mutually supportive way, and the coping process includes cognitive functioning as well as "normal" defensive strategies. Children are therefore able to mold and manipulate the environment assertively, to deal with its pressures successfully, and to comply with its demands passively and dependently.

What emerged from Murphy and Moriarty's studies was a profile of "good copers" who were cognitively capable, affectively expressive and effective, and attitudinally responsive in a wide variety of ways. These included good feelings about themselves (or "healthy" narcissism); good insights into interpersonal situations; realistic evaluations of the human and nonhuman environment; free-wheeling attentiveness; flexibility with regard to means and ends; integration in their thinking, feeling, and acting; free translation of ideas into action; and marked intuition, originality, and creativity. Observers could note that these children oriented themselves rapidly to situations; that they perceived lucidly; that they communicated without inhibition; that, when faced with lots of material in their activities, they were able to accept substitutions; that they could allow others to get close to them and reciprocated in a warm and friendly manner; that they accepted the pleasurable functioning of their bodies; and that they looked upon themselves and what they did positively. Their capacity to tolerate frustration, to handle anxiety, and to ask for help when they needed it set them apart from the more vulnerable children, who coped poorly on all these counts.

The patterns of recovery from transient setbacks were another distinguishing feature. When under stress, the "good copers" were prepared to retreat for a while into safety, to take time out to recuperate, to make use of self-comforting devices, to play traumatic experiences out, and, if necessary, to transform unpleasant reality through the medium of fantasy.

Quite typically, "good copers" also had parents who were models of resilience themselves and who were available, but not obtrusively so, with encouragement and comforting reassurance. The parents who coped well were able to help their children to understand the problems confronting them, to work through losses sustained, and to help with restitution and compensation. Fantasy, denial, regression, and repression all had places at certain times in the coping process, but the identification with the resilient caregivers was a critical factor. The adaptation of "good copers" was never a simple compliance with the dictates of adults, but rather a subtle amalgam of coming to terms with grownups while at the same time meeting their own needs as children.

The milieu that generates good coping processes provides a requisite amount of space, safety, and freedom. It furnishes the opportunity to explore novel environments, to draw upon inner resources, to reach self-generated conclusions, and to establish sound bases for assessing assets and liabilities that arise. The "facilitating environment" thus permits children to be active or inactive as the circumstance requires, to let off steam, and to discharge tensions without invoking catastrophic consequences. It is essentially a reliable setting that fosters reliability and self-reliance in the young individuals immersed in it. I am talking here of nothing out of the ordinary. It is both "average" and "expectable," but this very element of ordinariness encourages the development of a solid realism that is based on the adults' respect for the children's growing individuality—the buttressing quality of a well-put-together environment where the parents set clear limits but yet expect the children to grow up in their own way. An interesting feature of the parents of "good copers" as noted by Murphy and Moriarty was that they did not resort to rigid sex-typing, so that the children were able to resort, without shame or discomfort, to both "masculine" and "feminine" modes of coping.

Murphy and Moriarty (1976) have therefore provided an assessment precedure—the Comprehensive Coping Inventory (CCI)—that allows the diagnostician to make an assessment of coping with a certain degree of confidence. It covers cognitive, motoric, affective, and self–ego coping capacities. These are clearly identified and itemized, so that by the time of completing the inquiry, the tester does obtain a comprehensive picture of a child's ability to fend off excessive stimulations by a number of means: diverting the stimulations from the setting; withdrawing himself from active engagement; postponing the need for immediate response; turning to newer and more manageable situations; restructuring the environment when this is possible; accepting both good and bad elements as part of everyday reality; and, in general, working toward maintaining optimal conditions of integration, security, and comfort.

As depicted by Murphy and Moriarty (1976), the resilient child is above all an active, humorous, confident, and competent child who is prepared to take risks, although not unrealistically; can alter his approach flexibly; and, as a result of repeated successful coping experiences, has reason to feel confident of both inner and outer resources. In their description of Rachel, the authors summarize the qualities of the "good coper" when confronted with a new experience:

> A remarkable flexibility and resilience enable her to respond freely once she is out of the immobilizing, awesome, or frightening new experience; a capacity for deep, sensuous delight and gratification and for sensitive, non-verbal, interpersonal communication through smiles and shining eyes contributes to a genuine relationship; a capacity for resourceful manipulation and problem solving leads to constructive use of the play opportunity; *a capacity for representation and symbolization of disturbing experiences and fantasies* helps her to tolerate the frustration and stress. (Murphy & Moriarty, 1976, pp. 109–110; italics added)

In their longitudinal research, Murphy and Moriarty extracted two global variables in the area of coping: Coping I, related to the capacity to deal with opportunities, challenges, frustrations, and threatening aspects of the environment; and Coping II, concerned with efforts to maintain "internal integration" through the management of relations to the environment. However, as might be expected, there was a certain degree of overlap between the two coping processes. The many aspects of coping outlined by the authors are roughly classifiable into techniques, devices, and dispositions, but they add up to the coping resources available to the ego in its attempt to solve difficulties and problems confronting it. Although the authors speak of "coping styles," as one may speak of defensive characteristics, they recognize that these must be viewed in relation to the situation and to the developmental stage of the child, since time brings new challenges, new resiliences and new vulnerabilities. In general, the resources gradually increase with age.

This work has added a richer dimension to the ego and its resilience, since the ego is not considered in isolation but always in relation to the caregiver. The parental egos play a crucial role in structuring the child's ego. The parents of "good copers" are good copers themselves and provide models of resilience to their children. There is an easily discernible interrelationship between the child's coping capacities and those of the parents, the family, and the community in which they are all located. Parents who cope well have a distinctive profile: They enjoy their children, provide them with a holding and facilitating environment without obtruding on their autonomy, support their efforts to care for themselves, furnish a reassuring background, and are highly receptive to the "assumptive worlds" developed by the children.

There are drawbacks to building up an authentic picture of the child's ego and its robustness or vulnerability, since it requires a longitudinal perspective—a long-term study of daily life within the setting of the family and its social orbit, carried out by highly skillful and trained observers who, through working together over the years, begin to show a high degree of concurrence in their judgments. The CCI is not really a workable instrument for the short-term investigator or clinician: It covers too much ground, with consequently some degree of redundancy, and it demands hair-splitting judgments that can only be acquired through prolonged use. Yet it is the best such instrument that we have to date, and it will remain a stimulus to further coping work until it can be refined for everyday research and clinical application.

In fact, the CCI is so comprehensive that it covers every area of autonomous functioning, running the gamut to encompass the cognitive, the motoric, the emotional, the integrative, and the psychological aspects of the self. Coping verges on the areas of competence and creativity.

Fraiberg (1959) has provided two interesting illustrations of the comprehensive nature of coping, which have been paraphrased for this presentation.

Tony was a small boy with generalized fears of the strange, the unfamiliar, and the unknown. His approach to dealing with this was mainly an investigative one. "If he could find out how something worked, if he could locate the causes for events, he felt himself in control and lost his fear." His favorite toy at the age of 2 was a pocket-sized screwdriver that he carried with him everywhere and with which he managed to unhinge doors, tables, and chairs. Since he was afraid, like many small children, of the vacuum cleaner, he took it to pieces to find where the frightening noise came from. With his handy instrument, he imperiled himself by removing plates from wall outlets, and when his parents put a stop to this research, he was furious. Warnings only served to increase his need to locate the source of danger and to find out "why." As he grew older, he not only wanted to take dangerous things to pieces, but also to reassemble them and make them work again. At the age of 4, he had an emergency appendectomy, which was a frightening experience. Relatives brought him toys, but what he wanted and asked for was "an old alarm clock that doesn't work," and he occupied himself during his convalescence repairing it. In working through the psychologically traumatic experience of the surgical operation for which he was unprepared, he took apart the alarm clock and made it work again, just as the doctor took him apart and made him work again. "In this way he employed a well-established sublimation, mechanical investigation and construction, to overcome a frightening experience." Yet the anxiety provided a powerful motive "to fix something" so that the little boy could go beyond his age-appropriate capacities and accomplish something that had not been possible before. During latency, he continued his scientific interests in the basement, inventing new projects. Small explosions unsettled the family from time to time. There was never any question, at this point, that he would grow up to become a scientist, and eventually he became a physicist. (pp. 23–27)

Jennie, aged 2 years, 8 months, had an imaginary animal companion—a laughing tiger, the latest of a steady influx of an invisible menagerie. What was special about the laughing tiger was that he did not roar, bite, or scare children. He just laughed. He also had to learn to mind what Jennie said and to understand that he could not have everything his own way. For months, he had his place at the dinner table, but after Jennie's third birthday he disappeared, and nobody missed him. He first came into existence when the little girl was very afraid of animals who might bite and even eat up small children. Even little dogs in the neighborhood scared her. The question confronting her was how to deal with these threats. She could have stayed close to her parents and cling to them, avoided going outside the house because of a possible encounter, or kept awake at night so as not to encounter animals in her dreams. All these would have been poor solutions based on avoidance and dependency. What Jennie planned to do was to cope with it herself, using her own best resources. "There is one place where you can meet a ferocious beast on your own terms and leave victorious. That place is the imagination." Jennie had transformed a ferocious beast into an easily controlled creature who shrank into his corner after one word from his mistress. This transformation was paralleled by Jennie's own domestication, in which her primitive impulses were brought under control.

Another solution to creating a nice tiger is to become a tiger and out-roar the enemy. Coping with such fears is part of normal development, and the normally developing child develops a variety of strategies to overcome them. When such imaginery fears, however, become real fears, as when a parent becomes psychotic or abusive, the child can no longer overcome his fears through imaginative play, and a world view develops in which the surroundings are populated with dangerous people against whom one must constantly defend oneself. Fantasy play for the purpose of dealing with actual threats may then become more than a drama in the nursery theatre: It is carried into the child and becomes part of his personality, and he then constructs elaborate defenses that not only protect him but paralyze his initiative. If the coping is to remain healthy, the imaginative play must preserve the boundaries between fantasy and reality, and the rules of the game that ensure this must be adhered to. Under such conditions, the child's contact with the real world is strengthened by these periodic excursions into fantasy and allows him to tolerate the frustrations of reality and accede to its demands. At a very early age, the child discovers that his intelligence and his ability to acquire knowledge would also help him to combat his fears. (pp. 16-19)

Vulnerability, even at its most hypervulnerable, is not necessarily a message of doom, since individuals can bounce back and achieve a significant degree of nonvulnerability. Seemingly invulnerable individuals may also reveal unsuspected weaknesses under certain circumstances or during certain phases of development. Murphy and Moriarty (1976) make this point very clearly: "In our use of vulnerability, *there is no completely invulnerable child*—we are concerned with the degree and locus of vulnerability in relation to the intensity and quality of the stress. When the child's most vulnerable area is confronted by severe stress for that area, some degree of breakdown is likely to occur" (p. 346). They note that among the children they studied, "Some loss of their best functioning occurred in all [of them] in the face of one or another experience evidently felt as threatening or stressful" (p. 346). When coping is successful, some sense of invulnerability grows within the child, and the same is true in the face of failure—the sense of vulnerability may become chronic. Accumulated stresses, if not overwhelming, may challenge the child to get the better of them or get used to them. The reduction of stress reactions may be brought about by familiarization, negative adaptation, or the development of specific skills through which the child "learns to conquer."

Ego Competence and Resilience

"Every interaction with another person can be said to have an aspect of competence . . . in extreme cases, interpersonal acts may have virtually no purpose beyond the testing or display of competence" (White, 1963, p. 73). As mentioned in the preceding section, interpersonal competence, along with other types of competence, can be included in any comprehensive inventory of coping skills, but recent work has tended to highlight the more essential aspects of competence and to investigate it as a singular phenomenon in itself.

White (1959) has been prominent in defining the concept that he sees as the capacity, fitness, or ability to carry on transactions with the environment that result in the maintenance, the growth, and the thriving of the organism; in the human instance, this capacity is largely based on learning. White also speaks of the "sense of competence," which does not correspond exactly to actual competence as estimated by others. He points out that the sense of competence has been widely recognized in a clinical negative form as evident in feelings of helplessness, inhibition of initiative, or attitudes of inferiority. From the positive viewpoint, the sense of competence is closely associated with a buoyant self-confidence and realistically perceived self-esteem. The interpersonally incompetent individual sees himself as ineffectual in his human group, unable to obtain a hearing from them, and powerless to influence them to any significant extent. What he lacks is what Erikson (1950) has referred to as a "lack of sending power" (p. 207), but he also lacks a clear receiving station, as a result of which people remain inscrutable and the human environment is like a mysterious puzzle-box to which he does not have the key.

The growth of interpersonal competence and the correlate of interpersonal confidence continues throughout the life cycle, constantly feeding on successful interactions and peaking critically at certain developmental points. Important facilitating factors include parental pleasure and interest in the child's growing initiative and autonomy, as well as acquisition of sufficient language to issue commands, offer defiance, and express feelings and engage in play with peers, with roles mutually decided upon. The mutual interplay of interpersonal competence and confidence contributes to feelings of relative invulnerability in the face of difficult or disturbing human relationships.

What has been referred to as academic or scholastic competence has less to do with native intelligence as manifested in a test of IQ, aptitude, or achievement (although these are all important contributory factors) than with a mental set that allows the individual to concentrate on the problem at hand, analyze its component parts, and set about energetically and confidently to solve it. It therefore includes organizational skills, a finely tuned critical faculty, and an equanimity of mind that frees the individual temporarily from distractions. Once again, successful undertakings help to breed confidence and thus sustain fresh operations. Piaget's (1950) concept of "operational thinking," in fact, captures much of the essence of academic competence.

As with other ego functions, competence beyond the developmental stage may make its appearance precociously when small children are left to their own resources. Motherless children, for example, begin to care for themselves and their bodily wants like little mothers. The concern for their health that had been the mother's business in the past is taken over after separation or bereavement, so that the self-caring function of the ego is strikingly enhanced. Its "forced competence" may disappear when the child is reunited with the mother, but if this is delayed indefinitely or becomes impossible, a persistent hypochondriasis may develop. Being compelled to look after younger siblings may also precipitate adultomorphic parental behavior, but this is often associated with heightened ambivalence.

One of the most interesting facets of competence has been termed "representational" (Anthony, 1984) and has to do with the child's capacity to make what Jaspers (1963) called "meaningful sense" out of the chaotic and traumatic events that confront him. Representational competence is concerned with how far the child acquires understanding of what is going on around him, the assumption being that such acquisitions help the child to master the stress. Burlingham and Anna Freud (1942) noted this phenomenon in small children during the years of World War II:

> It can be safely said that all the children who were over 2-years at the time of the London "blitz" have *acquired knowledge* of the significance of air raids.

They all *recognize* the noise of flying airplanes; they *distinguish* vaguely between the sound of falling bombs and anti-aircraft guns. They *realize* that the house will fall down when bombed and that people are often killed or get hurt in falling houses. . . . They fully *understand the significance* of taking shelter. Some children who have lived in deep shelters will even *judge the safety of a shelter* according to its depth under the earth. . . . The children seem to have no difficulty in understanding what it means when their fathers join the Forces. (p. 157; italics added)

This understanding of catastrophe plays a crucial role in permitting the child to react emotionally in an appropriate manner and in offering him outlets that might help to deal with the experience. The child's conception of what is going on may be represented inwardly in forms that reflect the developmental stage, and these representational roles were carefully documented by Piaget in his studies (Piaget, 1929). The representations also include the thinking of the child, his rudimentary notions of causality, his understanding of relationships, and the theories with which he explains them. As he gets older, so do his representations become more sophisticated. Murphy and Moriarty (1976) quote the representations of a 14-year-old-boy, Karl, who might have been musing on the contents of this chapter:

"As you encounter one stressful experience, it strengthens you like a vaccine for a future crisis. One acquires a callousness and builds up a sort of reserve. When you are young, there is a natural ability to survive a crisis; you aren't as deeply involved; even though a minor crisis may seem great, or is exaggerated, it disappears quickly. As one grows older, the natural ability to live ahead and forget, diminishes, but experience in living gives you a maturity that takes the place of your natural ability to survive—you have to bounce back or you couldn't go on." (p. 263)

Here Karl is offering us an immunization model of resilience. He perceives it as developing over time, with different resources supplanting one another with age. Is he right, however, that working through a crisis strengthens a person to meet future crises, or do different individuals respond differently? Is he right that youths have "a natural ability" to survive because they are not as deeply involved (the Meursault phenomenon)? Is he right that older people live more in the here and now, and are therefore more likely to react more intensely to the present crisis? Karl balances the "natural ability" to survive against the maturity of experience, so that both youth and age, for different reasons, are able to bounce back.

Perhaps the highest degree of representational competence is to be observed in creative individuals, writers, artists and musicians, whose sensitivity and vulnerability to stresses are compensated for by this intriguing and somewhat mysterious function.

Ego Creativity, Vulnerability, and Resilience

A great deal has been written both scientifically and nonscientifically about the mysterious process of creativity, much of it speculative. First of all, there is a widely held belief that creativity is a natural ingredient of early life, and that creative adults either retain this infantile component intact or return to it as a wellspring from time to time to refresh and sustain their imaginative and inventive powers. It is also held that the equally mysterious disappearance of creativity in the average person is a consequence of having it trained out of him as a defensive latency, coupled with a stern demand on the part of teachers for factuality. At this point, the spontaneous, the intuitive, and the imaginative are frowned upon as regressive phenomena and ruled out of order. The well-recognized "third-grade slump" sets in, and nothing unique is ever again seen except for a pathetically few eccentric children. Who are these odd ones who stand out from the group and persistently feel themselves at variance with it? In the first place, they are a minority and have neither the numbers, the forcefulness, nor the organization to take on the majority. Second, they are so unsure of themselves, so lacking in confidence, and often so impractical that they tend to keep themselves out of the way and out of the limelight as far as possible. And third, they are invariably victimized as punishment for their idiosyncrasies. As a result, they feel unsafe and insecure in the conventional environment and are burdened by a sense of vulnerability.

The prodigious development of a creative capacity can be regarded, in its less engimatic tenor, as a superior level of competence and, as such, as part of the autonomous equipment of the ego. A disproportionate number of creative individuals who have contributed invaluably to the culture of societies appear, to the clinical eye, to be highly vulnerable to the risk of mental disorder. With this group, vulnerability is deep-seated and long-lived. From the very beginning, they seem to lack the "protective shield" and the constitutional buffering between themselves and the world around. The hypersensitivity that permits such free exchange between outer experience and the psychic interior may conduce to two outcomes: "breakdown" when the primitive content takes over and allows the milieu of irrationality and unrealism to pervail without constraint, and an upsurge of creative productivity, delicately controlled by the ego. However, this regression "in the service of the ego" is accompanied by some relinquishing of defenses, which imperils the ego. The attenuation of the primary buffering system can therefore be compensated for by an enhanced ego creativity that rehabilitates the battered psyche and brings it back into meaningful contact with the fearsome outside environment. However, when

the creative energy is expended, there may be a lapse into hypervulnerability and ego disintegration. Thus, many creative artists and writers
manifest cycles of vulnerability and resilience determined by the ebb
and flow of the creative urge.

Virginia Woolf (see Woolf, 1977) represents a striking example of
this syndrome. Both vulnerability and creativity were scattered liber-
ally through her family through the generations. Her sister became a
gifted painter, her brother a successful psychoanalyst, and she herself a
writer of genius. She was always an introverted child much given to
fantasies and storytelling, but following an attack of whooping cough
at the age of 6, she became even more different from other children and
quieter. She described herself as a "skinless" individual like her father,
and all through her early life, she suffered from an appalling sense of
vulnerability. She was constitutionally delicate and responded to the
smallest physical ailment with great intensity. She was also painfully
excitable and nervous, and her fear of people was such that if spoken to,
she blushed vividly. Within the family home, she felt relatively safe, but
as soon as she left the house, the ordinary things of life horrified her.
During the latter part of childhood, she experienced what she called
"breakdowns in miniature," but at 13, she had her first significant
breakdown. She developed the impression that she had "no outer protection" and seemed unable to become "part of real life"; she felt that
she belonged "outside the loop of time." Ordinary people around her
seemed to live in the real world, but she fell into "nothingness." But she
was able to tap the private inner world replete with images, memories,
and fantasies, and her representational competence was of such a high
order that she could construct fascinating literary accounts of them. If
the process went too far and control was lost, she became psychotic,
but while she was engaged in the creative transformation of these
inner resources into words that translated the experience accurately,
she was free from her sense of vulnerability and gloried in her creativity and in the recognition she was accorded as a creative writer.

Another writer, Franz Kafka (see Kafka, 1974), also carried a
burden of persecution and victimization within him that transformed
the everyday world into a denizen of monsters that could only be
exorcised through the power of verbal representation. He described a
memory of himself as a small child taking a nap in the afternoon on
a warm summer's day and drowsily listening to his mother calling to a
neighbor from the balcony in terms that were quite commonplace:
"What are you doing, my dear? It is so hot." "I am having tea outside."
However, it was this quite ordinary exchange that haunted Kafka for
much of his life. It seemed to him that somewhere out there beyond
him there was a world of ordinary people interacting in an ordinary
way, whereas he was encircled by an environment characterized by

menace and threat. Later in his life he remarked, pathetically, "I have always wanted to see things as they are before they show themselves to me. . . . I am, as it were, specially appointed to see the phantoms of the night." His "skinlessness" was exquisitely excruciating. The largest threat from the outside was his father, whom he depicted as an ogre so dreadful and disagreeable that he could only cringe and hide as far away as possible to escape the abuse, the threats, the irony, the sarcasm, the spitefulness, the cruelty, and the malicious laughter and teasing. "And what happened inside? I became a glum, inattentive, disobedient child intent on escape mainly into my own self." Like Woolf, Kafka was aware of the extent to which his creativity preserved him from his hypervulnerability.

The third example is that of Hans Christian Andersen (see Andersen, 1847), whose sense of vulnerability stayed with him throughout his life. From an early age, he was aware that he had no barrier against the minor predicaments of everyday life and was habitually tense and hypersensitive. He was a solitary boy who rarely played with other children. He identified himself closely with his psychotic grandfather, a wild-eyed man with an artistic element who was the butt of the village. His father was also a solitary person who gradually became delusional, and all through his life, Andersen felt that he would become psychotic or kill himself. His main interest was in his little puppet theatre, and this was where he began to create his stories. His "skinlessness" was only too obvious. He was described as "a sensitive plant *but able to unfold and withstand the most inclement weather."* His own reason he gave for his survival was that he was supremely capable of withdrawing into fantasy away from actual reality, thus transforming an unkind and often belligerent world into a fairy story. He said that he had learned how to abreact and pour out the details of his "case" in endless representations, metaphors, and flashes of self-knowledge. During the act of creation, he achieved a few glorious moments of relief, but once the writing was over, he relapsed into a constant sense of aching depression and deprivation. Like Woolf, his "breakdowns in miniature" came when his creative energy ran out, and like Kafka, he would often ask, "Why can I never enjoy the present like other people?"

Although creativity appears to stave off, at least for a while, some of the perils of vulnerability, it does not make for true resilience: There is an *illusion* of powerfulness, of immunity from stresses, and of well-being. It constitutes a pseudoresilience, and there is a price attached to it. Jung (1930) had this to say about it: "There is rarely a creative man who does not have to pay a high price . . . the human element is frequently bled for the benefit of the creative element and to such an extent that it even brings out the bad qualities—ruthlessness, egotism, vanity—and all this in order to bring to the human I at least some life-strength, since otherwise it would perish of sheer inanition" (p. 231). Successful creativity does bolster the ego, but the self-absorption does detract from good object relations if true resilience is a product of good relations; and if good mental health is based on a viable mother–infant relationship, then creativity represents one of the many varieties of self-repair that enables the human organism to recover from periods of malfunctioning.

The Vulnerability–Invulnerability Spectrum

The concept of a continuum of susceptibility is in keeping with the principle of continuity that is currently favored over the "discontinuous" hypothesis in regard to both normal and abnormal development. The principle of continuity assumes that all attitudes and responses found in behavior pathology are in some way related to and derived from normal biosocial behavior; that there are no radical changes apart from steady accretions and higher intensities of response; that the dividing lines between so-called "stages" are artifacts of theory; and that dominant stage theories, specifying qualitative shifts, are responsible for various "developmental profiles" that confine the individual within a certain response set. Accretion viewpoints are based on calculation and therefore are favored by researchers, whereas stage theories have supplied an endless variety of constructs that have helped to illuminate and illustrate the various vicissitudes of development that observers, particularly clinical observers, encounter in their day-to-day work. It is possible, however, to make the best of both worlds—to acknowledge the principle of continuity, while at the same time slicing the data in such a manner as to extract qualitative differences between the highest and lowest scorers for any measured assessment. This can be done for the vulnerability continuum, thus differentiating characteristics of the hypervulnerables from those who are highly resilient.

With this type of data analysis, one can parcel out four categories of individuals (see Table 1-2). First, there are the hypervulnerables, who succumb to even "ordinary" and expectable life stresses. Second, there are the pseudoinvulnerables, who are vulnerable or extremely vulnerable individuals who have been "blessed" with an overprotective environment (particularly the maternal portion of it), and are relatively unchallenged and thriving until the environment fails, and they fail along with it. Third, there are the invulnerables with acquired resilience, who are exposed to cumulative traumas, but "bounce back" after each stress that they experience; with each successful rebound, they become increasingly resilient. Finally, there are the nonvulnerables, who seem robust from birth onward and continue to thrive and prosper

Table 1-2. Risk, Vulnerability, and Resilience

Vulnerability axis (V)	Risk axis (R)	
	High (H)	Low (L)
High (H)	HRHV (1)	LRHV (2)
Low (L)	HRLV (3)	LRLV (4)

Note. Cells: (1) hypervulnerables; (2) pseudoinvulnerables (unchallenged); (3) acquired resilience or capacity to "bounce back"; (4) Nonvulnerables (inherent robustness operating within "average expectable environment"). Predictions of breakdown or immunity are offset by degrees of acquired defensiveness, coping skills, and competence.

within any "average expectable environment." This analysis has several shortcomings, in that it fails to take into account factors of acquired defensiveness, coping skills, competence, and support from external sources. For this reason, predictions of breakdown or psychoimmunity may fail unless the degree of vulnerability or invulnerability is extreme and directly manifest to the observer.

The Topeka group (Murphy & Moriarty, 1976) has come up with a Vulnerability Inventory based on the concept of a continuum and derived from the theoretical or experiential viewpoint of different researchers; some of these have stressed constitutional factors, some linguistic ones, and some ego-functional ones, but all have taken special note of "developmental vulnerability." The Vulnerability Inventory is largely based on data stemming from normative studies and tries to evaluate (again beyond the resources of human assessors) the primary (constitutional or early infantile) and secondary (acquired) vulnerabilities.

The primary vulnerabilities include sensory–motor deficits, deviant body morphology, unusual sensitivities, integrative and adaptive difficulties and imbalances, temperamental deviances, inherent dispositions to passivity, inhibitions, low "sending power," insufficient impulse control, and an incapacity to read caretaker's cues. The secondary vulnerabilities are acquired over the period of development and dispose the child to anxious preoccupations regarding the functioning of his body, the maintenance of his relationships, the management of ambivalence, and the inability to bear frustration. As a consequence, the child is easily fatigable, unable to relax, and unable to handle energy resources.

The vulnerability begins to show a cumulative effect: Mistrust grows, communication flags, imitation and identification are weak, the affect range is narrow, postponement and delay are intolerable, and social capacities are poorly developed. At this later stage of childhood, the clinical aspects of vulnerability begin to manifest themselves. The maladjustment is overt; dependency is increased at the expense of autonomy; and the deficiency in self-control is evident in the need for a greater exercise of external controls. On the clinical side, the child appears persistently anxious and depressed, is highly prone to regress or retreat in the face of minimal stress, and is unable to recover from transient setbacks. On the nonclinical side, certain features show themselves: a striking lack of spontaneity, an absence of positive coping attitudes, and a minimal capability for "representational competence." There is an increasing spread of vulnerability to sensory–motor, emotional, cognitive, and communicative areas.

The concept of the vulnerability spectrum is well summarized by Murphy and Moriarty (1976):

> Along the continuum of vulnerability, children may be distributed in different numbers: few if any are so robust, so completely lacking in small as well as moderate or major handicaps as to be totally free from some zone of vulnerability. *Most children have a checkerboard of strengths and weaknesses,* or an "Achilles heel," or a cluster of tendencies that interact in such a way as to produce one or another pattern of vulnerability as well as strength. Given an infant of greater or lesser initial adequacy, decreases in invulnerability depend on outcomes of interaction between this child and its environment and the extent to which these outcomes compensate for early deficiencies or allow for progress in mastery. Increases in vulnerability are seen when the interaction between the child and the environment results in new limitations or difficulties, new threats to homeostasis and to integration, new obstacles to learning, increased difficulties in mastering anxiety or negative expectancies. Secondary vulnerabilities often develop from self-defeating defense mechanisms, which in therapy can be revived by substituting others that support effective coping. . . . [S]econdary vulnerabilities resulting from developmental damage or from emotional reactions to the frustrations arising from handicaps have been increasingly avoidable as the difficulties of children with specific disease defects, or damage, have been recognized early, and expert ways of helping them have been developed. (pp. 202–203; italics added)

The concept of a vulnerability continuum, together with the recognition of primary and secondary vulnerabilities, has therefore led to greater therapeutic and preventative optimism for change. One can look forward to shifts in vulnerability from infancy into childhood, and this progression offers important clues to possible sources of resilience or lack of it. Better coping skills begin to emerge in parallel with healthy defenses, or else the small child becomes increasingly inhibited as a measure of avoidance or a greater need for rigid control. Integration and disintegration are concomitant processes to these.

Most observers and investigators are now agreed that vulnerability and resilience are best studied and assessed during infancy, and it is to this phase that research has now turned.

The Significance of Infancy for Vulnerability and Resilience Studies

The capacity to cope with early risks and primary vulnerabilities provides observable indices, but, of course, no access to self-reflection and verbal communication. "It is unfortunate that our limited capacity for exploring the inner life of the infant . . . does not give direct clues to the outcomes of changes in vulnerability (Murphy & Moriarty, 1976, p. 133). Older children have ample opportunities to note the parental capacity to mobilize extra resources at times of family stress, but with infants, it is the experience with failing mothers that begins to dominate their responses but that cannot be specified directly. A mother under stress can become a multimodel of stimulus distress, which shows itself in her facial expressions, the tone of voice, the touching, the carrying, and the caring. The poorly facilitating and clumsily holding mother builds up a vague load of "disappointment" in the baby, especially if she deals with the infant according to her own interests and needs. This type of mother is depriving even when she is manifestly giving.

The notion of "fit" has increasingly crept into the literature as a primary phenomenon in terms either of inherent temperaments (Thomas, Birch, Chess, Hertzig, & Korn, 1963), or of "preadaptedness" (Hartmann, 1951) as a more dynamic and acquired index of attunement. Poorer "fit" is seen when the mother is temperamentally so different from her baby that she cannot provide what the infant demands. For example, a vigorous mother may lack the gentleness required by an infant with unusual sensitivity, and an unforthcoming mother may find an energetic, robust baby too much for her, although both types may be basically good enough mothers. Today, one would assume both genetic and epigenetic factors in the determination of "fit," with the further assumption that the "misfit" tends to escalate with experience and to generate conditions of risk and vulnerability. The situation of "misfit" is not only stressful for the infant, but makes the mother feel inferior and unsure about her parental competence. Highly sensitive babies may also create circular patterns of reaction, especially in the breast-feeding situation, where their lower thresholds may lead to a greater intolerance with nursing frustrations. This was more likely to happen with male babies in the Topeka studies, but with such a small sample it is not possible to make any generalizations. However, from the point of view of mortality and morbidity, there was a well-founded sex difference. There were good correlations between the robustness of girl babies, the ease of the mothers' deliveries, and success in breast feeding (Murphy & Moriarty, 1976, pp. 66–67). There was a general tendency for robust mothers to have robust babies who nursed well and contributed to the success in breast feeding. Furthermore, as a mother had further pregnancies, later-born babies experienced greater ease in being delivered and responded more robustly. It was also apparent in these studies that mothers seemed more aware of baby girls' needs, more skillful in handling them, more respectful of their autonomy, and more generally empathic than was the case with boy babies.

As a rule, optimal mothering in terms of sensitivity to the infant's needs, attentiveness to him, and acceptance of him—all variables furthering nurturance—is positively correlated with early resilience. The most striking feature of good nurturance is the seeming ease with which it is brought about by both members of the dyad. Thomas *et al.* (1963) delineated a group of "easy" babies whose development took a noticeably smooth course. Their mood was generally positive, their physiological functioning regular, their reactivity consistently mild, and their adaptation to new situations unusually rapid. They also contributed to the mothers' sense of maternal effectiveness, skill, and well-being, thus establishing a cycle of positive interactions from very early on. The interaction of the basic temperament of the infants with the environmental setup generated mainly by the mothers produced a harmonious "fit" between mothers and babies. It is surprising how actively such infants manage to affect their own experiences, so that even at 1 month of age, the robust infant initiates four out of five interchanges with the mother (Korner, 1971). The vulnerable infant, in contrast, is far less active, has far less "sending power," cries more frequently and for longer periods, is less easily pacified, and requires much more caretaking. All these observations presuppose the operation of both innate and experiential factors in the genesis of individual differences in infant behaviors. Not only do the babies show differences from the beginning, but their mothers may behave differently with different babies and differently at different times, depending on how they are feeling toward the babies or on how the babies are feeling toward them.

Resilience is also a function of age. Certain coping capacities are important for preparing the groundwork of resilience, especially those related to the management of stimulation from the environment. Good initial coping still involves the capacity to return to equilibrium shortly after arousal, the capacity to obtain a desired object or posture, the capacity for self-comforting, the capacity to delay responses, and the capacity to become interested in novel stimuli.

Vulnerable infants—that is, those manifesting low activity, poor functional stability, a slow tempo of decline from disturbance, high reactivity, and a tendency to be easily frustrated in general—show poor stress management, poor self-regulation, and slow recovery rates. Resilient babies manifest across-the-board proficiencies, having excellent physiques, stable vegetative functioning, high drives, good vocalization, and sound developmental balance. (This is in keeping with Terman's [1925] findings with gifted children, which demonstrated the correlation between mental, physical, and social development, indicating a tendency for well-endowed children to be well endowed in all basic spheres.)

It must be constantly born in mind that both resilient and vulnerable infants are functioning in a dyadic relationship, and that their mothers' response to them is all-important for their future mental health and development. Babies favored by their mothers are likely to thrive, while neglected ones will probably continue to fail cumulatively. The style of adaptation is determined by experience interacting with basic temperament and maturational level. The basic defenses are laid down at this time, and as the infants turn into children, one finds one polar type moving into obsessiveness, inhibition, overcontrol, isolation, rationalization, and an avoidance of new or strong stimulation; at the other pole are children who respond quickly, impulsively, affectively, and with a defensive tendency to externalize, displace, and act out.

Freud was well aware of the way in which resilience emerged out of the mother–infant dyad when he talked about self-confidence breeding success in the maternal favorite, helping him to overcome difficulties. According to Freud, it would seem that the future hero is born in the cradle rocked by an ever-loving, attentive mother.

Risk, Vulnerability, and Resilience during the Course of Development

The psychoanalytic concept of "trauma" has already been discussed, but it can also be understood in terms of cumulative trauma over the period of development (Kahn, 1963). The traumas gather connections so that eventually a traumatized personality development occurs. Associated with this is a second concept of phase-specific trauma, implying that there are developmental periods that are at high and low risk at different stages. If the trauma is inflicted at a certain time, when the child is preoccupied with certain specific anxieties to which the trauma has some degree of relatedness, its impact is intensified. In short, a child may be vulnerable to a particular traumatic event at one stage of his development and nonvulnerable for the same event at another developmental stage.

Development is largely an interactive process, and the individual undergoing it is by no means a passive receptacle for stimulations that write themselves onto the *tabula rasa* of his passively waiting brain and mind. From the start, the infant is actively accommodating to the world (Piaget, 1950); from the start, his mind is not a "bucket," but a "searchlight" actively exploring a "horizon of expectations" (Popper, 1972, p. 347); from the start, he is not a simple tape recorder on whom experiences are registered like sounds, but a busy painter "who begins with a blank canvas and paints continuously, or, to put it in other words, conceives and organizes the external world within his mind as a creative activity" (Kagan, 1969, p. 104), and the world models that he constructs are continuously in the process of change throughout development.

If this interactional viewpoint is accepted, not only does growing up become an active, constructive, and increasingly autonomous process of getting to know oneself and one's milieu; the phenomena of risk, vulnerability, and resilience also become active and ever-changing constructions.

Following this line of thought, Kagan (1969) puts forward two hypothetical cases. In the first, a happy, socially alert, secure, curious, creative, and spontaneous 3-year-old child is growing up successfully within a benign environment that holds and facilitates his development. He is then suddenly transferred to a different type of milieu, where he is inconsistently punished and constantly exposed to violence, cynicism, failure, and derogation. On a follow-up, 10 years later, the chances are that the strengths and assets present at the age of 3 will have been extinguished (possibly in the same way that Pavlov's dogs lost their conditioned reflexes following the Leningrad floods). The resilient individual will have been transformed into a vulnerable one, and the basic resilience will have been lost from the developmental account, which thus will present an erroneous picture of developmental history. Recent work, however, tends to negate this hypothesis. The early resilience will not be "extinguished"; although it may go underground for a while, it will later present itself as surprising and unexpected strengths in the behavior of the older individual.

In a second hypothetical case, Kagan reverses the story and has the 3-year-old removed from a powerfully toxic environment to a benevolent one. He suggests that 10 years later, this child as an adolescent will be substantially different from his siblings who have remained in the destructive environmental context. From the point of view of vulnerability and resilience, the nature of the difference will be difficult to predict, since without careful investigation during infancy and early childhood it is not possible to assess the individual's primary levels of vulnerability and resilience irrespective of experience. Thus, it is quite possible that the child will turn out to be more vulnerable and less resilient than his unfortunate brothers and sisters.

In a real instance, Kagan tells the history of a 14-year-old girl who had spent most of the first 30 months of her life in a crib in a small bedroom with no toys. The mother, who had felt unable to care for a fourth child, had locked her in this room and instructed an 8-year-old daughter to look after her. When she was removed to a foster home at the age of 2½, she was severely malnourished, retarded in weight and height, and so intellectually backward that she was untestable. She was therefore a child at high risk and apparently highly vulnerable. She remained with the foster family for 12 years; when she was re-examined, her full-scale IQ was within normal range, and she performed normatively on a wide battery of tests. *More crucially, her interpersonal behavior was not significantly different from that of an average rural adolescent.* However, many other cases have been reported when cognitions have more or less recovered, but the child has remained socially and emotionally abnormal. Both outcomes are possible. For Kagan, the developmental–environmental interactions make for unpredictability. In the context of this presentation, the outcomes would be more predictable if these crucial assessments of defense, coping, competence, and creativity were made. It is only through careful longitudinal studies of these factors that some of the mystifying developmental outcomes can be clarified. This is not to deny the complexity of prognostication over extensive periods of time or to underestimate the difficulties in all human predictive work.

The Effect of Powerful Environments

Bloom (1964) has discussed the impact of powerful environments on individuals interacting with them. Today, now that we are somewhat less shackled by the all-exclusive role attributed to heredity, the environment is being more carefully and meticulously studied as a significant codeterminer of the extent and kind of change induced in individuals. There are two important unknowns in this consideration— behavioral manifestations and personality traits, both of which vary considerably in their stability. MacFarlane (1963), in her Berkeley studies, traced the course of "normal" symptomatic behaviors from infancy to adulthood; she found that many of them were evanescent, appearing and disappearing during the course of development, but that some temperamental traits were invariant. This would conduce to a wide range of differential responses to the same "powerful" surroundings. A second problem has to do with the fact that it is difficult to secure reliable change measures regarding the environment, which responds diffusely as a stressor. One cannot predict, therefore, that all the individuals in a particular powerful environment will change or will change in some uniform way.

There is still another consideration related to this presentation: Individuals who live within a particular powerful environment will vary in their vulnerability and resilience and will thus respond differentially to it. This raises the question as to whether circumstances do exist, as might be in the case of massive natural disasters, when individual differences will cease to show their effect. Bloom (1964) has this to say:

> We have found a few instances in which very powerful environments bring about very similar changes in the large majority of individuals. Such powerful environments represent rather extreme instances of abundance or deprivation and apparently involve most individuals in very similar ways. That is, they are relatively uniform in preventing individuals from securing the necessary nutriments, learning experiences, or stimulation necessary for growth or they are so powerful in reaching all with the appropriate nutriments, experiences and stimulation that all (or almost all) individuals are affected in similar ways and to similar extents. In such powerful environments, *only relatively few individuals* are able to resist the effects of the environmental pressure. (p. 212; italics added)

To exercise such an influence, the environment would need to be all-pervasive, totally engulfing the individual in a situation that presses him from every angle toward a particular type of development or outcome. "It is the extent to which a particular solution is overdetermined that makes for a powerful environment" (Bloom, 1964, p. 212). Within this frame of reference, the "relatively few individuals" referred to by Bloom would correspond to "invulnerables."

Powerful environments also tend to affect the individual most during a rapid phase of growth, when he is generally at his most vulnerable. If one examines clinic termination rates for children in the United States (Rosen, Bahn, & Kramer, 1964), the peaks coincide roughly with growth velocities. This finding brings into the picture the concept of the "developmental environment" (Anthony, 1975), which specifies that development takes place within a succession of environments, some of which may be "average" and "expectable" and others highly powerful, pathogenic, and unpredictable. If change within the developmental environment occurs too rapidly, a state of "future shock" may be precipitated. Again, it is hard to predict without measures of vulnerability and resilience how individuals will respond. Those coming from a stable, constant, and consistent background may overreact to change as a stressor, although, at the same time, the environmental constancy may have induced sufficient resilience for them to withstand this. Individuals emerging from rapidly changing environments may be expected to respond to powerful environmental shifts resiliently, but their uncertain environments may have brought about high degrees of vulnerability, so that they may be among the first to succumb to disastrous occurrences.

One thing is fairly clear from the research: As individuals reach a virtual plateau in adult life, they appear to become less at risk from radical environmental change, although it is possible that the vulnerability may increase again sharply with old age.

Some Tentative Conclusions

In this overview, I have emphasized the dynamic nature of vulnerability and invulnerability, their close ties to innate factors operating genetically, their sensitivity to environmental circumstances, and the vicissitudes that they undergo over developmental time. The resilient can become vulnerable if, as Freud put it, they are subjected to "too searching a destiny," and the vulnerable can become resilient and develop competences, coping capacities, and creativities that were not apparent at the earliest stages. The "mother's undisputed darling" can succumb to chronic setbacks in a world that is indifferent to mothering him or to meeting the intensity of the mothering needs to which he has become accustomed.

On the other hand, the "ugly duckling" with little or no "sending power" may become "immunized" by the early challenges and be gradually changed not only into an attractive swan, but a highly robust one. This enhancement of resilience and this acquisition of new resources often occur in the third year of life, when the basic coping capacities are integrated and when self-management is established. There is always a combination of internal and external resources working together that furnishes the invulnerable child with the necessary resilience to overcome life's stresses.

Hans Christian Andersen has been cited as a highly vulnerable individual who underwent this transformation and described it in various stories. In his case, the transformation involved the constructive use of fantasy in the restorative rebound process, with additional help from language skills, symbolic functioning, the use of play and dramatization, and the identification with significant figures with whom he came into contact. Mediating adults in the outside world helped this imaginative child to develop competences that did not interfere with the development of his own autonomy and mastery. Although a "dreamer," he was active in externalizing his fantasies and making use of them in the service of creative productions. Although his setting was impoverished, his parents allowed him ample opportunity and privacy to enact his make-believe activities in a little theatre that they constructed for him and encouraged him in this activity.

In Andersen's case, fantasy played a central role in generating and maintaining vitality, counteracting his extreme vulnerability. It was through this mode that unpalatable reality could be altered and assimilated into the inner representational system, and the symbolic dramatizations allowed him to select bits of experience to incorporate into a scenario over which he had ultimate control. Fantasy also gave Andersen the opportunity for life experiences that were blocked from direct expression, thus reducing some of the misery and loneliness of his life. It was through fantasy, too, that he was able to work on his personal integration, bringing together his talent, his intelligence, his temperament, and his will to succeed. He himself thought that persistence was his saving grace. Finally, fantasy brought him fame and fortune, and this also played a part in carrying his fragile ego through to the end, although not without depressive crises en route from which he always bounced back.

Murphy and Moriarty (1976) have furnished a longitudinal account of resilience replacing vulnerability:

> As a baby, Helen was striking in her quick expression of discomfort to stimulation. She was a thumb sucker even in utero. On the Gesell scale, her adaptive resources were low. She began to experience a series of gastrointestinal difficulties and upper respiratory infections; her autonomic reactivity was reflected in flushing and coldness in her hands and feet. She was rated as of "low functional stability," and was evaluated as *one of the most vulnerable infants in the project* because of the early digestive difficulties, the proneness to infection, the autonomic lability, the low responsiveness to outside interests, the easy fatigability and the poor adaptive resources. She seemed much less skillful than other infants in gratifying her needs. Her mother was not a gratifying mother and gave little time to what she referred to as a "very dumb" baby. In addition, Helen was not physically attractive and seemed to lack "sending power." (p. 297; italics added)

The assessment would seem to be damning, and one might have predicted that Helen would end as a chronically disabled adult, with little in the way of achievements and a great deal in the way of ailments. She was such an odd-looking and sickly infant that adults rapidly became impatient and disenchanted with her. This merely aggravated her brash, demanding behavior. One might understand her caretaker's giving up on her, but the extraordinary thing was that she did not give up on herself and gradually developed a strong if not naive philosophy that "bad things could turn into good things." We will now jump the gap and see her years later.

> She had become a lovely and healthy teenager. She was strongly religious, felt a deep sense of support from God and was very emotionally responsive to church rituals. She found a task within the church that made her indispensable to the pastor. She began to believe that bad people can also turn into good people and so one should be tolerant and accepting of everyone, even those who differed from one's self. She was, thus, able to take people as they were without needing to reform them. At college her resilience increased further. She won a musical scholarship and became an outstanding collegiate. After graduation she married and taught music in the public schools. No one who saw her later as a happy mother and wife would have correlated this picture with the early image of a highly vulnerable baby. (p. 332).

The sense of incorporating something larger than oneself has provided strengths for hypervulnerable children in the St. Louis Risk Research Project (Anthony, 1984), where several children who seemed at risk within a disadvantageous milieu climbed to success and health through intense affiliations with religious groups, especially those on the fringe of established religions. In the more esoteric sects, eccentricities and vulnerabilities seem more acceptable, more tolerated, and better supported by the faithful community; furthermore, purpose and meaning are added to lives that are lived somewhat tenuously.

What confront the investigator of outcomes are the apparent paradoxes, and these are to some extent explicated by the current work on vulnerability and resilience. Elsewhere (Anthony, 1978, pp. 7-8), I have spoken of "a new scientific region to explore" and told a story of resilient development under almost hopeless odds:

Mary was a child of a "poor white" family living in a dilapidated and dirty two-room apartment in the inner city. She had been the seventh of nine children, prematurely born with a congenital dislocation of the hip that was so inadequately treated at the city hospital that she developed a permanent limp. She was hospitalized several times in the first 2 years of life for "chest trouble" from which she almost died. Between 2 and 5 years of age, she was placed in a foster home with three of her siblings because the family living quarters had been condemned as overcrowded and unsanitary. The health visitor reported that the children were constantly exposed to the crude sexual behavior of the parents, especially when the father was drunk, which was fairly frequent. His unemployment, which seemed to be permanent, made him irritable, short-tempered, and brutal. He was brought before the court several times for physically abusing the children, particularly Mary, whom he called "the cripple." The mother was chronically depressed and tired and seemed to have little feeling left inside her for her husband, her children, or herself. A social worker reported that she herself felt depressed every time she made a home visit.

When Mary was referred as a child at risk, I was struck by her immediate friendliness. The warm, comfortable, and trustful reaction took me completely by surprise, since I was expecting almost the reverse. She was only 9 years old, and yet her experience of life had been dark and dismal. I found myself curiously unsure of how to approach her, but she put me at ease and I soon found myself talking to her with less guardedness than I usually use in a first interview. She herself was quite open when she spoke of her life at home, where sometimes "everyone got in the way" and she had "to keep an eye on the little ones because someone might stamp on them, not knowing they were there." Her dad was "grumpy," but one expected this because he did not have a job. "If he hits us, it hurts a little but then we do something else and we don't feel it anymore." I asked her about her mother and once again she answered with a depth of understanding that was surprising. "We haven't got much money and we all have to eat. I try not to eat too much. Sometimes your stomach hurts and you want to eat more. We don't have too much clothes and some of them have big holes, but the holes are not in bad places so you can still wear them." I asked her if this made her feel sad and received once again a very matter-of-fact reply, "It doesn't make me feel sad because I am used to it. But it does make my mom feel sad and she cries sometimes. I help out in the house as much as I can."

I wondered how she spent her spare time. Her eyes lit up as she said enthusiastically, "I am collecting money for the poor children in India. They are starving. They haven't anything to eat and they go to bed hungry. They are always sick and their stomachs get big." I asked what she would want if some kind fairy gave her three wishes, and she considered it very seriously. "First, I want to grow up soon. Then I want to become a nurse. Then I want to go and look after the poor children in India." And what did she want for herself? Her answer was characteristic for her as I had come to know her in this short time, and yet so uncharacteristic for this age of child. "I think I've got everything I want but [and here her eyes sparkled] I have a good wish for you if you like. How would you like to go to Disneyland?" I asked whether she had ever been on vacation, but it turned out that she had never actually left the neighborhood except to visit her mother in the hospital and to come to the clinic.

In risk research, one tries to put such human conditions on a rating scale and reduce them to a set of numbers that can be statistically manipulated. One even attempts to add the stresses together so as to derive a score or to arrange them hierarchically in order of disadvantage. The clinician, taking a holistic view, tends to be affronted by such reductions, but one has to also realize the researcher's predicament when confronted with such an unwieldy mass (or mess) of fantasies, feelings, facts, fictions, and fears and doing his best to quantify the material and institute proper scientific controls.

The paradoxes are evident to the most naive observers, who may resort to transcendental explanation to account for them. In another work (Anthony, 1974b), speaking of what I termed "the syndrome of the psychologically invulnerable child," I commented:

> There are many inequalities into which children are born in this unfairly constituted world—inequalities of rank, of riches, of opportunities, of basic endowment—all of which have been with us for so long a time that they are more or less taken for granted. One of the most significant inequalities for the future well-being of the individual is the inequality of risk, that is, the uneven distribution of stress through the population of children. This means that for some the world is secure, stable, and predictable; they are born into acceptance, concern, and care; they are planned for, hoped for, and welcomed. For others, the reverse is true. Life for them is short, sharp, and brutish. They have parents who hate them from conception, reject them from birth, batter them as infants, neglect them as toddlers, and institutionalize them or have them fostered at the drop of a hat. Nevertheless, two children from the same stock, the same womb, the same propitious or unpropitious environment may end it quite differently with one falling psychologically ill and the other apparently blossoming. A super child may come out of the ghetto and a sad and sorry child from the well-to-do suburbs. Why and how? By what mysterious process of psychological selection is the one destroyed and the other preserved? Admittedly, the two worlds may not be so different beneath the surface; a seemingly indulgent household in a superior neighborhood may camouflage as many cruelties and crudities as an overcrowded tenement apartment. Exposure is clearly not the whole story; vulnerability and mastery also play integral roles in determining the response to stress. (p. 533)

Certainly adversity itself is not the whole story: that it can also conduce to resilience and mastery has been documented by Goertzel and Goertzel (1962) in their study of the childhoods of more than 400 famous 20th-century men and women. They found that over three-quarters of them were highly stressed as children by poverty, broken homes, rejection, overpossessive mothers, estranged or domineering parents, and handicaps such as blindness, deafness, crippling conditions, small size, chronic physical illness, and speech defects.

Segal and Yahraes (1978) speak of "children who will not break" (p. 282)—that fascinating group of children who have been identified and defined as "the invulnerables" and who, despite disadvantages of every description, manage to achieve emotional health and high competence. Instead of falling victims to despair, degradation, and deficit, they not only remain unscarred, but can function at remarkably high levels. Segal and Yahraes feel that "the study of so-called invulnerability may be among the most important research projects underway in child development today. If we can discover what the factors are (other than genetic) that make the difference between prevailing over and succumbing to adversity, we can hope to learn how to impart these capacities to the children who need them" (1978, p. 288). If one could find out what makes the small percentage of "supernormals" rise to greater heights, we might be able to incorporate these ingredients, whatever they turn out to be, into every childhood. It is for this reason that Garmezy (1971) refers to them as "the children of the dream" (p. 114). As Segal and Yahraes put it: "People like Garmezy and Anthony emphasize the positive side of the risk statistics, and indeed these new studies are exciting and hold out great hope. We need to know what it is that makes children prevail, as well as what makes them succumb" (1978, p. 285).

Some observers have pointed to the importance of a crucial and constant figure in the life of the child confronted with adversity. This is what the Russian author Maxim Gorky (1915) wrote of his grandmother:

> Until she came into my life, I seemed to have been asleep, and hidden away in obscurity; but when she appeared, she woke me and led me to the light of day. Connecting all my impressions by a single thread, she wove them into a pattern of many colors, thus making herself my friend for life, the being nearest my heart, the dearest and best known of all; while her disinterested love for all creation enriched me, and built up the strength needful for a hard life. (1915)

Gorky's grandmother came to help the household when his father lay dying, and she remained as the bedrock on which he built his life successfully amidst great disadvantages and hardships.

The idea of invulnerability, like the idea of immortality, has haunted the human race since the beginning of recorded history and has given rise to many and varied interpretations of mysteries appertaining to origin and extinction, to the relationship of the natural to the supernatural order, and to the apparent immunity from the disasters of illness and injury granted to certain individuals (Anthony, 1974b). The greatest curiosity about myths of invulnerability is that they are repeated in various similar forms in cultures widely separated in time and space. One set of stories relates invulnerability to the care and devotion of the mother, who works in a number of ways to make her offspring immune from injury or death. A second set of stories attributes the extraordinary resilience to an inherent robustness that allows the gifted individual an inordinate capacity to cope with dangers that threaten to overwhelm him in ways that help to enhance his resilience. Still a third group of stories tells of initially vulnerable individuals who gradually develop resources that help to overcome the vulnerability and eventually create invulnerability. The vulnerable ones bounce back against all odds, and this experience helps to harden them against all misfortune. The myths of the Scandanavian god Balder, the Greek heroes Achilles and Hercules, and the Indian man–god Krishna all exemplify a seeming invulnerability. It is not total, and the drama is enacted around some tiny locus of vulnerability that is concealed but eventually discovered. The buffering system operates in all these myths in terms of constitutional, maternal, familial, ego-based, and community-derived factors, as it does in the human material described and discussed in this overview (see Figure 1-1). This paradigm summarizes the various ways in which vulnerability develops or fails to develop into resilience. However, the concept of the buffering system suggests some degree of passivity on the part of the organism, unless one takes careful note that the operations of the system involve both passive and active processes, as outlined in Table 1-3. It will be noticed that the individual deals with stress, trauma, and overwhelming change with increasing activity and increasing use of inner and outer resources.

In spite of tragic endings to the mythological "invulnerables," many subsequent writers have been tempted to convey the more wishful idea that resilience has its own rewards. For instance, Daniel Defoe (1722) told the charming tale of "The Fortunes and Misfortunes of the Famous Moll Flanders, Who was Born in Newgate [a prison], and during a Life of continu'd variety for Threescore Years, besides her Childhood, was Twelve Year a Whore, Five Times a Wife (whereof once to her own Brother), Twelve Year a Thief, Eight Year a Transported

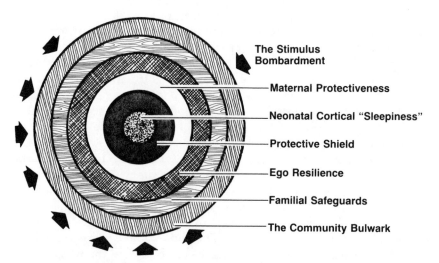

The Stimulus Bombardment

Maternal Protectiveness

Neonatal Cortical "Sleepiness"

Protective Shield

Ego Resilience

Familial Safeguards

The Community Bulwark

Figure 1-1. The buffering system of the human organism against undue excitation.

Table 1-3. Dealing with Stress, Trauma, and Overwhelming Change

1. Stimulus barrier and threshold level of response.
2. Habituation: "inoculation" effect.
3. Defensive and coping ego functioning.
4. Enhancement of competence: scholastic, interpersonal, representational.
5. New creative, inventive, playful, and imaginative activity.

Felon in Virginia, at last grew Rich, liv'd Honest, and died a Penitent" (p. iii).

Are there "types" of "invulnerability" that can be diagnosed with prospective or retrospective longitudinal research and with long-term psychological treatment? The state of the field is such that only a very tentative "typology" can be attempted at this stage, with the understanding that future work will revise it radically or even discard it in the light of field and laboratory studies of resilience. One has to take it for granted that "invulnerability" is a partial and dynamically changeable state in constant interaction with a changing environment.

The following is an incomplete list of types that have been so far described:

1. First, there is the "invulnerable" who has a "sociopathic," uninvolved approach to the world and is strategically estranged from it. The type has been picked up in epidemiological research (Hinkle, 1974), in literature (Camus, 1954, in the character of Meursault), and in risk research (Anthony, Chapter 6, this volume; Bleuler, 1978). I have spoken of early-developing defenses of suppression, isolation, and distancing from objects. Bleuler takes exception to labeling these individuals schizoid. As he puts it, "What appeared to be a form of Schizoid Autism [in children of schizophrenic parents] in an erotic situation, *without knowing their internal suffering*, was actually the understandable, rather dramatic reaction of a warm-hearted, sensitive human being" (1978, p. 380; italics added). In his opinion, therefore, the "stranger" reaction overlies strong positive interactional feelings. In my own experience, the affect may or may not be blunted, but there would seem to be a "basic fault" (the emotional "Achilles heel") in establishing a groundwork of intimacy and generativity within object relationships. The individual may be alienated or emotionally responsive, but the crucial element of intimacy is missing. They do not, cannot, or will not get close to the object because of early experiences of suffering at the hands of primary objects. Whether the narcissism dominating their way of life is primary or secondary has still to be deciphered by treatment in depth (but this, of course, is strenuously avoided and rejected by these individuals).

2. There is also the "invulnerable" who leads a charmed life because of the overprotectiveness of the mother (the Achilles and Balder myths); actually, such an individual is a pseudoinvulnerable, because he is largely unchallenged by the actualities of life. One such person remarked, "I was born in a caul and therefore nothing can harm me," and behind this comment was his deep-seated belief that he was symbiotically tied to his all-powerful mother whose magical powers would ensure that nothing bad would ever happen to him. In my discussion of "the syndrome of the psychologically invulnerable child" (Anthony, 1974b), I quote a fairly typical case:

> When he was an infant, his mother could never leave him for an instant, and she still feels worried and unhappy when he is out of her sight. . . . she breastfed him for 13 months and spoonfed him for the first five years. She dressed him in the morning although he was now eight and watched from the window while he walked to school. When out together, she always insisted on holding his hand. She was afraid to let him run upstairs since he got out of breath, and he was not allowed to visit in other homes because of possible infection. She never allowed him to play with other children because they were rough and might hurt him. He was allowed no outdoor sport for fear of injury. (Levy, 1966, p. 28)

Such children, because of the high degree of maternal care, enjoy a good measure of health, but as a consequence they remain psychologically attached, dependent, avoidant, and self-centered. They tend, however, to break down when they leave the magical ambience of the mother and may, in disposed cases, develop schizophrenia.

3. Another group of "invulnerables" who are also pseudoinvulnerable tend to be accident-prone from the endless risks that they take, especially when an audience is around. These "heroes" suffer from overdeveloped counterphobic defenses and marked exhibitionistic drives to be conspicuous (A. Freud, 1949). For a while at least, their propensities may serve the aim of adjustment to the community and may result in good performances of very difficult tasks carried out unselfishly, but there is a compulsiveness about their behavior that makes their condition highly brittle. When the difficulties or dangers increase beyond a certain point, the underlying phobic tendencies erupt into the open, or their exhibitionism may become socially disruptive and unacceptable. They are therefore "pseudoheroes," who glory in demonstrating their prowess but invariably and inevitably are shown up eventually as essentially needy and timid. Psychoanalysts would see their behavior as a variant of the castration complex.

4. The true "invulnerables" are also true heroes who tend to leave the scene of heroism self-effacingly. Instead of breaking down when the going gets rough, they perform better than ever. The developmen-

tal history is characteristic, with an onset in infantile robustness coupled with strong "in-the-world" feelings and attitudes. Under the unobtrusive aegis of resilience parental models, they constantly explore the environment and practice their growing skills. They seem inherently endowed with a wide range of competences, and their normal defenses, coping skills, and creativity grow with age. They typically represent outer experience clearly, unequivocally, and authentically. Their creativity tends to be "healthy" and outer-directed, but they are not afraid to explore the inner world. Their object relationships are soundly based and enduring. In mythology, one thinks of Hercules, whose resourcefulness and resilience developed in the face of challenge and adversity to the point that he underwent an apotheosis. As a group, therefore, these true "invulnerables" display a high degree of competence in spite of (or sometimes because of) stressful environments and experiences. They are interpersonally skillful, popular with peers and adults, well regarded by themselves and others, active on their own behalf, characterized by a strong sense of personal control, responsible for their own actions, and (for the most part) self-regulatory. They are reflective rather than impulsive, and keep a good hold on their emotions, although they can exercise the full range of normal feelings. Their eagerness to learn, their curiosity, and their involvement with the total scholastic experience endear them to teachers. As Whitehorn (quoted in Segal & Yahraes, 1978) put it, they "work well, play well, love well and expect well" (p. 285).

5. A special subgroup of "invulnerables" comprise those who have bounced back and continue to rebound from high risks and vulnerabilities. They frequently begin life as frail, weak, and ailing infants and children; despite this fragility, they gradually develop a seemingly implacable resolve "not to be broken" and demonstrate an extraordinary degree of persistence in their continuous struggles with adversity. In the service of survival, they can display a high degree of creativity, which tends to be inner-directed and agonizingly expressed. Their capacity to transform intolerable reality through fantasy is of a high order and, at its best, gains the lasting attention of the world. Their creative activity relieves their overwhelming sense of vulnerability, but as it abates, they become susceptible to breakdown. It is a lifelong struggle by often very miserable people, but society benefits from it. On a more humdrum level, they may find *lebensraum* for themselves that fits their capacities and provides them with absorbing vocations. Bleuler's Vreni (see Anthony, Chapter 6, this volume) is a good example of constructive but not creative thriving. Developing a philosophy of life or a religious outlook may also be highly affective in making the vulnerable resilient. Helen (Murphy & Moriarty, 1976; see pp. 37–38, this chapter) came to believe, with a growing conviction, that "good

things can come out of bad things" and that "bad people can become good people." In the St. Louis Risk Research Project (Watt, Anthony, Wynne, & Rolf, 1984), esoteric religion has been seen to furnish vulnerables with strength and support from the religious community and to give meaning and substance to their lives. Very often there is some charismatic or inspirational person who helps to "turn them on" and sustain them, and the effect may be long-lasting. Occasionally, some chronic disaster (handicap or illness) may help to organize the often disorganized life of the vulnerable one and give it structure and, indirectly, increasing resilience (see Anthony, Chapter 6, this volume).

This brings to a close this tentative typology that may help to stimulate further thought and investigation. There is so much promise bound up with this group. As Segal and Yahraes (1978) put it, they constitute "our best research hope" (p. 297). And in an even more rhapsodical vein, Garmezy (1971) declares that "with our nations torn by strife between races and between social classes, these 'invulnerable' children remain the 'keepers of the dream' " (p. 114). Were we to study the forces that move such children to survival and adaptation, the long-range benefits to our society may be far more significant than our many efforts to construct models of primary prevention designed to curtail the incidence of vulnerability.

REFERENCES

Andersen, H. C. (1847). *The true story of my life*. London: Longman, Brown, Green, Longman.

Anthony, E. J. (1958). An experimental approach to the psychopathology of childhood autism. *British Journal of Medical Psychiatry, 31*, 211–225.

Anthony, E. J. (1970). The impact of mental and physical illness on family life. *American Journal of Psychiatry, 127*, 138–146.

Anthony, E. J. (1974a). A risk–vulnerability intervention model. In E. J. Anthony & C. Koupernik (Eds.), *The child in his family: Children at psychiatric risk* (International yearbook, Vol. 3). New York: Wiley.

Anthony, E. J. (1974b). The syndrome of the psychologically invulnerable child. In E. J. Anthony & C. Koupernik (Eds.), *The child in his family: Children at psychiatric risk* (International yearbook, Vol. 3). New York: Wiley.

Anthony, E. J. (1975). Influence of a manic–depressive environment on the child. In E. J. Anthony & T. Benedek (Eds.), *Depression and human existence*. Boston: Little, Brown.

Anthony, E. J. (1978). A new scientific region to explore. In E. J. Anthony, C. Koupernik, & C. Chiland (Eds.), *The child in his family: Vulnerable children* (International yearbook, Vol. 4). New York: Wiley.

Anthony, E. J. (1984). The St. Louis Risk Research Project. In N. F. Watt, E. J. Anthony, L. C. Wynne, & J. Roth (Eds.), *Children at risk for schizophrenia: A longitudinal perspective*. Cambridge, England: Cambridge University Press.

Bergman, P., & Escalona, S. K. (1949). Unusual sensitivities in very young children. *Psychoanalytic Study of the Child, 3–4*.

Berlin, I. (1953). *The hedgehog and the fox: An essay on Tolstoy's view of history*. New York: Simon & Schuster.

Bleuler, M. (1978). *The schizophrenic disorders*. New Haven, CT: Yale University Press.

Bloom, B. S. (1964). *Stability and change in human characteristics*. New York: Wiley.

Bornstein, P. E., Clayton, P. J., Halikas, J. A., Maurice, W. L., & Robins, E. (1973). The depression of widowhood after thirteen months. *British Journal of Psychiatry, 122*, 561–566.

Burlingham, D., & Freud, A. (1942). *Young children in wartime: A year's work in a residential war nursery*. London: Allen & Unwin.

Campbell, A., Converse, P. E., & Rodgers, W. L. (1976). *The quality of American life*. New York: Russell Sage Foundation.

Camus, A. (1954). *The stranger*. New York: Knopf.

Caplan, G., & Killilea, M. (Eds.). (1976). *Support systems and mutual help: Multidisciplinary explorations*. New York: Grune & Stratton.

Cohen, F., & Lazarus, R. S. (1973). Active coping processes, coping dispositions and recovery from surgery. *Advances in Psychosomatic Medicine, 35*, 375–389.

Defoe, D. (1722). *Moll Flanders*. Harmondsworth, England: Penguin, 1978.

Dohrenwend, B. S., & Dohrenwend, B. P. (Eds.). (1981). *Stressful life events and their contexts*. New York: Prodist.

Engel, G., & Schmale, A. H. (1972). Conservation-withdrawal: A primary regulatory process of organismic homeostasis. In R. Porter & J. Knight (Eds.), *Physiology, emotion and psychosomatic illness* (Ciba Foundation Symposium 8). Amsterdam: Elsevier/Excerpta Medica.

Erikson, E. H. (1950). *Childhood and society*. New York: Norton.

Fenichel, O. (1945). The psychoanalytic theory of neurosis. New York: Norton.

Fraiberg, S. (1959). *The magic years*. New York: Scribner's.

Freud, A. (1949). Certain types and stages of social maladjustment. In *The writings of Anna Freud: Vol. 4. Indications for child analysis and other papers*. New York: International Universities Press, 1968.

Freud, S. (1922). Beyond the pleasure principle. *Standard Edition, 18*, 1–64. London: Hogarth Press, 1955.

Freud, S. (1937). Analysis terminable and interminable. *Standard Edition, 23*, 209–253. London: Hogarth Press, 1964.

Freud, S. (1925). *General works, 12*, 26. London: Imago Publishing.

Friedman, M., & Rosenman, R. (1974). *Type A behavior and your heart*. New York: Fawcett Crest Books.

Garmezy, N. (1971). Vulnerability research and the issue of primary prevention. *American Journal of Orthopsychiatry, 41*(1), 101–116.

Goertzel, V., & Goertzel, M. G. (1962). *Cradles of eminence*. Boston: Little, Brown.

Gore, S. (1981). Stress-buffering functions of social supports. In B. S. Dohrenwend & B. P. Dohrenwend (Eds.), *Stressful life events and their contexts*. New York: Prodist.

Gorky, M. (1915). *My childhood*. Harmondsworth, England: Penguin, 1966.

Hartmann, H. (1950). Comments on the psychoanalytic theory of the ego. In *Essays on ego psychology*. New York: International Universities Press, 1964.

Hartmann, H. (1951). Technical implications of ego psychology. In *Essays on ego psychology*. New York: International Universities Press, 1964.

Hinkle, L. E. (1972). An estimate of the effects of "stress" on the incidence and prevalence of coronary heart disease in a large industrial population in the United States. In *Proceedings of the International Society on Thrombosis and Haemostasis*. Stuttgart, West Germany: Shattaur Verlag.

Hinkle, L. E. (1974). The effect of exposure to culture change, social change, and changes in interpersonal relationships on health. In B. S. Dohrenwend & B. P. Dohrenwend (Eds.), *Stressful life events*. New York: Wiley.

James, W. (1890). *The principles of psychology.* New York: Dover, 1950.

Jaspers, K. (1963). *General psychopathology.* Chicago: University of Chicago Press.

Jung, C. G. (1930). Psychology and poetry. In *The collected works of C. G. Jung: Vol. 10. Civilization in transition.* Princeton, NJ: Princeton University Press, 1964.

Kafka, F. (1974). *I am a memory come alive* (N. N. Glatzer, Ed.). New York: Schocken Books.

Kagan, J. (1969). Continuity in cognitive development during the first year. *Merrill–Palmer Quarterly of Behavior and Development, 15,* 101–119.

Kellam, S. (1974). Stressful life events and illness. In B. S. Dohrenwend & B. P. Dohrenwend (Eds.), *Stressful life events.* New York: Wiley.

Kahn, M. M. (1963). The concept of cumulative trauma. *Psychoanalytic Study of the Child, 18,* 286–306.

Koos, E. (1946). *Families in trouble.* New York: King's Crown Press

Korner, A. (1971). Individual differences at birth. *American Journal of Orthopsychiatry, 41,* 608–619.

Kroeber, T. C. (1963). The coping functions of the ego mechanisms. In R. W. White (Ed.), *The study of lives.* New York: Atherton Press.

Langer, S. (1942). *Philosophy in a new key.* New York: North American Library of World Literature.

Levy, D. M. (1966). *Maternal overprotection.* New York: Norton. (Originally published 1943)

MacFarlane, J. W. (1963). From infancy to adulthood. *Childhood Education, 39,* 336–342.

Murphy, L. B., & Moriarty, A. E. (1976). *Vulnerability, coping and growth.* New Haven, CT: Yale University Press.

Piaget, J. (1929). *The child's conception of the world.* London: Routledge & Kegan Paul.

Piaget, J. (1950). *The psychology of intelligence.* London: Routledge & Kegan Paul.

Popper, K. (1972). *Objective knowledge.* Oxford: Clarendon Press.

Rapaport, D. (1960). The structure of psychoanalytic theory. *Psychological Issues, 2* (Monograph 6).

Redl, F. (1969). Adolescents—Just how do they react? In G. Coplen and S. Debovci (Eds.), *Adolescence: Psychosocial Perspectives.* New York: Basic Books.

Rotter, J. B. (1966). Generalized expectancies for internal versus external control of reinforcement. *Psychological Monographs, 80*(1, Whole No. 609).

Rosen, B. M., Bahn, A. K., & Kramer, M. (1964). Demographic and diagnostic characteristics of psychiatric clinic outpatients in the U. S. A. *American Journal of Orthopsychiatry, 24,* 455–467.

Schmale, A. H. (1972). Giving up as a final common pathway to changes in health. *Advances in Psychosomatic Medicine, 8,* 20–40.

Segal, J., & Yahraes, H. (1978). *A child's journey: Forces that shape the lives of our young.* New York: McGraw-Hill.

Terman, L. M. (1925). *Genetic studies of genius.* Stanford, CA: Stanford University Press.

Thomas, A., Birch, G., Chess, S., Hertzig, M. E., & Korn, S. (1963). *Behavioral individuality in early childhood.* New York: New York University Press.

Toynbee, A. (1972). *A study of history.* New York: McGraw-Hill.

Watt, N. F., Anthony, E. J., Wynne, L. C., & Rolf, J. E. (Eds.). (1984). *Children at risk for schizophrenia: A longitudinal perspective.* Cambridge, England: Cambridge University Press.

White, R. W. (1959). Motivation reconsidered: The concept of competence. *Psychological Review, 66,* 297–333.

White, R. W. (1963). Sense of interpersonal competence. In R. W. White (Ed.), *The study of lives.* New York: Atherton Press.

Woolf, V. (1977). *Moments of being* (J. Ferrone, Ed.). New York: Harcourt Brace Jovanovich.

The Development of Competence   II

Competence—the capacity to effectively resolve problems presented in daily life, leading to a sense of mastery and positive self-esteem—has received less careful study than factors associated with origins of limitations in coping processes, or psychopathology. The chapters in this section focus on the determinants of competence. First, Seifer and Sameroff discuss the complex interaction of temperament and experience in early childhood. In Chapter 3, Earls, Beardslee, and Garrison report epidemiological findings regarding adaptability, positive response to environmental stress, capacity for work, and self-initiation; Earls and his colleagues find that life context may be more important than attributes of the person as the primary determinant of competence. Murphy then reviews findings focused on characteristics of the children she has followed in the longitudinal Coping Studies at the Menninger Foundation. Her perspective is further documented in Moriarty's discussion of the development of competence, across infancy and the preschool years, of a boy in the Coping Studies sample who initially showed sensory deficits and learning problems.

2

Multiple Determinants of Risk and Invulnerability

RONALD SEIFER
ARNOLD J. SAMEROFF
Brown University

The development of competence in infants and young children is an area that has attracted much attention in recent years. The appeal of such studies is obvious. By examining the development of children in their first years, we may be able to understand the genesis of many psychological characteristics before the effects of family and larger environmental contexts have had an impact on the young child. There has also been a hope that the relative simplicity of the infant's psychological system would allow us to understand more fully the intricacies of human development in a straightforward manner. Unfortunately, this has not been the case. Models for describing and explaining competence during the first years of life are no less complex than models for explaining adult behavior and must account for a multitude of factors that are often not considered in developmental research. A further complicating factor is the tenuous relationship between competence during early childhood and competence in later life (McCall, 1979).

Perhaps the most basic issue that creates problems is the definition of "competence" itself. As with many such questions, there are two complementary issues: definition of "competence" on the one hand and of "incompetence" on the other. Historically, we have been more successful in defining the latter; models of mental illness, psychological disturbance, and developmental disability are well defined. However, the qualities that define a competent, well-developed child are more elusive to specify in a manner that encompasses all children one wishes to classify as competent (B. L. White & Watts, 1973; R. W. White, 1959).

A second issue of importance is the definition of research models used to study competence and incompetence. One approach is to identify children who clearly fall into one or the other of these categories, and then to examine their psychological functioning. The problems with such approaches have been discussed at length—for example, in connection with the study of schizophrenia (Mednick & McNeil, 1968). Briefly, when examining individuals at the end of a developmental path—for example, competent adults—one loses the ability to study the developmental process. One cannot distinguish between qualities that lead to the end result (etiological factors) and those that are caused by or are merely associated with that outcome.

These issues have produced a high level of interest in risk models. Two factors are particularly important in such models. First, populations are studied prospectively, so that findings are not contaminated by knowledge of developmental outcome. Second, populations are selected so that a greater number of outcomes of a particular type will be found. Given that psychologists have been more effective in defining incompetence (i.e., poor outcomes), risk models (as the name implies) have most often concentrated on populations where children are vulnerable to a particular disorder at rates greater than those in the general population.

In the context of this emphasis on risk for unfavorable outcomes, there has been a growing interest in the converse issue of what determines *favorable* outcomes in individual children who are defined as vulnerable to a particular disorder by virtue of their individual, family, or social status. These at-risk children who show good outcomes are often called "invulnerables" (Anthony, 1978). Thus, we have what appears to be a relatively simple research model. One may define populations at risk, follow the children prospectively to determine their developmental outcome, and examine differences between the true vulnerables (those who in fact turn out poorly) and the invulnerables (those who turn out well).

Unfortunately, the real-life situation is not so neat. The major problem lies in current understanding of "risk" and "vulnerability," the foundation on which models of invulnerability are based. Stated simply, most risk models are based on a single factor that defines child vulnerability, such as parental mental illness (Garmezy, 1974), preterm birth of the child with associated medical problems (Field, Goldberg, Stern, & Sostek, 1980), or parental social status (Ramey, Farran, & Campbell, 1979). However, we are becoming increasingly aware that such simple models of vulnerability are inadequate to explain the development of at-risk children who have been studied prospectively during the past two decades (Sameroff & Seifer, 1983; Sameroff, Seifer, & Zax, 1982; Werner & Smith, 1982; Zeskind & Ramey, 1978). What are needed are models that encompass the complexity of developmental processes so that one may properly understand the interplay of risk factors and protective factors in young children.

In the sections to follow, we present data indicating the complex interplay of factors that affect the development of children during their first 4 years of life. These children were part of the Rochester Longitudinal Study (RLS), which examined infants who were at risk for emotional disorder because their mothers suffered from mental illness (Sameroff et al., 1982). We also discuss the theoretical and research context in which these data are examined. The emphasis in our presentation is on the nature and definition of "risk" and "vulnerability." The discussion of vulnerability also has obvious implications for the definition of "invulnerability."

Rochester Longitudinal Study

We have been conducting a longitudinal study that investigates the role of parental mental illness, social status, and other family cognitive and social variables that might be risk factors in the early development of children from birth through 4 years of age. The RLS (Sameroff et al., 1982; Sameroff & Zax, 1978) was one of many studies begun in the last 15 years that were explicitly concerned with the impact of parental schizophrenia on the development of children (Garmezy, 1974). The RLS differed from most of these other studies in three ways. First, the age range of children studied was younger; most other studies focused on school-age children, while we were concerned with infants and preschool children. Second, the RLS studied a variety of other diagnosis groups in addition to schizophrenia, in order to explore issues related to mental illness in general, as well as schizophrenia in particular. Many other studies had only normal controls, or only a single mental illness control group. Third, the sample was heterogeneous on many family variables, in particular socioeconomic status (SES) and race. The strategy of almost all other high-risk schizophrenia studies has been to remove race or social class factors from their designs by matching subject groups on demographic variables or by choosing subjects from limited social status samples.

The results of the RLS to date have been that the offspring of women with severe and chronic mental disturbance suffered from a variety of deficits in social, emotional, and cognitive functioning (Sameroff, Barocas, & Seifer, 1984; Sameroff et al., 1982). These deficiencies, however, could not be related to any specific maternal psychiatric diagnosis, including schizophrenia. Particularly striking was that the differences found between children with mentally ill mothers and normal mothers were frequently mimicked by differences between children from lower social status homes and higher social status homes. The interplay between the risk factors that were associated with having a mentally ill parent and having a poor parent required a careful developmental analysis.

In an assessment of the social and adaptive competence of the children in the study, we (Seifer, Sameroff, & Jones, 1981) compared groups from families that differed on mental illness and social status dimensions when the children were 30 and 48 months old. The measure used was the Rochester Adaptive Behavior Inventory (RABI), which assesses global competence in addition to competence in a number of specific domains. At 30 months, children from families with mentally ill mothers differed from those whose families had no parental mental illness, and children from lower social status families differed from children in higher social status homes on most of the same dimensions. Both groups of at-risk children were less cooperative, more timid, more fearful, and more depressed, and engaged in more bizzare behavior, than their comparison groups. However, at 48 months there was a separation between the risk groups' behaviors. The children of mentally ill mothers continued to show the same differences from children of healthy mothers as they had at 30 months, but some of the differences among children in different social status groups became less pronounced.

The effects on preschool children's social–emotional functioning of having a parent with social–emotional problems may be more pervasive and long-lasting than the effects of having a low social status parent. Alternatively, the risks associated with social status and maternal psychopathology may be different in kind. The impact of social status may be merely to delay the common achievements of childhood. In contrast, mentally ill mothers may provide a qualitatively different child-rearing environment that distorts their children's development in kind, rather than in timing.

Of equal interest is the necessity for a developmental analysis in such areas. If the children had only been assessed at one point in time, we would have reached far different conclusions based on evaluations made only at 30 months or only at 48 months. A further caution is that while one can attempt to separate the effects of social status and mental illness, they are correlated in the real world. The prevalence rate for schizophrenia, for example, is eight times as high in the lowest-SES group as in the highest (Hollingshead & Redlich, 1958). When women were recruited as lower social status controls in the Rochester study, one-fourth of those randomly selected from an obstetrics clinic showed emotional disturbance during a psychiatric interview.

Parental Social Status as a Risk Factor

Social status also had a major impact on the cognitive competence of the children in the RLS. Child mental development was assessed at 4, 12, 30, and 48 months of age, using the Bayley Scales of Infant Development at the three early ages and the Wechsler Preschool and Primary Scale of Intelligence (WPPSI) at 4 years. Figure 2-1 shows the Bayley Mental Development Index (MDI) and WPPSI verbal IQ scores for three groups of subjects: whites from SES levels I, II, and III (Hollingshead, 1957); whites from SES levels IV and V; and blacks from SES levels IV and V. At 4 and 12 months there were no differences in the group means, but by 30 and 48 months there were large effects. Golden and Birns (1976) found a similar lack of differences before the second year in both standardized and Piagetian cognitive tests, with major differences thereafter. In Broman, Nichols, and Kennedy's (1975) report of the Collaborative Perinatal Project sample of over 20,000 children, while there was a trivial correlation between Bayley MDI scores and SES at 8 months of age, there was a strong relation in their 4-year assessment. The data from all of these studies indicate that SES has an impact on the development of intellectual growth after the first year. As children grow older, those from higher-SES families thrive more and more, while lower-SES children become more stifled.

A continuing theme that appears in the results of risk studies based

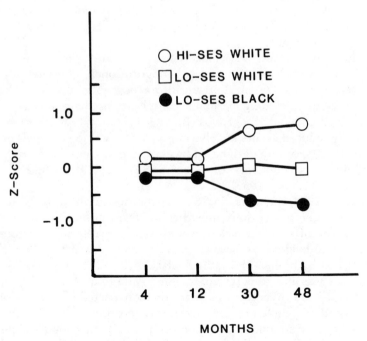

Figure 2-1. Mean standardized IQ scores at 4, 12, 30, and 48 months for three social status groups: high-SES whites, low-SES whites, and low-SES blacks.

on biological factors in a number of areas is that the developmental outcomes are either determined or moderated by social status variables, which are of equal or greater importance than the risk variables themselves. What is so pervasive about these social variables that they intrude into the analysis of every longitudinal study? Hess (1970) discussed the concept in his analysis of SES influences upon socialization in terms of differences with respect to the prestige of occupations, power to influence the institutions of the community, economic resources, and educational opportunity. Different levels of SES give children experiences that are both different and unequal with respect to the rewards of the society. Hess also discussed the relationships between social structure and early experience of children in terms of a number of questions, such as the conditions of the external social and cultural world in which a child lives, the adaptive consequences that adults in the environment acquire in their interaction with the system, the specific forms in which adult orientations appear in interaction with children, and the behavioral outcomes of these experiences in children. These questions assume a linkage between the culture and the behavior of adults who act as socializing and teaching agents for their children.

An attempt to relate these issues to the role of SES in the etiology of schizophrenia was undertaken by Kohn (1973). He argued that "social class is related to schizophrenia primarily because the conditions of life built into lower social class position are conducive to that disorder" (p. 68). The conditions of most concern to Kohn were stress and conceptions of reality.

The case for stress was made by Rosenthal (1970) in his interactive model for schizophrenia, in which a constitutional vulnerability is potentiated by environmental stress into a psychotic illness. Biological vulnerabilities, including perinatal complications, have a higher frequency in the lower-SES groups (Birch & Gussow, 1970). Stress from externally induced events are also more frequent at lower levels of SES (Kohn, 1973). For any designated level of stress, mental disturbance is found in more members of lower-SES groups than higher ones (Langner & Michael, 1963).

Kohn (1973) explains this SES difference in the rate of mental illness by arguing that there must be important differences in the way people from different classes deal with stress. Stressful situations for lower-SES individuals are less alterable by individual action than those experienced by higher-SES individuals. Furthermore, lower-SES individuals are less able to perceive, to assess, and to deal with complexity and stress. Kohn hypothesizes that "the constricted conditions of life experienced by people of lower social class position foster conceptions of social reality so limited and so rigid as to impair people's ability to deal resourcefully with the problematic and the stressful" (1973 p. 73).

If Kohn is correct, then one can conceptualize the differences in developmental outcomes for children in terms of the ability of the children's families to mediate between the children and the environment. Better conceptions of reality, or what we have called "parental perspectives" will permit families to reduce the impact of stress on children and also to provide the children with optimal growth experiences; worse parental perspectives will prevent families from moderating the effects of stressful life experiences on the children or from providing special experiences for children with special needs. Psychological assessments of parental beliefs, attitudes, and values have produced a variety of measures that reflect rigidity and limited conceptions of reality. One can test to see whether parental perspectives, combined with estimates of stressful life events, explain the variance in developmental outcomes associated with social status. One would then have evidence regarding the psychological consequences of the sociological variable of social status.

Analysis of Single Risk Factors

In our previous analyses comparing children from various groups of mothers, we demonstrated that both parental mental illness and family social status factors were directly related to child performance.

Characteristics of the Sample

The 215 members of the RLS who were examined at 48 months were heterogeneous on many dimensions. On social status, all five of Hollingshead's (1957) classes were represented. The sample was about 65% white and 35% nonwhite. Virtually all of the blacks were from the lower SES levels, IV and V. About 75% of the women were married at the time of the prenatal assessment. Mothers' ages when their children were born ranged from 15 to 40 with a mean of 24.4, and about 25% of the women were having their first child.

Child Competence

Two measures of child competence were used that indexed cognitive and social–emotional competence. The first was the verbal scale of the WPPSI IQ test (Wechsler, 1967), which has four subscales: comprehension, vocabulary, similarities, and information. The second measure was the global rating from the RABI, which is derived from a 90-minute parental interview that assesses a child's social–emotional competence in the areas of family life, social interaction, and solitary behavior (Seifer *et al.*, 1981).

Maternal Mental Illness

The diagnosis, chronicity, and severity of the mothers' illness were determined (1) by psychological interviews conducted during the prenatal period and again when their children were 30 months of age; and (2) from records of mental health contacts and hospitalizations kept in a county-wide registry. Four diagnostic comparison groups were formed: women with schizophrenia, women with neurotic depression, women with personality disorder, and a no-mental-illness group. In addition to this categorical measure, we examined two other dimensions of mental health. The severity-of-illness dimension had four categories that were determined from the psychological interviews: (1) no illness; (2) no illness at birth, but some illness at 30 months; (3) mild illness at birth; and (4) severe illness at birth. The chronicity of mental illness dimension also had four categories: (1) no illness; (2) diagnosis made at one interview or one previous mental health contact, but not both; (3) diagnosis made at one interview and one to three previous mental health contacts; and (4) four or more previous mental health contacts or hospitalization.

   Effects of these factors on child outcomes may be summarized briefly. On measures of intelligence at our final two assessment periods (30 and 48 months), no two diagnostic groups differed. However, severity of illness was inversely related to intelligence at both age periods, while chronicity of illness was related only at 48 months. On measures of social–emotional competence, there was only one diagnostic-group difference: The children of depressed mothers were doing worse than those of healthy mothers. However, severity and chronicity of illness had significant effects at both age periods (Sameroff *et al.*, 1982, 1984).

Family Social Status

The RLS sample was heterogeneous on measures of race and SES. Our race measure had two categories: white and black. The SES measure was a modification of the Hollingshead (1957) two-factor system. The original Hollingshead measure uses only the head of household's occupation and education; the modification was to include the mother's education as well. Prior to computation of the index of social position, the mother's and head of household's education were averaged to create a family education score. This was considered preferable to the more recent Hollingshead (1974) scale, which uses occupation and education of both parents. The categorizations that resulted from our modification of the two-factor scale made more intuitive sense than those resulting from either of the Hollingshead schemes.

Social status was related to both intellectual and social–emotional competence at 30 and 48 months (see Figure 2-1). On intelligence measures at both ages, the high-SES whites performed much better than the low-SES whites, who in turn did better than the low-SES nonwhites. On the RABI measure, the high-SES whites were better adjusted than the low-SES nonwhites at 30 months (with the low-SES whites in between), while at 48 months the high-SES whites were better adjusted than both low-SES groups (Sameroff *et al.*, 1982, 1984).

While the effects we found for family mental health and social status are important, these results do not fully address the issue of what psychological processes were responsible for the individual and group variation observed in the children's development. On the one hand, these measures are global indices of a child's environment and do not address the mechanisms of transmission. On the other hand, these factors are not independent (see above) and might be expected to have additive, overlapping effects. As the next step in addressing the complex interactions of risk factors, we examined these two risk factors along with three additional groups of measures that might explain the broad social status and mental illness effects.

Analysis of Multiple Risk Factors

In view of the problems of analyzing single risk factors, described above, we began to examine the RLS data in terms of the interplay among the various risk factors. Two additional steps were taken. The first was to broaden the scope of the variables examined. In addition to social status and mental illness, risk factors of parental perspectives, family stress, and maternal anxiety were added. The second was to examine all of these risk factors combined in the same set of analyses, in order to directly compare both the unique and the overlapping properties of each factor. We considered such an examination of the complexity of risk as a necessary prerequisite to the identification of invulnerable children.

Parental Perspectives

Parents' beliefs about children and the developmental process were viewed as important factors in the relationship among mental illness, social status, and stress. We chose three measures for this dimension that reflected rigidity versus flexibility in attitudes, beliefs, and values that parents had in regard to children. The Concepts of Development Questionnaire (CODQ) (Sameroff & Feil, 1985) evaluates parents' understanding of development on a scale ranging from "categorical" to "perspectivistic." At the "categorical" end, child development is seen as a determined expression of single causes such as constitution or environment. At the "perspectivistic" end, child behavior is seen as the outcome of complex, transactional processes.

The Parental Values Scale (Kohn, 1969) is a measure of the degree to which parents value conformity versus independence in their children. At the "conformity" end are items such as obedience and cleanliness, while at the "independence" end are values of self-control and curiosity.

The "authoritarian/control" factor of the Parental Attitude Research Instrument (PARI) was used. This factor accounts for most of the variance in the PARI and reflects acceptance of parenting attitudes that consolidate control in the parent and minimize the importance of child-directed behavior (Schaefer & Bell, 1958; Zuckerman, Ribback, Monaskin, & Norton, 1958).

These three scales were standardized and summed with unit weight, so that "categorical," "conformity," and "authoritarian" were in the same direction.

Family Stress Factors

The basic method of measuring individual experience of stress is through the use of life events inventories. This method makes an accounting of the number and type of events experienced, but not the individuals' interpretation of those events. Data regarding life events were collected throughout the course of the RLS. These data were reduced using a scale patterned after that of Holmes and Rahe (1967). The variable used in the present analyses was the total number of negative events that occurred from birth until the child was 4 years of age. Events such as divorce, illness, and loss of job were included in the scale (Rosenzweig, Seifer, & Sameroff, 1985).

A second family factor that is related to child competence, especially cognitive competence, is birth order. We used as a measure of birth order whether the child was the firstborn or a later-born child (Zajonc, Markus, & Markus, 1979).

Maternal Anxiety

Where the diagnosis, severity, and chronicity measures of maternal mental illness tapped clinical symptoms, anxiety measures were thought to be more sensitive to variation in the subclinical range of functioning. Three measures of anxiety were combined to form a single scale. These were the total score from the Institute for Personality and Ability Testing (IPAT) Anxiety Scale Questionnaire (Cattell & Scheier, 1963), administered at 30 months; the neuroticism scale from the Eysenck Personality Inventory (Eysenck & Eysenck, 1969), administered at 48 months; and the total score from the Malaise Scale (Rutter, Tizard, Yule, Graham, & Whitmore, 1976), also administered at 48 months. The three scores were standardized and summed with unit weights.

Analysis Plan

The general questions addressed in these new analyses of the RLS data were these: How much of the mental illness or social status variance could be explained by the more specific measures, and how much did the mental illness and social status measures overlap in explaining child competence? Specifically, the analyses (1) determined direct relations between the risk factors and the criterion measures, (2) tested the relative predictive power of the risk factors, and (3) determined the unique variance associated with individual risk factors after the effects of all other predictors were partialed out.

A series of hierarchical multiple-regression (HMR) analyses were performed (Cohen & Cohen, 1983) to address these issues. The HMR approach allows one to examine the effects of sets of variables as predictors entered in regression equations in a planned stepwise manner. The variance explained on the step(s) associated with the predictor variables reflects the relationship between the predictors and the criterion after partialing covariates that are entered on previous steps (i.e., the unique variance associated with the predictors). By systematically permuting the steps on which sets of variables are entered, one may test specific hypotheses such as those described above.

Four regression equations were examined for each of two child competence measures: WPPSI IQ and RABI global rating. There were

four sets of variables entered in each of the regression equations:
(1) mental health (severity, chronicity, and anxiety), (2) parental perspectives, (3) family factors (life events and family size), and (4) social
status (SES and race). A series of HMR analyses was performed so that
each set of variables was entered on the first step (to determine its
direct effect) and on the final step (to determine its effect after all other
predictors were partialed out). These HMR results are summarized in
Tables 2-1 and 2-2. The explanatory power of each set of predictors is
discussed below.

Effects of Risk Factors on Intelligence

The direct relationship between each set of risk factors and the children's intellectual competence was significant (see the first column of
Table 2-1). However, the size of the effects varied by a factor of 5. The
most powerful effect was for social status which explained almost 40%
of the total IQ variance. The next largest effect was for parental
perspectives (about 25% variance explained), followed by family stress
(about 12% variance explained); the smallest effect (about 8% variance
explained) was for maternal illness.

When each predictor set was entered into the HMR equation on
the final step, thereby partialing out the effects of the remaining risk
factors, the situation changed in two ways (see the second column of
Table 2-1). First, the amount of variance explained was much smaller.
The largest effect was still for social status (13% variance explained)
and the smallest for mental illness (0.5% variance explained). The
second change was that maternal mental illness was no longer a significant predictor of child outcome after social status, parental perspec-

Table 2-1. Summary of Hierarchical Multiple-Regression Equations for WPPSI IQ
Scores

Risk factor	Entered first	Entered last	Remaining variables
Mental illness	.081**	.005	.374**
Perspectives	.249**	.012*	.206**
Social Status	.397**	.132**	.058**
Family stress	.125**	.029**	.330**

Note. Each table entry is the change in R^2 associated with the regression step in question.
*$p < .05$.
**$p < .01$.

Table 2-2. Summary of Hierarchical Multiple Regression Equations for RABI Global Rating Scores

Risk factor	Entered first	Entered last	Remaining variables
Mental illness	.156**	.081**	.050**
Perspectives	.068**	.010	.138**
Social Status	.099**	.013	.107**
Family stress	.042*	.003	.164**

Note. Each table entry is the change in R^2 associated with the regression step in question.
*$p < .05$.
**$p < .01$.

tives, and family stress were partialed out. The remaining three sets of risk variables did remain significant, although both parental perspectives and family stress accounted for less than 3% additional variance.

Although the size of some effects was large, there was no single risk factor that accounted for all of the significant variance in the IQ scores. That is, when the variance explained by the remaining risk variables was examined after partialing out any one set of risk factors, the effect was significant in all cases (see the third column of Table 2-1). The total amount of variance explained by all risk factors entered simultaneously was just over 45%.

Effects of Risk Factors on Social–Emotional Competence

Each of the risk factors was directly related to the RABI measure of social–emotional competence (see the first column of Table 2-2). While these results were similar to those for intelligence, the size of the effects for social–emotional competence was much smaller, and the relative ordering of the risk factors in terms of size of effect was much different. Maternal mental illness explained the largest portion of variance in RABI scores (about 16%), followed by social status (about 10%), then by parental perspectives (about 7%), and finally by family stress (about 4%). The smallest and largest effects differed by a factor of 4.

When the risk variables were entered in the HMR equations on the final step, the situation changed markedly (see the second column of Table 2-2). Only one of the risk factors, maternal mental illness, remained significant when all other predictors were partialed out. It explained about 8% of the variance.

While only one of the risk variables was significant when the remainder were partialed out, there was no risk factor that used up all of the significant predictive variance (see the third column of Table 2-2). The smallest amount of variance left over after one predictor set was entered was about 5%, a figure similar to that for the intelligence results. The total variance explained by all risk factors was 26%, little more than half that explained in the intelligence HMR equations.

Rethinking Models of Vulnerability

The analyses presented above are consistent with the idea that (1) there were multiple risk factors operating in our sample and (2) that these factors operated jointly in a complex manner. These findings are also consistent with those of other work (Werner & Smith, 1982) and are indicative of the necessity to examine multiple risk factors in unison rather than single risk factors in isolation. There are many implications of these findings for studies of invulnerability. First, if the research program described at the outset (where one compares subgroups from populations with similar initial risks whose outcomes are good vs. poor) is to have meaning, the initial definitions of "risk" and "vulnerability" must be sound. Existing studies may be just beginning to scratch the surface of what in fact determines risk in young children. In order to examine the concept of "invulnerability," it is necessary to have a well-established definition of "risk." This will only be accomplished when there is full and careful consideration of the multiplicity of and interactions among various risk factors.

A related problem is a conceptual distinction that is implicitly made between what are called "risk factors" and other psychological processes or environmental constraints. There is currently no criterion by which a particular variable is determined to be a risk factor, a protective factor, or merely a measure that is related to the outcome in question. The current situation is that individual researchers make informed, but arbitrary, choices in this matter. However, when investigators with different points of view examine the same populations, conflicts are bound to arise.

For example, risk factors commonly studied are parental mental illness or social status. But when one examines the particular psychological components of these summary descriptions, should each one be considered a risk factor, or simply a psychological process that may exacerbate or ameliorate the presumed risk? In our data presented above, we examined parental cognition as a potential risk factor. However, this variable lies outside the realm of those generally assumed to increase vulnerability. Should this be thought of as a risk variable (as we have thought of it), or merely as a characteristic of the mother that has some effect on child outcome?

Another example from our study involves what is often considered a straightforward example of a risk factor: maternal mental illness. However, we were faced with two major complications. First was the need to decide what are the critical aspects of child risk. In terms of clinical symptoms, severity and chronicity of maternal mental illness were better predictors of poor outcomes in young children than diagnosis. Second, a variable that taps subclinical aspects of mental health—namely, anxiety—was also strongly related to child competence. Thus, a factor often treated as a simple index of risk has its own complex internal structure that must be considered.

Still another example is from the Werner and Smith (1982) 20-year prospective study of a cohort of children born on the Hawaiian island of Kauai. They conceived of risk in terms of perinatal factors and examined variables such as high SES and good family support as potential protective factors. Others with the same data might have chosen to identify SES as the primary risk index, with good perinatal status as the protective characteristic that produced vulnerable versus stress-resistant children.

This issue of defining "risk" might be a trivial matter, except for the fact that what determines vulnerability or invulnerability is dependent upon the initial determination of risk. To some extent, this is a logical dilemma. One could assume that any factor shown to affect child outcome adversely should be considered a risk factor. But then there would be no possibility of finding a set of measures that consistently differentiate vulnerables from invulnerables, since anything that differentiates children with good outcomes from those with poor outcomes would be considered a risk factor. At the other extreme, one might rigidly restrict the conception of risk factors to a small set of measures. But in this case a different type of problem arises. If in the RLS we had considered only parental mental illness to be a risk factor, then we could have concluded with certainty that SES and race are the essential factors that differentiate vulnerables from invulnerables. However, we consider this form of analysis relatively uninformative, since it fails to account for variables at different levels of individual, family, or societal organization as potential risk factors. In sum, to accomplish the goal of identifying factors that protect at-risk children from poor outcome, it is necessary to define the meaning of "risk" somewhere between two extremes. At one pole is a rigid set of single factors, and at the other is an operational definition that includes any factor related to poor outcomes in children.

Contexts of Development and Levels of Organization

One potential solution to the dilemma of how to define "risk" is to entertain a predetermined conceptualization of the developmental process. Doing this would enable investigators to make rational decisions about what aspects of development are to be defined as risk factors (and, by implication, the potential identification of invulnerables) and what aspects are to be reserved for the characterization of stress-resistant children.

One such general approach to understanding human development has been suggested by Sameroff (1982, 1983). It is proposed that a systems model of hierarchies of organization may best define the components of developmental processes. The three levels of most interest for the present question of defining "risk" would be the individual organism, the immediate family, and the cultural context that the family inhabits. Sameroff asserts that the interplay of all three levels must be considered if one is to understand developmental processes and outcomes.

In the case of research on risk factors, there is conflict as to which level produces the primary vulnerability. Those studying perinatal complications such as preterm birth implicitly assume that the risk resides in the constitution of the organism. The area represented most in this volume, parental mental illness, presumes that the risk resides in family contributions (when genetic models are excluded). Finally, another area represented in this volume, social context, assumes the risk to be in the cultural milieu of children and their families. The data analysis we have presented in this chapter is an attempt at simultaneous examination of all three levels of organization. We believe that this multiple-systems approach is an essential component in the definition of "risk" and "vulnerability," and, by extension, of "invulnerability."

What is still lacking is a criterion by which to include a particular measure, at any of these levels of organization, as a risk factor. At the level of individual children, existing studies have concentrated on early biological insults, for which outcomes are extremely variable. Those studies examining illness at the level of the family have focused on a relatively stable characteristic of the parent in question. Again, the range of child outcomes is large. Finally, at the level of social context, very general and relatively stable factors define the risk. As in the other domains, the range of outcomes for children from different cultural contexts is quite large.

Some general themes appear in these determinations of risk: General factors are used (1) that produce a large range of child outcomes, (2) that are stable defining characteristics of an individual, and

(3) that do not involve explicit psychological processes. One task for future research in risk and invulnerability is to more clearly stipulate such qualities that determine a risk factor.

Summary

A common research paradigm for studying invulnerability has been articulated that examined at-risk children in terms of whether they had poor versus good outcomes. Such a strategy relies on well-defined concepts of "risk" and "vulnerability." We have identified problems with existing definitions of "risk," and presented data that highlight the complexity of interactions among risk factors. These findings have been discussed in the context of understanding development in terms of hierarchical levels of organization. Existing studies of vulnerability have located risk at the level of the individual, the family, and the cultural context. However, at all of these levels, there is no clear criterion for differentiating a risk factor from any other psychological variable. Tasks for future work are to further refine the definition of "risk" to overcome these conceptual difficulties, to account for the interplay among risk factors at different levels of organization, and to determine criteria by which a particular variable should be considered a risk factor. When these tasks are accomplished, the problems of identifying invulnerable children—and, conversely, vulnerable children—should be greatly reduced.

ACKNOWLEDGMENTS

The research reported here was supported by grants from the National Institute of Mental Health and the W. T. Grant Foundation.

REFERENCES

Anthony, E. J. (1978). A new scientific region to explore. In E. J. Anthony, C. Koupernik, & C. Chiland (Eds.), *The child in his family: Vulnerable children* (Vol. 4). New York: Wiley.
Birch, H., & Gussow, G. D. (1970). *Disadvantaged children*. New York: Grune & Stratton.
Broman, S. H., Nichols, P. L., & Kennedy, W. A. (1975). *Preschool IQ: Prenatal and early developmental correlates*. Hillsdale, NJ: Erlbaum.
Cattell, R. B., & Scheier, I. H. (1963). *Handbook for the IPAT Anxiety Scale Questionnaire* (2nd ed.). Champaign, IL: Institute for Personality and Ability Testing.
Cohen, J., & Cohen, P. (1983). *Applied multiple regression: Correlation analysis for the behavioral sciences*. (2nd ed.). Hillsdale, NJ: Erlbaum.

Eysenck, H. J., & Eysenck, S. B. G. (1969). *Personality structure and measurement*. San Diego: Robert R. Knapp.

Field, T. M., Goldberg, S., Stern, D., & Sostek, A. M. (Eds.). (1980). *High-risk infants and children: Adult and peer interactions*. New York: Academic Press.

Garmezy, N. (1974). Children at risk: The search for the antecedents of schizophrenia. Part 1. Conceptual models and research methods. *Schizophrenia Bulletin*, No. 8, 14–90.

Golden, M., & Birns, B. (1976). Social class and infant intelligence. In M. Lewis (Ed.), *Origins of intelligence: Infancy and early childhood*. New York: Plenum.

Hess, R. D. (1970). Social class and ethnic influences on socialization. In P. H. Mussen (Ed.), *Carmichael's handbook of child psychology* (Vol. 2). New York: Wiley.

Hollingshead, A. B. (1957). *Two factor index of social position*. Mimeograph. (Available from the author, Sociology Department, Yale University, New Haven, CT)

Hollingshead, A. B. (1974). *Four factor index of social status*. Mimeograph (Available from the author, Sociology Department, Yale University, New Haven, CT)

Hollingshead, A. B., & Redlich, F. C. (1958). *Social class and mental illness: A community study*. New York: Wiley.

Holmes, T. H., & Rahe, R. H. (1967). The Social Readjustment Rating Scale. *Journal of Psychosomatic Research, 11*, 213–218.

Kohn, M. L. (1969). *Class and conformity: A study in values*. Homewood, IL: Dorsey Press.

Kohn, M. L. (1973). Social class and schizophrenia: A critical review and reformulation. *Schizophrenia Bulletin*, No. 7, 60–79.

Langner, T. S., & Michael, S. T. (1963). *Life stress and mental health*. New York: Free Press.

McCall, R. B. (1979). The development of intellectual functioning and the prediction of later IQ. In J. Osofsky (Ed.), *Handbook of infant development*. New York: Wiley.

Mednick, S. A., & McNeil, T. F. (1968). Current methodology in research on the etiology of schizophrenia: Serious difficulties which suggest the use of the high-risk group method. *Psychological Bulletin, 70*, 681–693.

Ramey, C. T., Farran, D. C., & Campbell, F. A. (1979). Predicting IQ from mother–infant interactions. *Child Development, 50*, 804–814.

Rosenthal, D. (1970). *Genetic theory and abnormal behavior*. New York: Wiley.

Rosenzweig, L., Seifer, R., & Sameroff, A. J. (1985). *The impact of stressful life events on high risk families*. Unpublished manuscript.

Rutter, M., Tizard, J., Yule, W., Graham, P., & Whitmore, K. (1976). Research report: Isle of Wight studies, 1964–1974. *Psychological Medicine, 6*, 313–332.

Sameroff, A. J. (1982). Development and the dialectic: The need for a systems approach. In W. A. Collins (Ed.), *Minnesota Symposium on Child Psychology* (Vol. 15). Hillsdale, NJ: Erlbaum.

Sameroff, A. J. (1983). Developmental systems: Contexts and evolution. In P. H. Mussen (Ed.), *Carmichael's handbook of child psychology*. Vol. 4, Section 1. *History, theory and methods* (W. Kessen, vol. ed.). New York: Wiley.

Sameroff, A. J., Barocas, R., & Seifer, R. (1984). The early development of children born to mentally-ill women. In N. F. Watt, E. J. Anthony, L. C. Wynne, & J. Rolf (Eds.), *Children at risk for schizophrenia: A longitudinal perspective*. Cambridge, England: Cambridge University Press.

Sameroff, A. J., & Feil, L. (1985). Parental perspectives on development. In I. E. Sigel (Ed.), *Parental belief systems: The psychological consequences for children*. Hillsdale, NJ: Erlbaum.

Sameroff, A. J., & Seifer, R. (1983). Familial risk and child competence. *Child Development, 54*, 1254–1268.

Sameroff, A. J., Seifer, R., & Zax, M. (1982). Early development of children at risk for emotional disorder. *Monographs of the Society for Research in Child Development, 47*(7, Serial No. 199).

Sameroff, A. J., & Zax, M. (1978). In search of schizophrenia: Young offspring of schizophrenic women. In L. C. Wynne, R. L. Cromwell, & S. Mathysse (Eds.), *The nature of schizophrenia: New approaches to research and treatment.* New York: Wiley.

Schaefer, E. S., & Bell, R. Q. (1958). Development of a parental attitude research instrument. *Child Development, 29,* 339–361.

Seifer, R., Sameroff, A. J., & Jones, F. (1981). Adaptive behavior in young children of emotionally disturbed women. *Journal of Applied Developmental Psychology, 1,* 251–276.

Wechsler, D. (1967). *The Wechsler Preschool and Primary Scale of Intelligence.* New York: Psychological Corp.

Werner, E. E., & Smith, R. S. (1982). *Vulnerable but invincible: A longitudinal study of resilient children and youth.* New York: McGraw-Hill.

White, B. L., & Watts, J. L. (1973). *Experience and environment: Major influences in the development of the young child.* Englewood Cliffs, NJ: Prentice-Hall.

White, R. W. (1959). Motivation reconsidered: The concept of competence. *Psychological Review, 66,* 297–333.

Zajonc, R. B., Markus, H., & Markus, G. B. (1979). The birth order puzzle. *Journal of Personality and Social Psychology, 37,* 1325–1341.

Zeskind, P. S., & Ramey, C. T. (1978). Fetal malnutrition: An experimental study of its consequences for infant development in two caregiving environments. *Child Development, 49,* 1155–1162.

Zuckerman, M., Ribback, B. B., Monaskin, I., & Norton, J. A. (1958). Normative data and factor analysis on the Parental Attitude Research Instrument. *Journal of Consulting Psychology, 22,* 165–171.

3

Correlates and Predictors of Competence in Young Children

FELTON EARLS
Washington University School of Medicine
WILLIAM BEARDSLEE
Harvard Medical School
WILLIAM GARRISON
Washington University School of Medicine

As is traditional in epidemiological studies, the aim in the project to be reported on in this chapter has been to establish reliable and valid grounds for distinguishing young children with clinically significant levels of behavior disturbance from the general population (Earls, 1980a, 1980b, 1982; Earls *et al.*, 1982). Attention has also been given to examining social circumstances and temperamental characteristics of the children as correlates and as potential causes of childhood psychiatric disorder (Earls, 1981, 1983; Garrison & Earls, 1982a, 1982b). From the beginning, however, the ultimate purpose has been to determine the causative roles of both stressful life events in families and temperamental characteristics of young children in the genesis of the common types of psychiatric disorders in children. Children as young as possible have been examined, on the assumption that the hypothesized causal factors might occur early in life, and that through a prospective, longitudinal design their impact on later development might be determined.

The initial study on the prevalence of psychiatric problems in children was devoted to examining 3-year-old children (Earls, 1980a). The age of 3 is generally when children begin to be seen in psychiatric clinics, and about the age when most child psychiatrists have experience in diagnosing and treating children. To date, that aspect of the project has been completed, and a follow-up study of those 3-years-olds at school age has been achieved (Garrison, Earls, & Kindlon, 1983; Garrison & Earls, 1985). Simultaneously, a vigorous effort has been made to collect comprehensive information on family life events and the children's temperaments from new samples of children between birth and 2 years of age living in the same study area, in an effort to establish a solid foundation on which to conduct an even more thorough-going prospective study.

Because we chose to study children quite early in development, several issues particularly germane to this phase of the life cycle were encountered. First, there was the obvious concern with the temporal stability of behavioral characteristics during a time of rapid growth and development. Second, it is commonly believed that children are more resilient than adults, and that young children may be more resilient than older ones. Thus, the effects of a stressful environment may be relatively less harmful to an infant or toddler than to a child of school age. Third, there was an awareness that the questions most fundamental to the epidemiological pursuit were overly narrow in their conceptualization. By studying the impact of stressful events, which occur to some extent in all families, on the development of psychiatric disorders, which occur in only a few children, there were several missed opportunities to address a broader range of questions. In fact, early in the course of this work it became clear that there was no simple, linear relationship between family stress and behavior problems in young children. The possibility was even raised that high levels of stress might exert a protective effect for some children, presumably by fostering the development of successful coping strategies. It was equally apparent that parents differed in how they transmitted the effects of stressful family experiences to their children, and that this too was a major factor in understanding how behavior disorders originated. Finally, it was clear that a measure of "host resistance" was necessary to complete the research design. The characterization of infants' and young children's temperaments was an approximation of this concept that had already been used in the prevalence study (Earls, 1981).

Taken together, these issues suggested that the focus of the study should be expanded to include an emphasis on adaptive and competent behavior. This chapter presents results from an epidemiological survey of 3-year-olds carried out in 1978, and some preliminary data from a 3-year follow-up study of the same children. Because the study sample represents a total population, this new emphasis on health and competence puts the study in a position to generate findings that are free of the typical biases attending sample selection procedures in child psychiatry. The results permit inferences to be made about the proportion of well-adapting children and the variability in measures of competence, just as past results from this project have permitted similar inferences to be made about disordered behavior.

In the course of the study, a number of different psychological constructs have been used that (for purposes of this analysis) all reflect aspects of healthy adjustment. At the beginning of the project, these constructs were used for the purpose of characterizing deviant behavior. In the present exploratory analysis, the risk was taken of assuming that the absence of deviant behavior was equivalent to healthy adjustment. As will be seen, by the time of the follow-up examination, a more direct approach to the measurement of competence had been found. Throughout this analysis, primary interest has been in a comparison of social characteristics and personal assets of children as either correlates or predictors of above-average adaptation and competence in young children. The results of these exercises are interpreted here within a framework of current conceptualizations of social competence, coping, and resiliency.

Methods

Details of the sample have been provided in previous reports (Earls, 1980a; Earls, 1983). In 1978, the total population of 3-year-old children living in a rural, demarcated community in the northeastern sector of the United States was surveyed. Of 110 children identified through a family register, 100 participated; the parents of the remainder refused participation. Methods included separate and independent interviews with mothers and fathers and blind assessments of the children at play (Earls et al., 1982). The interviews with each set of parents covered a wide range of topics related to the family environment, the parents' health, and the child's health and behavior. A home-based play session was also conducted, taking about 1 hour to complete. It combined elements of unstructured free-play technique and structured procedures. The free-play portion involved a portable sandbox and a group of miniature toys; it lasted 20 minutes. Following a brief transitional period, the child was administered selected items from the McCarthy Scales of Developmental Activities (McCarthy, 1974).

These data contained several indices reflecting the behavioral adjustment of the children: a score tallying the number of behavior problems reported by the parents, derived from the Behavior Screening Questionnaire (BSQ; Richman & Graham, 1971); temperament scores derived from the nine categories proposed by Thomas and Chess (1977); and several scores derived from observations of the children's play behavior (Earls & Cook, 1984). These three sets of variables, shown in Table 3-1, were all rated on ordinal scales. In addition, both clinical and statistical techniques were used to combine and summarize these data in second-order analyses. One of the clinical approaches, described in detail elsewhere (Earls, 1982; Earls et al., 1982), produced judgments about the severity of behavior problems, need for intervention, and prognosis for the children.

Table 3-1. Key Study Variables

BSQ items	Temperament categories	Play observation variables
Eating problems	Activity	Play involvement
Soiling	Rhythmicity	Anxiety
Sleep problems	Adaptability	Organization of scene
Activity	Approach–withdrawal	Theme development
Concentration	Threshold	Vitality
Dependency/attention seeking	Intensity	Language
Moods	Mood	Physical activity
Worries	Distractibility	Self-esteem
Fears	Persistence	Ability to adapt/cope
Relationships with peers/sibs		Efforts to cope
Temper tantrums		Construction
Difficult to manage		Anger
		Happiness
		Number of objects used
		Trusting of examiner
		Imaginative play
		Maintenance of interest

A statistical analysis of play observation data reported by Block and Block (1979) has produced a typology of personal characteristics of children. Since the play technique used by these investigators was adapted for use in this study, similar data were obtained, and this allowed use of a similar typology to classify the children's personal characteristics. The item pool from which the typology was derived is the California Child Q-Sort (Block & Block, 1979); the typology, which is a characterization of resiliency and control, is shown in Table 3-2. These Q-Sort data exist in addition to the 22 play observation variables contained in Table 3-1.

In the analysis that follows, two strategies have been used. From data collected when the children were 3 years old, the absence of behavioral problems as reported by the parents (i.e., low BSQ scores) and clinical ratings denoting the absence of any clinical concern about the children's emotional development were used as criteria. Personality characteristics, as measured in the temperament questionnaire and observed by two blind examiners in the play session, were correlated with these measures of good adjustment. Social factors pertaining to the home environment and parent mental status variables were also included in this correlational analysis.

Table 3-2. Four-Factor Personality Typology Based on Items from the California Q-Sort

Resilient undercontroller	Resilient overcontroller
Physically active	Open and straightforward
Vital, energetic	Empathic
Tends to arouse liking	Neat, orderly
Curious, exploring	Obedient, compliant
Recoups after stress	Calm, relaxed
Emotionally expressive	Seeks to be independent
Brittle undercontroller	*Brittle overcontroller*
Reverts to immature behavior under stress	Fearful, anxious
Is eager to please	Tends to brood
Restless and fidgety	Inhibited, constricted
Rapid shifts in mood	Shy, reserved
Unable to delay gratification	Tends to withdraw
Overreacts to minor frustrations	Rigidly repetitive under stress

Note. Q-Sort adapted from Block and Block (1979).

Because of the indirect nature of this approach—that is, because it was assumed that the absence of symptoms was an index of social competence—a clinical review of the cases was made by one of us (W. B.), who had not been involved in any aspect of the data collection. This was done as a conscious effort to isolate from the children's play behavior and from parents' reports those characteristics that indicated adaptive behavior and good coping skills. The strategies involved in doing this were governed more by a thorough review of the literature on competence (Bemporad, Beardslee, & Earls, 1982) than by any one theoretical persuasion.

By the time of the follow-up of these children in 1981, a more direct approach to the measurement of competence, applicable to young children, had been discovered. The measuring instrument known as the Pictorial Scale of Perceived Competence and Acceptance for Young Children (Harter, 1981) was developed from a theoretical perspective articulated by Harter (1978) and is similar to the language based scale for older children (Harter, 1982). The methods used at follow-up involved (1) self-reports from the children on perceived competence; (2) administration of intelligence and achievement tests; (3) teachers' reports of children's competence and classroom behavior; and (4) parents' reports of children's behavior problems. Data from the children and teachers were collected in school classrooms. A previous analysis on the applicability of this instrument for use in this population found that of the four subscales (cognitive competence, physical competence, peer acceptance, and maternal acceptance) included in this instrument, the children's self-ratings of cognitive competence agreed well with the teachers' ratings of the same and with achievement scores (Garrison *et al.*, 1983). The other subscales were found to possess less agreement with measures external to them. The analysis reported here represents an initial step in exploring some of the social and temperamental antecedents of competence in young school-age children. All of the predictor variables are taken from the parent interviews and play sessions done when the children were aged 3.

In summary, the methods involved efforts to identify in the same total population sample the most socially competent children at two points in time. In the preschool period, an indirect index of competence was derived, and other variables were correlated with it. A case-by-case review of the children selected using this approach added a measure of validity to the approach. At the second point in time, 3 years later, a more direct measure of competence was achieved, and the predictive significance of home environment and temperament variables from the preschool period for the children's level of competence at school age was analyzed.

Results

Quantitative Analysis of Symptomless Children

Twenty 3-year-old children, 12 boys and 8 girls, had BSQ scores of 3 or less; these represented the lowest-scoring children in the sample of 100. Although 41 symptoms were reported by the parents of this group, only 1 of these symptoms was rated as present to a degree significant enough to interfere with a child's emotional adjustment. The most frequent symptoms reported were (1) fears (55%), (2) poor sibling relationships (40%), and (3) temper tantrums (35%). It should be reiterated that although these were the most frequent symptoms, they were of little or no clinical significance because all of these children received clinical ratings in the normal range.

All these children were described by their parents as having "easy" temperaments, and 90% of the children were classified as ego-resilient on the California Q-Sort. The play characteristics most highly correlated (all p's $< .01$) with this group were (1) high play involvement, (2) high initiation of play, and (3) the development of clear themes during the course of the play session.

A number of home environment variables were examined, but none were found to be closely associated with this group. Of these children, 10% had mothers who reported depressive symptoms, and 15% had parents who were separated. Both these figures were similar to those found for the total sample. The social class distribution, the number of working mothers, the percentage of children in nursery school, and the average number of stressful events experienced by the families in the year prior to the interview were all very similar to proportions observed in the sample as a whole.

Case Review of Symptomless Children

STRESS

The clinician reviewing these records (W. B.) found that many of the children were under high stress, despite their low BSQ scores. A number of the stresses were in areas though to be harmful to the children, such as birth of siblings, marital separation of parents, depression in mothers (severe enough in some cases to require psychiatric treatment), and the absence of fathers for long periods because of work. Social isolation was also described in a number of mothers. A child of a parent with the most severe illness of any one in the entire sample was among the low-scoring children.

PARENTAL DESCRIPTIONS OF CHILDREN

Throughout the material, the parental descriptions of these children were filled with positive words and phrases. There was a kind of undifferentiated, unqualified positive regard expressed for them. However, they were not "Pollyannaish." Indeed, in a number of instances, general anger, general dissatisfaction, anger toward a spouse, somber mood, or dissatisfaction regarding a living situation were expressed, while talk about a child was quite different. Words like "lovable," "considerate," "affectionate," "pleasant," "happy," "calm," "warm," "easy," "confident," "imaginative," and "courageous" occurred frequently in their descriptions. The children's activeness, imagination, and energy were valued, as was their capacity to spend time alone. For example, one mother commented that her son was an active child who liked "to talk, sing, draw, and roughhouse." These children then, seemed spared from the frustrations and difficulties that their parents encountered in a variety of life circumstances.

PLAY CHARACTERISTICS

The free-play session involved three phases: (1) initial engagement, (2) the development of symbolic themes represented in the child's verbalizations and toy constructions, and (3) termination. The most obvious general characteristic evident in this group was the ability to handle transitions well. Almost all the children engaged rapidly with the play situation and with the examiner. This was impressive, given the facts that the examiner was a stranger and that the session took place in the children's own homes, where there were many distractions. Throughout the entire 1-hour session these children maintained an affective relationship with the examiner, demonstrated by the fact that they communciated their feelings and thoughts to the examiner.

These children displayed an ability to initiate and construct themes, which rendered their play coherent and intelligible to the examiner. A vignette taken from a play observation summary serves to illustrate this phenomenon:

> His first attention was given to the transportation toys. He named, asked about, examined parts and details of, and was attentive to their opening parts, use, and function, and then lined them up here and there in the sandbox.

Thus, the child began by making sense of the sandbox situation, both by engaging the examiner and by defining the objects within it. This child and many others proceeded to enact sequences of play in which characters (primarily family members) were clearly identified doing different tasks or constructing an interesting scene. A salient characteristic of the play sequences was their coherence. In a coherent play sequence, the child produced an overall conceptualization for the actions and events taking place. Objects were used appropriately, and the sequence had a clear beginning and ending in these instances. When environmental distractions occurred—for example, a father's coming in or leaving the house, or the entry of a sibling into the room—this event was often reflected in the child's play. It was obvious that in such coherent sequences the child was able to incorporate environmental events, instead of becoming fragmented or disorganized. The most difficult transitions confronting the children were at the beginning and ending of the free-play phase. In all but one case, these transitions were encountered without difficulty by the children.

It is interesting, given these observations, that the internal meanings of various toy constructions—for example, speculations about relationships to parents extracted from the play behavior—were much less salient than the children's capacity for relationships and for coherent thought development in organizing the play material.

Two other qualities deserve special note. One is the self-initiated quality of the play. These children defined the limits of what they wanted to do and then carried it out, rather than passively waiting for directions or following the lead of the examiner. The other characteristic is that the descriptions repeatedly showed that these children demonstrably enjoyed the play. Many commented, "This is fun." Others, through gestures and facial expressions, displayed exuberance, warmth, and enthusiasm while playing.

Prediction of Competence and Risk

Several classes of predictor variables from the assessment of the children at age 3 were correlated with the four subscales of the Pictorial Scale of Perceived Competence and Acceptance Scale, administered when the children were between 6 and 7 years old. Both children's and teachers' reports were used as outcomes. Because of the large number of correlations done, only those that were significant at the .01 level are reported. The results are shown in Table 3-3.

Of the demographic variables, social class and social support predicted teacher-rated cognitive competence and peer acceptance in the expected directions, but not the children's self-reports of the same measures. On the other hand, family size predicted the children's ratings of their cognitive competence and maternal acceptance, but not the teachers' ratings of cognitive competence (teachers did not use the maternal acceptance subscale). Only a few other variables were found

Table 3-3. Predictors of Competence at Follow-Up

Predictor variable	Outcome variable[a]		r
Social class	Cognitive competence	(T)	−.30
	Peer acceptance	(T)	−.34
Family size	Cognitive competence	(C)	−.37
	Maternal acceptance	(C)	−.34
Social support	Peer acceptance	(T)	.35
Number of activities father engages in with child	Physical competence	(T)	.31
Recent death in family	Peer acceptance	(C)	−.31
	Maternal acceptance	(C)	−.36
	Peer acceptance	(T)	−.35
Father reports stress at work	Peer acceptance	(C)	.30

[a]Pictorial Version of the Perceived Competence Scale for Young Children, teacher's version (T) and child's version (C).

from all the other sources of data, and these in themselves were not sufficiently robust to produce statistical confidence. It is important to point out that the temperament and play observation variables were not found to be predictive, with two exceptions. The play variable "organization of scene" was significantly correlated with teacher-rated peer acceptance, and the temperament variable "threshold" was correlated with teacher-rated cognitive competence. Other temperament and play observation variables were related to indices of clinical disturbance at follow-up, as were several demographic and family environment variables (Garrison, Earls, & Kindlon, 1984). In the prediction of competence alone, however, the data show that demographic and home environment factors are more important than ratings of personal characteristics of a child, either as observed by an examiner or as reported by a parent.

The distribution of reading, spelling, and math scores, teacher- and self-reported perceived competence scores, and the total number of behavioral symptoms reported by teachers were examined for these 20 children at follow-up; *t* tests for each of these variables revealed no significant differences in comparison to the remaining sample.

Discussion

In exploratory fashion, the results presented in this chapter represent efforts to expand the range of objectives included in an epidemiological study that was initially devoted to estimating rates and examining correlates of behavioral disorders in young children. Using data about 3-year-olds, we have employed quantitative and qualitative approaches to attempt to isolate personality and home environment characteristics of those children whose parents described them as being relatively free of behavioral symptoms. The two analytic approaches were in agreement in presenting a picture of a group of highly adaptable preschoolers. Since the present purpose is to explore data and generate hypotheses about competence in young children, it is useful to attempt a synthesis of these analyses here.

It was surprising to find that characteristics of the children's home environments were not correlated with an absence of symptoms in the preschool period. Rather, personal–social qualities of the children predominated at this age, and of these, four characteristics best represent the range of data collected: adaptability, response to environmental stress, capacity for work, and self-initiation.

Since the initiation and termination of the play session were the most striking points at which to observe a child's adaptability, two aspects of this dimension were isolated: engagement and disengagement. By "adaptability–engagement" is meant the capacity of a child to engage actively, enthusiastically, and wholeheartedly in a variety of endeavors, including play, learning, and relationships. This was evident in the play session primarily from the high degree of initial engagement in spontaneous play, but also from the rapport between the parents and children in a number of daily contacts in the home. The parents' descriptions of these children made it clear that the parents enjoyed and derived pleasure from these contacts.

"Adaptability–disengagement" refers to the capacity of a child to move from one kind of activity to another without undue difficulty. The ending of a play sequence within the context of the overall play session, or the completion of the entire session, occurred without distress. More broadly, these children were reported by their parents to handle transitions and leave-taking easily. Analytic theorists would posit that appropriate leave-taking is possible only when some kind of internalized remembrance of the person being left exists. The observations reported here did not approach the level of what is going on inside a child's mind, but rather the manifestations in behavior and the consequences of leave-taking. What is striking is that the capacity for successful termination was quite variable in the entire population of 3-year-olds, making this group of 20 children all the more remarkable.

Response to stress in the environment was viewed not only in the play situation, but in the overall lives of these children. Many had faced significant stresses, yet it was striking that these children had handled these difficulties well. This was evident in that they had not begun to manifest behavioral symptoms, as reflected in high BSQ scores generally; they also had not shown specific symptoms, such as sleep or eating disturbances, which are often indicative of a stress response.

It seems reasonable to assume that children's relationships with others, their cognitive development, and their capacity to actively engage in play are roughly equivalent to the capacity for work in adults. These children clearly demonstrated an intense and high degree of involvement in play, either in the presence of others or alone. In fact, many parents commented on the children's capacity to amuse themselves when alone.

Perhaps the most striking characteristic of all was how strongly these 20 children initiated interactions in the play session. They actively engaged the examiner, named objects, chose particular action sequences, and then carried them out. This attribute was correlated with initiation in many other areas, in that they displayed the capacity to become rapidly and spontaneously involved in these other areas. The self-initiated behavior, in conjunction with the obvious exuberance and enjoyment of the children in such activities, suggests that there was high self-esteem present. It can be speculated that the children's inner sense of themselves was reflected in these dimensions of outward activity. Overall, then, these case reviews revealed positive dimensions that went far beyond the mere absence of symptoms.

Attempts to predict levels of competence from preschool to early school age were quite modest and suggested that demographic and family variables were most important classes of predictor variables than personal qualities. The fact that variables such as social class, family size, and family stressful events over a 3-year period predicted competence indicates that the social environment is a powerful determinant of healthy adaptation. In the preschool period the home environment is, of course, the primary social field of the child, so it is expected that family life variables exert a major influence. Since the Kauai longitudinal study of Werner and Smith (1979) has already demonstrated that demographic and family environment variables are more powerful predictors of psychosocial outcomes than perinatal stress variables over the first 2 years of life, the finding in this study that social variables are more important over time than personality or temperament variables is magnified. As a child enters the new social environment of the school, which brings with it new demands for cognitive performance and behavioral control, it may be that aspects of his home environment have not prepared him to make this transition easily. Most interesting is that high adaptability, the capacity for work and self-initiative, and good coping skills in this group of 3-year-olds selected on the basis of an absence of behavioral symptoms did not predict success in early school adaptation. The data can be interpreted to imply that personal assets, at least as measured in this subsample, are redefined as children mature from preschool to school age. If a more direct, developmentally sensitive measure of competence had been available for preschoolers, perhaps a different subsample of children would have been selected who had personal traits that remained stable over time. It should be emphasized that this finding may not be replicated when data from the entire sample are completely analyzed.

As a final check on the capacity to predict competence at school age, a separate analysis was done on symptom-free children at age 3. Evidence was not found to support the idea that these children possessed stable traits of easy temperament, above-average behavioral adjustment, or high competence over the 3-year follow-up interval. Again, this may simply be a reflection of the fact that a direct measure of competence was not used at age 3, or that a combination of maturational and contextual circumstances changed over the 3 years between initial assessment and follow-up to result in substantial changes in these children. This issue is the subject of a separate analysis currently being carried out in this project (Garrison & Earls, 1985).

The series of exercises reported here has served to underscore some problems and partial successes in measuring healthy adjustment on a population-wide basis. An important question remaining for longitudinal epidemiological studies to answer is how the stability of measures of competence and healthy adaptation compares with that of measures of behavioral problems and poor adaptation. To date, little emphasis has been placed on such a comparison. There is already good evidence that behavioral symptoms in 3-year-olds as reported by their mothers bear little or no association with teacher-rated behavioral symptoms by the time the children have entered school at 5 (Coleman, Wolkind, & Ashley, 1977). Suggested in the findings presented here is that measures of competence may fare similarly. As improved methods of assessing competence become available, this topic should become an important aspect in the design of epidemiological studies in child psychiatry and child development.

ACKNOWLEDGMENT

This work was supported by National Institute of Mental Health Grant No. MH-37044 and the John D. and Catherine T. MacArthur Foundation Mental Health Network on Risk and Protective Factors in Major Mental Disorders.

REFERENCES

Bemporad, J., Beardslee, W., & Earls, F. (1982). Mental health risk reduction for children. In A. D. Reinhardt & M. M. Faher (Eds.), *Promoting health through risk reduction*. New York: Macmillan.

Block, J., & Block, J. (1979). The role of ego-control and ego-resiliency in the organization of behavior. In W. A. Collins (Ed.), *Minnesota Symposium on Child Psychology* (Vol. 13). Hillsdale, NJ: Erlbaum.

Coleman, J., Wolkind, S., & Ashley, L. (1977). Symptoms of behavior disturbance and adjustment to school. *Journal of Child Psychology and Psychiatry, 18*, 201–209.

Earls, F. (1980a). Prevalence of behavior problems in three-year-old children: A cross-national replication. *Archives of General Psychiatry, 37*, 1153–1157.

Earls, F. (1980b). A prevalence of behavior problems in three-year-old children: Comparison of the reports of fathers and mothers. *Journal of the American Academy of Child Psychiatry, 19*, 439–452.

Earls, F. (1981). Temperament characteristics and behavior problems in three-year-old children. *Journal of Nervous and Mental Disease, 169*, 367–373.

Earls, F. (1982). Application of DSM-III in an epidemiological study of preschool children. *American Journal of Psychiatry, 139*, 242–243.

Earls, F. (1983). An epidemiological approach to the study of behavior problems in very young children. In S. B. Guze, F. J. Earls, F. & J. E. Barrett (Eds.), *Childhood psychopathology and development*. New York: Raven Press, pp. 1–15.

Earls, F., & Cook, S. (1984). Play observations of three-year-old children and their relationship to parental reports of behavior problems and temperament characteristics. *Child Psychiatry and Human Development, 13*, 225–232.

Earls, F., Jacobs, G., Goldfein, D., Silbert, A., Beardslee, W., & Rivinus, T. (1982). Concurrent validation of a behavior problems scale to use with three-year-olds. *Journal of the American Academy of Child Psychiatry, 21,* 47–57.

Garrison, W., & Earls, F. (1982a). Attachment to a special object at the age of three years: Behavior and temperament characteristics. *Child Psychiatry and Human Development, 12,* 131–141.

Garrison, W., & Earls, F. (1982b). Preschool behavior problems and the multigenerational family: An island community study. *International Journal of Family Psychiatry, 2,* 195–207.

Garrison, W., & Earls, F. (1983). Life events and social supports in families with two-year-old children. *Comprehensive Psychiatry, 24,* 439–452.

Garrison, W., & Earls, F. (1985). Change and continuity in child behavior from the preschool period through school entry. In J. E. Stevenson (Ed.), *Recent research in developmental psychopathology* (Journal of Child Psychology and Psychiatry Book Supplement No. 4). Oxford: Pergamon.

Garrison, W., Earls, F., & Kindlon, D. (1983). An application of the Pictorial Scale of Perceived Competence and acceptance within an epidemiological survey. *Journal of Abnormal Child Psychology, 11,* 367–377.

Garrison, W., Earls, F., & Kindlon, D. (1984). Temperament characteristics in the third year of life and behavioral adjustment at school entry. *Journal of Child Psychology, 13,* 298–303.

Harter, S. (1978). Effectance motivation reconsidered: Toward a developmental model. *Human Development, 1,* 34–64.

Harter, S., & Pike, R. (1981). The pictorial scale of perceived competence and acceptance for young children. Unpublished manual, University of Denver.

Harter, S. (1982). The Perceived Competence Scale for Children. *Child Development, 53,* 87–97.

McCarthy, D. (1974). *The McCarthy Scales of Children's Abilities.* New York: Psychological Corp.

Richman, N., & Graham, P. (1971). A behaviour screening questionnaire for use with three-year-old children: Preliminary findings. *Journal of Child Psychology and Psychiatry, 12,* 5–33.

Thomas, A., & Chess, S. (1977). *Temperament and development.* New York: Brunner/Mazel.

Werner, E., & Smith, R. (1979). An epidemiologic perspective on some antecedents and consequences of childhood mental health problems and learning disabilities. *Journal of the American Academy of Child Psychiatry, 18,* 292–306.

4

Further Reflections on Resilience

LOIS BARCLAY MURPHY
Menninger Foundation

My first discussion of resilience took place at a 1969 conference in Palo Alto, sponsored by the National Institute of Mental Health and, was reported in the volume *Coping and Adaptation* (Coelho, Hamburg, & Adams, 1974). However, my interest in resilience derives from a long history of experiences with people of all ages from infancy to the senior citizen stage, and I want to review some of the clues to understanding factors involved in resilience as I have noted them in some of these experiences.

As a child I was amazed at the way a baby would stop crying if someone merely held it up to a shoulder; evidently seeing the world from a different angle, plus the comfort of contact and the change of position, made the baby feel good and reduced discomfort. With my own children, I was equally surprised at the following incident reported by our 4-year-old daughter's nursery school teacher: A little boy accidentally hit her on the head with his shovel. Her scalp bled and she cried; then she stopped, saying, "Isn't it lucky that I have a red cap so the blood won't show?" Here a cognitive response, perhaps dealing with avoidance of an unpleasant appearance as she thought, competed with the pain and perhaps anger expressed on her initial upset.

In *Vulnerability, Coping and Growth* (Murphy & Moriarty, 1976, Chap. 10), we offered a series of illustrations of resilience of the children in our intensive "Coping Studies" of 31 children originally examined when they were young infants by Drs. Sibylle Escalona and Mary Leitch. In this chapter, I want to explore the experience of resilience further, drawing on observations over a longer time, with a wider range of people, and with a broader view.

A dictionary definition of "resilience" is as follows: "1. the power or ability to return to the original form, position, etc., after being bent, compressed, or stretched; elasticity. 2. ability to recover readily from illness, depression, adversity, or the like; buoyancy" (*Random House Dictionary of the English Language*, 1973, p. 1220).

As evidence for resilience, Heider's (1966) study demonstrated the decreased vulnerability of some children from infancy to the preschool level; related to this was the fact that some children were getting along better than expected, such as, for instance, Janice in Escalona and Heider's *Prediction and Outcome* (1959). Moriarty (1961) also reported on some children who showed improved cognitive functioning, while Rousey and Moriarty (1965) saw a high frequency of recovery from early speech difficulties. In addition, intensive studies of the recovery of individual children—for example, Susan's and Ray's recoveries from polio; Helen's recovery from prolonged and recurrent infections (Murphy & Moriarty, 1976, Chap. 11); and John's progress through the ups and downs of illness and frustrations related to defects (see Moriarty, Chapter 5, this volume)—have provided further evidence for resilience. Here I should like to consider resilience in the sense of recovery, and not necessarily instant recovery. There is a contrast between those who remain depressed after a major loss, injury, or illness, and those who recover even if—as with Sam (Murphy, 1962) and with Susan, Janice, and Helen (Murphy & Moriarty, 1976)—a long process of coping and help is involved.

When she was in her early 20s and exhausted from a demanding new job, my younger sister was diagnosed as hyperthyroid, and a thyroid operation was recommended. I asked her to get permission to spend the summer with us in the country, where she could relax, rest, walk, and paint, with complete freedom from responsibility. At the end of the summer, when she returned, her doctor said her thyroid functioning had returned to a normal level and there was no need for an operation. I considered this a happy example of resilience.

For another example, at the age of 65, on his first of three retirements, my father developed a gastric ulcer and an operation was recommended. I took a week's leave from my college teaching in the East and flew out to visit him in his Chicago hospital. Finding him uncomfortably situated with inadequate nursing, I arranged for him to be transferred to a private room, and stayed with him for a week. At the end of that time, his doctor said his condition had improved so much that an operation was not necessary. In this instance, "tender loving care" was the magic promoting recovery, while in my sister's case, rest and pleasure were the major factors involved.

The Coping Studies

It was a dozen years after this experience that our studies of coping and resilience began in Topeka; the planning for these studies began in 1952. We could not create, or were not willing to create, disturbances in the preschool children we were observing; we simply kept alert to sequences of behavior that included a loss of the children's normal level of functioning and recovery to that level. We were also interested in what babies and children did to prevent distress or disturbance. In fact, our broad concern included coping with all kinds of ordinary obstacles and challenges, and we hoped to find early beginnings of coping and resilience in the records of infant behavior bequeathed to us by Escalona and Leitch. We were not disappointed.

Coping in Infants

We saw young babies using a variety of ways to fend off what they did not want, or found distasteful, excessive, uncomfortable, or upsetting. They did this by various body adjustments and vocal protests. We also saw them reaching out for what they did want, and evoking responses from other people by a variety of sounds, movements, and expressive methods. Both of these autonomous self-protective and drive-satisfying processes were seen in different frequencies, and different patterns among individual babies served to motivate and to reinforce adaptive efforts that reduced upsets. These adaptive efforts in turn used available skills and stimulated development of new ones.

We also saw evidences of compliance with and response to mothers' techniques of handling the babies: For instance, some babies cooperated early with their mother's intention when she indicated that food was on its way. Coping with the frustrations, opportunities, and demands of the environment in the early months included both self-initiated and socially responsive behavior. It was oriented not only to getting satisfaction or pleasure and avoiding specific pain or discomfort, but to maintaining an equilibrium, achieving integration, and restoring a state of comfort after its loss.

At first the babies used chiefly their bodies, their voices, and their mouths as they selectively accepted, rejected, or terminated food, and as they turned away from or toward different sights, sounds, or materials in contact with their skin. As they gradually became able to coordinate their hands to reach objects, push them away, grasp them, bring them to their mouths, or put them into contact with other objects, their range of self-protection, experimentation, discovery, invention, and satisfaction was extended. Some babies experimented with sounds and nonvocal mouth activities, which provided built-in resources to counteract boredom—one of the major nuisances for babies limited to a crib or a room, and a major cause of "fussiness." (Perhaps one reason we hear less crying among babies in India, for instance, is that there is less likelihood of boredom when an infant is carried around on the mother's hip, from which a changing vista of sights and sounds is within range.)

Recovery and Support

We saw a range of patterns of recovery in infants and children: One child would snap back or bounce back from a defeat, whereas another would recover gradually, with effort. Four-year-old Darlene, who was afraid to jump from a height of about 1 foot above the ground, slowly worked up her courage and proudly shouted, "I jumped! I jumped!" after she actually managed to do it. She showed us that pride in resilient achievement may be proportional to the degree of anxiety or insecurity that precedes it. Children who took for granted their ability to jump were casual about it.

Variations in the stability of recovery were related to the dependability of support. Teddy was disturbed after his parents' divorce, but the integrity and unfailing support of his mother contributed to his recovery and his ability to master the sequences of his life in his own way. "I've had two lives, and I try to forget the first one." By contrast, Gordon's recovery after his parents' divorce was volatile in the unstable situation where his father took on one roommate after another. Where a child's disturbance is a reaction to the breakdown of his basic support system, his recovery requires consistency of input—which Richard received from his older sister.

The Role of Determination

Among adults, we often see the role of conscious determination or will. William James's intense commitment to and belief in the capacity of the will to overcome his chronic miseries is an example; so is Norman Cousins's successful autonomous program to cure his supposedly incurable disease. And in adolescence, Robin's stubborn determination to overcome the "weaknesses" that underlay her serious school retardation and deep despair is still another example. Are there parallels of "willpower" in infancy and childhood? Certainly determination was apparent in infant Ronnie's 35 minutes of struggle to get up on all fours, trying until he was exhausted, then collapsing on the floor to rest and suck his thumb, after which he struggled again. This went on until he actually succeeded. He did not give up when exhausted; he resiliently and determinedly continued his effort.

Vulnerability and Stress

Resilience needs to be considered in relation to vulnerability and to stress. While I cannot claim that the following is a complete picture of the stress experienced by the children in the Coping Studies during the preschool period, this summary provides a useful view of the stress we were able to record.

ECONOMIC STRESS

Seven of the families felt real economic stress; three of these felt chronically poor, while the others regarded their conditions as temporary or improvable. Although none of our children lived in slums, about a third of them lived in cramped or shabby homes, which were inadequate to provide privacy for individual members of large families. Nearly half the children had some problems connected with lack of independent sleeping arrangements—sleeping up to four children in one small room, sleeping in parents' room, and even lack of any consistent sleeping quarters. In a few cases, the children lived in poor neighborhoods, and some of these had very inadequate equipment for play. All but Janice, however, had outdoor space for activity, and most were free to roam the block.

RELOCATION

A third of the children moved to new towns during the first 10 years of their lives, and we have detailed records of the month-to-month struggle of two of these children to feel at home in their new localities.

ABSENCE OF MOTHER

At least 26 of the children had experienced absence of the mother—for hospitalization, birth of a baby, visit to relatives, vacation with husband or religious retreat (Daryl, Vivian)—during the preschool period. In addition, Sheila, her grandmother's favorite, felt deeply the loss of the grandmother's support when the family moved from the grandparents' home to an independent house. Six of the children had marked separation anxiety and anxiety about new situations at the beginning of the project, while an additional five showed mild anxiety from which they recovered in a short time. Sally showed separation anxiety only when her mother was ill; she recovered when her mother recovered.

RELATIVES' ILLNESS OR STRESS

Seventeen children had mothers who were at some time markedly depressed or ill; in half a dozen instances, emotional disturbance requiring psychiatric care occurred for a limited period. In some instances, the mothers appeared to be swamped at times by the burdens in their situations. Most mothers, however, seemed to be able to manage well during the entire period we have known them. Among the fathers, two were alcoholic at periods, two were hospitalized with diabetes, two had accidents, one had gastric ulcers, and two were unemployed for several months at a time. The majority of fathers were stable and devoted to their children, as well as supportive to the mothers. Seven children experienced the death of relatives, mostly grandparents; with Susan and Donald, death of the dog was a source of heartbreak. John (see Moriarty, Chapter 5, this volume) was most disturbed in the years that his two sets of grandparents divorced, but his parents' support helped him to regain his equilibrium.

PUNISHMENT

About half the children were disciplined by corporal punishment, in several cases with belts or paddles; deprivation, restriction, sitting on a chair, mouth washing, hand slapping, and other methods were also used. But the stressful effects of discipline were seen chiefly in children whose parents imposed unusual restrictions—in two instances, because of religious taboos. Restrictions typical of the culture (e.g., breaking things) were matter-of-factly accepted, along with the usual punishments.

ILLNESSES

All of the children had some illnesses. Approximately one-quarter of the babies had had colic, and seven had sufficient trouble with infections to undergo tonsillectomies; 11 children each had one or another acute illness (measles, rubella, severe ear infection, eczema, glandular fever, etc.). But only four suffered a prolonged developmental disturbance as a consequence of illness, and in all of these instances the children recovered normal functioning in time. For these four, the disturbing consequences appeared when too many illnesses came too fast (Helen); when an illness came in a setting of other stresses (Roy: broken arm, mild polio, sister with more severe polio, new baby within 10 months) or at a critical phase (Rachel: hospitalization for infantile eczema during period of development of locomotion, colic during first 3 months); or when an illness was prolonged and repeated (Tommy: loss of energy and drive during a period of long throat infection). As noted, however, all of these children recovered adequately after a period of regression; all had restitutive support from their mothers or grandmothers.

As would be expected, all of the children had some fears during the preschool period: many of them paralleling those described by Jersild in the 1930s on a New York sample, and Macfarlane on a California sample: new situations, strange people, thunder, other loud sounds and noises, dark, death, animals, bugs, storms, getting hurt, doctors, hospitals, fire engines, firecrackers, and so on. However, there were also the contemporary additions of hydrogen bombs and "shots" for immunization; locally stimulated fears such as tornadoes and kidnapping (Kansas City, 1953); and religiously stimulated fears such as hell and heaven, ghosts, and sin. With most children only one or two of these fears were noted, and as in the other studies the early fears were outgrown.

OTHER STRESSES

The everyday life of the normal young middle-class American children we studied in Topeka included, along with satisfactions, fun, and successes, a stream of mild to severe stress experiences in addition to those described above: starting school; demands for cooperation with unfamiliar tasks; time pressures; areas of limitations; frustration; threat of failure or humiliation; competition; sibling rivalry (keeping up with older siblings, being displaced by younger ones); growth irregularities (changing of body build); military absence of fathers; experiences of death; and pressure from parental authority.

In addition, the children had feelings of insecurity regarding the availability of a father or mother; unanswered questions about where babies come from and what parents do in bed; fears of body damage or loss; fears of the consequences of aggressive impulses; anxiety regarding accidentally breaking things; feelings of being little and perhaps helpless in a world of big people; puzzlements over differences between boys and girls; confusion about the fact that big people are both threatening and helpful, and uncertainty about which to expect at a given moment; worry about conflicts between adults; and fearfulness about saying what they wanted to say when they were angry or scared.

I have not included here many sources of stress appearing in larger cities that result from deprivation of social contacts and motor freedom—for instance, not being allowed to play with certain children or explore the city alone.

We also need to remember the peculiar situation of children. Adults have a considerable measure of control over their worlds; they can *choose* jobs, towns, homes, spouses, friends. By contrast, children may have almost no choice at all; they are stuck with their families, homes, neighborhoods, schools. A child's inability to exercise choice or control over his world can make him feel angry or helpless, or both. It can make him fight or give up; he may feel at a loss as to how to cope with the difficulties he faces. This in certain instances tends to push him into unrealistic ways of thinking and fantasy.

Stresses arise not only from children's situations, but from their own developmental patterns. Elizabeth Hellersberg (1957) has given especially careful attention to the role of uneven development in relation to difficulties in adaptation. She starts from this question: What accounts for the fact that the child with uneven development is more susceptible to insecurity, and more vulnerable to anxiety? Building on Karl Menninger's (1954) descriptions of reactions to stress, she emphasizes the fact that stress not only produces typical symptoms or "disintegrative responses," but also affects the process of growth itself. She sees the relation of uneven development and anxiety as a two-way affair: Some infants achieve an equilibrium slowly, and this makes their mothers anxious. The anxious relationship between such a mother and baby further retards the achievement of an equilibrium. As Sullivan pointed out, an irregular maturation pattern may be reinforced physically and psychologically: "Such a course of events can jeopardize the total integration of development, particularly when an inherited weakness of the organism is already present and patterns of uneven growth of various degrees of severity may be produced" (1953).

THE RELATIVITY OF VULNERABILITY

I find that it makes sense to discriminate between relatively vulnerable and invulnerable zones of the organism. We found no children in the Coping Studies who were totally invulnerable. There were more vulnerable and less vulnerable children, and in both groups there were more resilient and less resilient children—and children who recovered more quickly from certain kinds of disturbance than others. Whether we see a child as vulnerable or as resilient depends on the situation in which we see him. For instance, a few of the preschool children we studied, who were in general sturdy and resilient, were overwhelmed in the nude-body photograph situation directed by one of William Sheldon's assistants; to be naked in front of adults was intolerable to these few boys. (By contrast, some girls were charmingly exhibitionistic.) Here the meaning of the situation rather than physical pain was the source of their distress, which was too intense to be mastered.

Patterns of Recovery at the Preschool Level

I cannot discuss resilience here in relation to all of these zones of vulnerability in the children and in their environment; a few examples of recovery from stress will have to suffice.

A child's responsiveness to input by a caregiver includes experiences familiar to every mother. For instance, a toddler trips on the sidewalk and scrapes his knee; it stings and bleeds a little. He is upset and cries. Mother picks him up, saying, "Mommy will kiss it and make it well," and usually the crying stops with a resilient youngster. I think the loving contact probably does stimulate endorphins, which, as we now know, alleviate pain.

Two-year-old Molly was terrified by thunder; getting into bed with her mother or her big sister provided both tactual comfort and the reassurance evoked by a secure other person who was not afraid.

Annie, also 2, was silent, depressed, and wetting her panties the day after a big tornado ripped through Topeka, destroying many homes. Her teacher, whose apartment was demolished, had not come to Annie's center, but had sent word that she herself was safe at her mother's home. I sat down next to Annie and asked, "Are you worried?" She nodded. "Are you worried about your teacher?" She nodded again. "She is safe; she is with her mother, and she'll be here next Monday." Annie trustingly relaxed, and there was no more wetting.

Three-year-old Greg refused to go to the toilet in nursery school. His teacher brought him to "play with Mrs. Murphy's toys." After half an hour of playing, he threw a tiny rubber baby down the drain of the wading pool near which we sat. I said, "You know, some children are afraid they might be flushed down the toilet with their BMs. But that couldn't happen, could it? Children are much too big." After that there was no more trouble about going to the toilet. With both Annie and Greg, cognitive clarification relieved the child's anxiety.

Six-year-old Arthur was so bewildered and anxious in a first-grade class taught by a rather aggressive and tired teacher that he was nauseated every day before school. At his doctor's suggestion, his parents took him to a different school known for its excellent teachers. After the first morning there he said, "This teacher understands children so much better, I want to stay here until I'm 17!" There was no more nausea. In this instance, removing the sensitive child from an unbearable situation removed the symptom.

All of these children were resilient in the sense that they were trustfully and quickly responsive to the help that was offered. They had not internalized the problem; the symptom was not frozen and resistant to information or a changed situation.

Factors in Resilience

The Role of Developmental Phase in Vulnerability and Resilience

The potentialities for resilience are related to the state of the child as this is affected by health, and to the level of equilibrium as this is affected by the child's developmental stage. Thresholds for distress, pain, and disintegrative reactions to stress are lower when a baby is cutting teeth or has a cold or is colicky; fussiness is then more persistent, and it is more difficult to comfort the baby successfully. The more diffuse the baby's discomfort, the less resilient the baby is.

Critical phases of development are especially vulnerable to persistent emotional and behavior disturbances, from which the child does not recover as quickly as usual—"he isn't himself." At prepuberty, some children feel depressed; others are irritable and hard to live with. This leads to tension in the family as a whole, with circular disturbances as the parents' angry reaction to the children's upset adds to the children's stress. While Susan's mother said, "She's impossible to live with," Chester's mother punished him severely with belts, whips, or switches. With both children, resilience was much decreased from their earlier levels, along with the decrease in tolerance.

At this stage, biological changes, together with such worries as "How will I look? Will I be able to be on the team? Will I be popular?", bring anxieties increased by the environmental changes involved in transfers to junior high school, where "nobody will know me." Our Topeka 12-year-olds also worried about getting to be teenagers "because teenagers have such a bad reputation," and they felt concerned about "having to be more responsible for myself" and "having to give up kids' things." Under this complex biopsychosocial pressure, any specific stress—loss of a parent by death or divorce, injury in an accident, moving to a strange new community, failure in an examination— may be overwhelming. The child desperately needs understanding, warm support from a trusted adult or older adolescent. When Mary's father died near her 13th birthday, her devoted older sister drew closer to her and helped her to find a secure place in adolescent groups. When 12-year-old Richard and his father were injured in an auto crash that killed his mother, he sobbed interminably in the hospital until a young man from our research team brought him fascinating electronic toys. Then the tears stopped and he resiliently turned his attention to activities he enjoyed. Once out of the hospital, his older sister took over mothering responsibilities and helped him to feel more secure as a young adolescent.

Some children struggle at this stage with ad hoc coping maneuvers that may or may not succeed in their group. When my daughter was 13, her classmates invited to an evening party included boys who were tall, sophisticated, and skillful dancers; others, who had not yet started the growth spurt, were still little boys and preferred table games. One of these little boys seemed very much out of things. He came to me and announced boastfully, "Mrs. Murphy, I've had 24 cups of punch." Instead of retreating, he had made maximal use of the one resource he could use.

Marian, at this stage—irritable and even destructive at home, pressured in the popularity competition in junior high school—relaxed in a new school with less snobbish pressure, made many friends, and resiliently recovered her characteristic good humor. Here, as with Arthur at the beginning of his school career, an appropriate environmental change brough prompt recovery from internal disturbance.

I have discussed the complex biopsychosocial problems at puberty or preadolescence in some detail here because their expression is often so dramatic, while at the same time adults often fail to realize the multiple pressures on a child who is acting up. Comparable stressful interactions of the total physiological state of the child with pressures of environmental change or stimulation occur at other critical stages. For instance, Dr. David M. Levy (1945) found that a high proportion of children who had tonsil operations at the age of 2 developed persistent fears afterward, while only a small fraction of 5-year-old children developed such fears.

If we try to reconstruct the probable experience of the younger children as compared with the 5-year-olds, we have to include, first, the wide difference in the level of verbal comprehension. The 5-year-old is able to understand that the operation will help to prevent the tonsillitis that has so often kept him out of kindergarten and out of all the fun with other children, while the 2-year-old suffers an incomprehensible assault. The 5-year-old can understand the promise that his sore throat will "feel better tomorrow," while the 2-year-old has no such secure sense of time. But, more than this, the older preschool child can reduce his anxiety in playful repetitions of aspects of the experience that have disturbed him. In short, the 5-year-old has more resources to support recovery from the shock of the operation.

More fundamental even than these considerations, the 2-year-old is at an insecure transition stage. He can talk a little, but not enough to express his feelings adequately. He can walk and wants to be independent, but he is still insecure in many of his motor skills. By contrast, the 5-year-old who holds up his hand with fingers outstretched, proudly announcing "I'm 5!", has mastered many basic aspects of communication and mobility and is generally in a state of relatively secure equilibrium. He is not burdened by the underlying insecurity of the 2-year-old, which lowers thresholds for persistent anxiety and interferes with resilience. I see the 4- to 5-year-old stage with its zest for growth and pride in mastery as a propitious stage for resilience, in contrast to the earlier stage, in which resilience is threatened. Both energy and understanding contribute to resilience in older children. Children have more initiative and can use play more successfully in the service of resilience. Arthur played "put a cone on your nose" with his little sister after his operation, to come to terms with the stressful experience.

Varieties of External Stimulation Helping Resilience

Input from the outside to evoke resilience is not confined to physical comfort and restitutive love; a wide range of sensory stimulation can also turn the tide of feeling when a baby is upset. One infant always stopped crying when a record was started on the phonograph, and his favorite very rhythmic Czech folk dance most quickly changed tears to joy. For Andrew, a brightly colored mobile brought within the line of vision had the same effect. In short, recovery from an infant's mild distress is often initiated by a favorite pleasurable sensory stimulus to eye or ear.

In the world of children, "tender loving care" does not come solely from grownups who want to help them to recover from an upset. As I found in my study of sympathy (Murphy, 1937), even nursery school children come to the aid of, or give comfort to, a child who has had a fall or a bump or has been attacked aggressively by another child. Children can facilitate resilience in their companions. If the cruelty of school-age children to one another has been more impressive, we need to ask how this is related to the institutionalized competition and prestige hierarchies in our culture, as well as the brutality to which children are exposed directly and vicariously.

Among the settings in which I watched with fascination the resilient changes in young children were Head Start groups. Wild, frantic, disorganized Teresa baffled her teachers and threatened to disrupt the group. Deprived of adequate mothering by a hard-working single-parent mother, her overflowing energy had neither direction nor control. I suggested that her Head Start teacher hold her quietly and talk to her not about misbehavior, but about interesting things she would enjoy hearing. Since the group was still small and had an excellent teacher's aide, it was possible to give Teresa special attention for a few weeks. Teresa enjoyed this, quieted down, and soon learned to participate in singing games and other activities that gave direction to her energy. Instead of the wild child who entered the group, she became a stimulating leader. Her responsiveness implied that she *had* had enough mothering to respond to the restitutive mothering offered by her teacher, and to internalize her teacher's guidance and let it shape a new, more integrated self.

I had similar experiences with other children. Distraught Johnny came to Head Start making crazy gestures after weekends when his psychotic mother was at home on leave from the state hospital. In this instance a young teacher with a master's degree in education, who had been orphaned early, said, "I don't understand this lap business." So I spent time with Johnny myself, giving him the quiet mothering he needed, working puzzles with my arm around him. Here again, he had

had good enough earlier mothering to trust me and quiet down; to get absorbed in the puzzles we worked on together; and then to transfer the internalized constructiveness to building impressive structures with blocks.

With Cecily, the problem was different—her speech was unintelligible. I decided to try a direct approach: "Cecily, I really *want* to understand what you say. Couldn't you help me? I could hear better if you tried to talk more clearly." Cecily said, with perfect clarity, "But my mommy likes me to talk baby talk." I thanked her and told her that I liked to hear her talk big-girl talk because then I could really understand what she was telling me. Here again, there was a good enough foundation for relationship for her to respond trustingly to my sincere effort to improve communication. Her resilient recovery from what looked at first like a speech defect reflected her own caring about our relationship.

The Child's Resources Supporting Resilience

Our data from the Coping Studies indicated that it would be well worthwhile to undertake a study of changes in the following variables and their interaction with one another and with the environment, in relation to resilience:

1. Thresholds for and tempo of arousal of a disturbed state.
2. Tempo of decline from a disturbed state.
3. Use of protest, rejection.
4. Avoidance.
5. Capacity to adjust the body to a comfortable or acceptable position.
6. Capacity to use support (comfort, soothing) from others.
7. Capacity to find support (comfort) in own functioning (thumb sucking, rhythmic activities, play).
8. Capacity to find support in cognitive functioning (including watching, listening, exploring, manipulating).
9. Pleasurable versus unpleasurable vocalization, laughter.
10. Goal-oriented versus unfocused movement.
11. Ability to accept substitutes, to respond to restitution, and to respond to new opportunities.
12. Capacity to delay gratification.
13. Tendency to delay before action in response to a stimulus.
14. Tendency to "act to attain," to obtain objects, to change the environment.
15. Drive level.

16. Activity level.
17. Functional stability (autonomic nervous system, breathing, digestion, etc.).
18. Vigor, robustness.
19. Sensory thresholds or reactivity.
20. Pleasure and displeasure in response to sensory stimuli.
21. Balance in developmental levels.
22. Balance of stimulus response and management functions.

In looking at internal factors, we noticed one particular combination of these variables that was important for resilience—namely, the relationship between the tempo of decline of autonomic reactivity and the intensity of drive in the child. The summary presented in Table 4-1 illustrates variations in this relationship (which are worth studying more thoroughly than we were able to do). These variations reflect basic biological givens that help to shape the pattern of resilience.

Table 4-1. Variations in the Relationship between Tempo of Decline of Autonomic Reactivity and Intensity of Drive

Child	Score for tempo of decline	Score for drive
Resilient children—rapid decline, high drive		
John	1	1
Jo Ann	1	2
Karen	1	1
Diane	2	2
Terry	1	1
Stable children—rapid to moderate decline, low to moderate drive		
Vernon	1	4
Barbie	3	4
Children with conflict—slow decline, high drive		
Donald	4	2
Susan	4	1
Brennie	5	1
Children with serious adaptational difficulties—slow decline, high drive		
Steve	5	5
Cynthia	4	3?

Note. A score of 1 is high; a score of 5 is low.

Other patterns emerge from different combinations of the variables listed above: (1) intensity or severity of disturbance of equilibrium; (2) speed of arousal in different episodes or kinds of stress; (3) duration of different episodes of reaction to stress; (4) speed of decline (or recovery) from stress reactions. And I can add another variable that we found hard to study: perseveration of effects of disturbance, both negative (as in proneness to repeated disturbances) and positive (as in learning that difficulties can be overcome). We have to infer this variable from comparisons of data at successive major phases of the child's life, as in our study of Helen (Murphy & Moriarty, 1976, pp. 295–333).

At this point, the image of vulnerability presented here can be condensed into a model of organism–environment interaction (see Table 4-2).

Desensitization and Contributions of Early Coping

We must discriminate between useful learning of resilience by early mastering of stress and long-term disturbance from traumatic stress as we see this in children in clinics. In the Coping Studies we saw examples of mothers who allowed their babies to struggle for themselves, to protest discomfort and dislikes, and to learn to wait for postponed gratification. Such early experiences tended to contribute to the active

Table 4-2. Different Types of Organisms and Environments, and an Organism–Environment Model of Vulnerability

Organism
Balanced, cohesive, stable organism.
Unbalanced equipment: autonomic and/or affective reactivity high; motor functioning moderate; cognitive functioning limited.
Variable, unstable organism.

Environment
Consistent, supportive environment.
Marked to severe specific stress in generally supportive environment.
Unstable, inconsistent environment; recurrent stress.

Vulnerability
Variable motor and cognitive functioning in unstable, inconsistent environment.

coping capacities that supported resilience. But as David Levy's (1945) study of tonsil operations showed, the early experience of that distress and pain tended to lead to subsequent fearfulness. Frustration or pain that can be mastered in the early years can contribute to later resilience, as 14-year-old Karl commented (Murphy & Moriarty, 1976, Chap. 10); however, overwhelming, disorganizing, recurrent stress leaves residual anxiety that interferes with resilience.

A child's resilient struggle to recapture a sense of competence after an acute and debilitating illness was seen in Colin (Murphy, 1956). Between the ages of 2½ and 3, he had been a cooperative, trusting, friendly boy in nursery school. However, while sick, he had experienced some faint moments when he fell backward in his seat, and these upset him. When he returned to nursery school, he was for the first time extremely aggressive, as if he had to prove to himself that he was strong, not weak. His warm, firm, understanding teacher set clear limits, telling him that if he couldn't remember not to hurt other children he would have to play alone. "It's so hard to remember," Colin said, but he did develop adequate control in a few weeks. Here the trusting relationship with his warm teacher, his wish to cooperate, and his desire to play with the other children contributed to the development of his ability to handle his aggression constructively. The aggression, initially indiscriminate and destructive, had been mobilized to prove to himself that he had recovered from the weakness experienced during his illness. (There was no anger toward his teacher or anyone else as far as we could see.)

The same little boy was worried about his little sister's lack of a "tinkler." Here again he took action in play, putting a small bit of rubber band in the tinkler place on a tiny doll. And within the next year he developed a fantasy of being a doctor who could make things on his operating table. (Indeed, he eventually became a surgeon.) In this instance, we see again how fantasy contributed to resilient reduction of anxiety—not by repetition of an actual traumatic experience, as with Arthur, but by creative problem solving, which in Colin's case contributed to the direction of his life work.

Lack of Resilience

If resilience, the capacity for recovery from a disturbed state, depends on input or support from the outside, how do we distinguish it from lack of resilience? This question highlights the importance of openness and trusting responsiveness. We did not see little Daryl as a resilient child; tensely detached, she was unresponsive to our overtures, with no spontaneous delight in making use of new opportunities. She seemed distrustful. She had been a premature baby, much hovered over by her anxious mother and for months during infancy approached only by people whose faces were masked to prevent infection. On projective tests, examiners reported much more hostility in Daryl than the tests of other children showed.

Another child, less resilient than most of our normal well-mothered research group, was Gordon, an unstable boy. His own mother was in a mental hospital. His father had divorced her and then had a succession of involvements with other women. Gordon was unable to count on consistent mothering, unable to trust his father. A boy in a similar family remarked, "I guess I have to get used to a divorce every year"—an effort to come to terms with the instability of his life. And it should be noted here that, paradoxically, the same hypersensitivities that make a baby vulnerable to overstimulation may contribute to resilience when stimulation is optimal. The same child who gets anxious in reaction to a loud or cross voice may be soothed or delighted by a warm, resonant voice.

With most of our resilient children, trust and open responsiveness to the resources of a situation were prerequisites for the autonomy and initiative expressed in their capacity to select what they needed from the environment, to make active use of it (as Richard did in the hospital), and to change or restructure a situation (as some children did in tests, which they protested were *not* games"). We saw Erikson's sequences of the early life cycle in living form—trust, autonomy, and initiative, in particular.

A wide range of capacities developed during infancy contribute to resilience as they reflect the trust, autonomy, and initiative developed in the early years:

1. Trust and hope sufficient to withstand rebuffs and disappointment.
2. Nonverbal and verbal communication, imitation, identification.
3. Stable and yet flexible relationships; capacity to communicate, cooperate, and love in the setting of the relation with the mother.
4. Resources for discharge of tension, resolution of anger, and mastery of anger.
5. A range of affect, including capacity for fun, joy, interest in new experience, play, and creativity.
6. Capacity to satisfy needs, or expectation of being able to do so, along with a capacity for delay.
7. Ability to express drives along with socially acceptable motor efforts (thus avoiding hurting self or others, which arouses punishment and leads to conflict).

8. Capacity to exert effort, or capacity to struggle against obstacles, keep on trying after failure, and so on.
9. Capacity to "forgive and forget," tolerate frustration, renew positive relationships, or let go and begin new relationships.
10. Recovery following temporary regression or withdrawal—self-comfort, compensation, and so forth.
11. Ability to consolidate positive coping attitudes, resources with healthy defense mechanisms.
12. Clear verbal concepts of objects and space–time relationships in the immediate and broader environment.
13. Autonomy appropriate to the developmental stage and resources.
14. Balance of control and freedom.
15. Capacity to use the environment selectively, obtain substitutes, and structure or restructure the environment to achieve goals.

Conclusion

Resilience as I have conceived of it, in terms of recovery over a shorter or longer time, involves global aspects of the whole child—growth and growth drive, equilibration after disequilibrium. Different resources are mobilized in a given instance, depending on the particular strengths of the individual child, as well as on the pattern of stress or trauma and its relation to the child's vulnerability pattern. Resilience, like competence and adaptation as outcomes of coping, is an evaluative concept, not a unitary trait. The resilient child is oriented toward the future, is living ahead, with hope.

The child shares with other organisms a biological tendency to achieve wholeness—not as a static state, but as a dynamic, flexible balance that permits recoil or regression and rebound or progress. Biological rhythms of activity and rest provide a basic pattern for acceptance of restitution from the outside. The whole range of resources may be involved: biochemical factors, including hormones and endorphins; the interaction of cortical, subcortical, autonomic nervous system, and glandular activity; and psychophysiological forces. All these resources interact, mobilizing regenerative power. Residues of experiences of resilience after physical or emotional disturbance contribute both a sense of "feeling good" and also a consolidation of confidence, optimism, and ability to respond to or seek help when faced with threats in the future. The drive toward integration, then, utilizes selective combinations of other drives and capacities available at a given stage of the child's development.

I have seen processes of fending off intolerable pressures, shifting to more gratifying activity, temporary regression, biding one's time, containing and letting out fantasy, and sheer determined courage, among other endogenous patterns in children. I have also seen contributions from the outside—stimuli for pleasure and laughter; restitutive caring, sharing, and love; assistance in cognitive clarification; and other sorts of external support. Not to be overlooked are cultural maxims and assumptions such as those presented by the children's mothers: "Every cloud has a silver lining," "Tomorrow will be a better day," "If at first you don't succeed, try, try again," and "You have to take the bad with the good"; over time, these support positive expectations or acceptance of reality.

While everyone is familiar with critical phases as Erikson, Spitz, Bowlby, and others have discussed them, there has not been enough discussion of propitious phases, when children's energies are high and available for recovery. I have presented an example of this in Colin, and other examples can be found in the relatively stable period of latency, after early adjustments to school and a large group of peers have been achieved—or, for that matter, after any critical stage when its threats have been mastered.

Summary of Resilience

The recovery–resilience model presented here involves the following:
I. Biological and physical factors: resurgence of energy, vitality; tempo of decline of autonomic reactivity (somato-psychic); role of bodily stress reactions.
   1. Rest.
   2. Direct biochemical factors (vitamins, food, drugs).
   3. Thalamic–autonomic–hormonal factors.
   4. Prosthetics and props.
II. Psychological factors.
   1. Balance, ego cohesion.
   2. Reduction of pain, anxiety, or threat; discharge of anger; and so on.
   3. Containment of pain by differentiating life areas.
   4. Active introduction of pleasure, warmth, love: soothing, evocative contact.
   5. Demand, stimulus to recover—promises of results.
   6. Current models of recovery in the environment: family friends, culture.
   7. Expectation, fantasy; drive to recover, progress, grow.

8. Stimulation of action by the child (recovery of mastery, struggle capacity and potency).
9. Conditions supporting action, including symbolic support.
10. Integrative capacity, growth capacity, restructuring.
11. Reward for recovery.

But the resilience capacities of the child are also often related to the child's own prevention capacities, which involve coping with threat and dealing with tension at an early stage.

Coping with Threat

I. Means for coping with threat.
1. Action in relation to threat.
   a. Reducing threat: postponing, bypassing, retreating, shifting attention or interest, and so on.
   b. Controlling threat by changing or transforming limits.
   c. Balancing threat by changing relation of self to the threat or the environment in which it is contained.
   d. Eliminating or destroying threat.
2. Dealing with, avoiding tension aroused by threat.
   a. Discharging tension through action: releasing affect; displacing or projecting via fantasy (dramatics, painting, creative writing, etc.).
   b. Containing tension via insight, fantasy, defense mechanisms.
II. Sequence of coping with threat.
1. Preparing steps toward coping.
2. Coping acts.
3. Secondary coping (to deal with consequences of 1 and 2, using more drastic methods or retreating further).

The Optimistic Bias

While I have been reviewing resources contributing to resilience, I have not discussed failure in resilience or lack of resilience. Here, the individual's emotional orientation must be considered. An optimistic bias, even when latent, is often expressed in latching on to any excuse for hope and faith in recovery. (By contrast, a pessimistic bias is reflected in resistance to the opportunities, support, or other input that could contradict such a bias; the individual feels it necessary to do this in order to maintain consistency as a person.) Some children and adults, in other words, *want* to be resilient, and actively mobilize and respond to anything and everything that will contribute to recovery. We saw this in Helen, Susan, John, Chester, and other children in our Coping Studies. I am talking about a deep cognitive–affective bias that underlies the response to illness, frustration, disappointment, or other disequilibrium.

Now, when optimism is conceived of as a bias evoking resilience, the roots of optimism need to be defined. I have shown here that the roots of early coping skills lie in the baby's active protests and selectivity, and the young child's capacity to accept substitutes and restructure a situation. The roots of optimism also lie in infancy—in the repeated experiences of gratification of needs, of being able to count on life feeling good. The optimism and hope that come from the earliest satisfying, restorative experiences are reinforced in the next few years when separations are followed by reunions, frustrations bring support in coping, pain is followed by comfort, initiatives are backed up, and the child develops confidence that he and the environment will be able to manage any problem. There are ups and downs, downs and ups, and the growing child begins to feel that he can get out of the downs and help to make his life good. As Helen said at the age of 10, "Bad things can turn into good things."

ACKNOWLEDGMENTS

The studies on which I have drawn were supported by grants from the National Institute of Mental Health, the Gustavus and Pfeiffer Foundation, the Neumeyer Foundation, and the Menninger Foundation. In addition, some vignettes are quoted from records of children and adults that I knew personally. (All of the names of the latter have been changed to protect the individuals' privacy.)

REFERENCES

Coelho, G. V., Hamburg, D., & Adams, J. (Eds.). (1974). *Coping and adaptation*. New York: Basic Books.

Escalona, S., & Heider, G. (1959). *Prediction and outcome*. New York: Basic Books.

Heider, G. (1966). Vulnerability in infants and young children: A pilot study. *Genetic Psychology Monographs, 73*(1), 1–216.

Hellersberg, E. (1957). Unevenness of growth in its relation to vulnerability, anxiety, ego weakness, and the schizophrenic patterns. *American Journal of Orthopsychiatry, 27,* 577–586.

Jersild, A. T., & Holmes, F. B. (1935). Children's fears. *Child Development Monographs, 20.* New York: Bureau of Publications, Teachers College.

Levy, D. M. (1945). Psychic trauma of operations in children. *American Journal of Diseases of Children, 69,* 7–25.

Macfarlane, J. W., Allen, L., & Honzik, M. P. (1954). A developmental understanding of the behavior problems of normal children between twenty-one months and fourteen years. Berkeley, CA: University of California Press.

Menninger, K. (1954). Psychological aspects of the organism under stress. *Journal of the American Psychoanalytic Association, 2,* 67–106.

Moriarty, A. E. (1961). Coping patterns of preschool children in response to intelligence test demands. *Genetic Psychology Monographs, 64,* 3–127.

Murphy, L. B. (1937). *Social behavior and child personality.* New York: Columbia University Press.

Murphy, L. B. (1956). *Personality in young children: Vol. 2, Colin: A Normal Child.* New York: Basic Books.

Murphy, L. B. (1962). *The widening world of childhood.* New York: Basic Books.

Murphy, L. B., & Moriarty, A. E. (1976). *Vulnerability, coping and growth.* New Haven, CT: Yale University Press.

Random House dictionary of the English language. (1973). New York: Random House.

Rousey, C., & Moriarty, A. E. (1965). *Diagnostic implications of speech sounds.* Springfield, IL: Charles C. Thomas.

Sullivan, H. S. (1953). *The interpersonal theory of psychiatry.* New York: Norton.

5

John, a Boy Who Acquired Resilience

ALICE E. MORIARTY
Senior Psychologist, Menninger Foundation

Introduction

John was one of the children who was followed for a number of years through several studies at the Menninger Foundation in Topeka, Kansas. Though John had some marked sensory deficits, which contributed to difficulty and frustration in learning and fostered some dependency, he was a definite, vigorous individual with unusual warmth and resilience. In tracing his development, we saw intermingled coping strengths and weaknesses emerging out of his capacity to deal with physical vulnerabilities and the constant support from a warm but also uniquely stressful environment.

Even as early as 4 weeks of age, John was seen as a very positive, resilient little boy with considerable vigor; he was already able to express clear-cut preferences, such as for being held upright rather than laid supine. He could express protest by forceful crying. He recovered quickly from discomfort, utilizing support well, cuddling comfortably, and responding positively to physical contact or verbal communication.

In the preschool years, John's self-awareness was vivid and impressive, as described in an excerpt from a "Sensory Toys" play session at the age of 3 years, 7 months: "John is a roly-poly little mesomorph, bumbling as a baby Newfoundland, and as direct in motor response as any puppy could be. Objects exist for him to manipulate, to throw, to

Editors' note: This chapter was first written in August 1969

Author's note: This review draws upon concepts of ego development as discussed by R. Gardner and myself in *Personality Development at Preadolescence: An Exploratory Study of Structure Formation* (1968) and on concepts of intellectual functioning as presented in my *Constancy and IQ Change: A Clinical View of Relationships between Tested Intelligence and Personality* (1966). Most of the longitudinal data were collected in the Coping Studies at the Menninger Foundation; this series with L. B. Murphy, Director, followed S. Escalona and M. Leitch's Infancy Study. A full description of methods is available in the preface of Murphy's and my book *Vulnerability, Coping and Growth* (1976).

try to make work, or to make noise with. His face beams all over when he is pleased with a toy like the musical dog, and gives out a glowing warmth that is utterly contagious and irresistible. . . . He is so full of health, delight, warmth, and clear expressiveness that one feels bathed in a delicious sense of well-being."

At that time, John's emotional lability was shown in his ready pleasure with success, along with his quick discouragement with obstacles. He sometimes gave up, lost direction, turned to new goals, became scattered and aimless, or grew babyish and impatient. His unusually infantile speech and autonomic reactivity sometimes apparently interfered with sustained efforts when he became blocked or anxious. Yet, he was also socially amiable; he liked give-and take, cooperative, reciprocal, "live-and-let-live" relations; and aggression was low in comparison with his physical energy, appearing only when he was frustrated by failure in manipulation or communication. He could ask for and accept help, using it positively. He could be spontaneously assertive, yet he respected and yielded to limits without stubbornness or resistance.

At the age of 5 years, 5 months, following a winter of almost continuous infections of the eyes, ears, and throat, as well as a 4-week absence from kindergarten with measles, John's mother said that he was often disobedient and restless with restraints or restrictions. He frequently ran out of the yard, telling his mother, "I gotta run." He was also demanding of her time and that of his teacher, sometimes pushing other children aside or refusing to engage in group activities. Yet he was responsive to firmness and to gentle persuasion. When he understood the need for medication or treatment, for example, he behaved well and was pleased with whatever anyone did for him. As his mother put it, "Whenever it comes to standing up to the big things, he seems willing to take it."

He did this partly by seeking to understand through continuous questioning. According to his mother, he was "a proverbial question box. I thought he asked a lot of questions when he was smaller, but now he hardly gets one out until he has another started. He wants them answered to a degree that he fully understands all the whys and wherefores."

In this, as well as in his refusal to cooperate with babysitters, John was often a difficult and exhausting child. Yet he was capable of great warmth and of empathy for the feelings of other people, as well as for animals. He was devoted to a puppy with whom he was sometimes rough, but never intentionally so. The mother wrote, for example, "I wish I could describe his tenderness if I'm not feeling well; his outward signs of love—the quick hug or kiss, and after his prayers each night, the 'Mommy, I love you,' his 'Mommy, you're the best cooker in the whole wide world"; the little gift, be it a pretty rock (he fills his pockets with them) or a special toy brought to me with his 'just for you'; the pride he takes in his sister's weekly spelling tests; the sparkle in his eyes when he is pleased and interested; his chuckle at something funny. I could go on and on. At times he decides to be helpful and really is."

Later, when the puppy was accidentally killed, "John came running to the house crying as if his heart would break—but no tears since. We took Penny to the doctor but it was no use. She died later that night. John was so quiet the rest of the evening. He knew she was dead, but refused to cry. The next day he asked what happened to dead puppies— I explained the best I could and told him that his daddy had buried her. Then he said he wasn't sorry that Penny was gone because if she were here she would just be pulling at his clothes all the time—and he didn't mean a word of it. We changed the subject and no more has been said. He loved her so much he couldn't keep his hands off her. We plan to find another dog for him."

In the latency years, John developed considerable sensitive understanding of family economic limitations (he wanted but did not expect an expensive train for Christmas, for example); in the prepuberty years, he was aware, but not especially resentful, of the fact that some children had more social privileges than he. He also foresaw and accepted a future that would be modified by the needs and wishes of his own wife and family. He was able to deal constructively with some limits in his own activities because of poor eyesight.

At the age of 14 years, 6 months, our psychiatrist saw John as a poised and direct child. He still had many realistic self-doubts, but he had many friends and was a comfortable part of his peer group. On the whole, he seemed to be leading a remarkably rich life at an age-appropriate level. From the long view of John's continued development, therefore, we saw him as a child who, despite some very stressful experiences and incomplete integration, was remarkably reasonable and capable of perspective in a self-evaluation that was predominantly positive and realistic.

The resilience with which John dealt with the frustrations of sensory deficits, speech problems, and learning difficulties can only be understood by examining his strengths and weaknesses over the course of his development in relation to an environment that was highly supportive, although, for a child of his sensitivity, it was also in some respects pressured.

John in the Infancy Years

Encased in several layers of unusually beautiful yellow wool blankets, 4-week-old John's chubby little face with bright blue eyes "emerged as if from a cocoon." The baby was stylishly groomed in a long attractive white nightgown, yellow spun rayon jacket, white knit sweater and cap, and felt cowboy boots! This garb, combined with the fact that John slept during most of the 4-hour observation period, meant that the range of observable behavior was less than that for most infants in the Escalona–Leitch study. However, that which was observed, supplemented by later observations in the home, gave reliable evidence that he was a vigorous, active, assertive baby with high sensory and autonomic reactivity, differentiated social responsiveness, and a distinct capacity for self-expression through motor and preverbal channels. While he was an infant who could communicate needs, preferences, and protests, his intensity of experiencing also left him vulnerable to frustrations and occasional disintegrative reactions.

When awake, John was almost continuously active. His legs and arms, separately or as a part of generalized body activity, were in almost constant motion—squirming, quivering, flexing, rubbing, kicking, waving, clenching, fisting. Usually these movements were relatively smooth and suggested muscular strength, though there was some lack of coordination, along with occasional tense, stiff, or jerky movements.

John's high activity level was not surprising to his mother, who had experienced him as so active *in utero* as to be embarrassing when "he scooted all over my abdomen" in such a way as to cause "people to stop talking and look." She added that she had felt she "might spank him when he was born, just on general principles." Nor was it surprising to her to see him "gulping down his feeding" when still in the hospital—an observation consistent with his eager anticipation of his bottle, his greedy, noisy eating, and his loud burping during the experimental session.

Of equal intensity was John's sensory responsiveness. For example, he seemed interested in looking and seeing, hearing, or feeling everything, though he was sometimes uncomfortable with strong stimulation. He raised his head and moved his hands when observers approached; he turned his head toward the window during his bath; he slowed his pace of eating when sounds occurred; he could be quieted by soft music or his mother's voice, as well as by her patting, rubbing, or holding him; he cried when wet or when his armpits, nose, or arms were washed; he was sometimes startled in response to touch; and he frowned when bright lights were turned on. All of this, of course, reflected marked alertness to external stimulation, which made him vividly aware of the world in which he lived, but also subject to discomfort at times.

Paralleling his sensory responsiveness was marked autonomic reactivity. For example, observers repeatedly noted deep flushing, especially when he was actively moving, crying, or having a bowel movement: "Whenever he moved very much or cried, his face flushed red, and a couple of times when he was crying very hard, it seemed to me that it turned almost purple. A few times, I noted that this flushing extended over his entire head, and it may well be that this happened each time. However, when he stopped moving, his face returned to its normal coloring rather rapidly." His breathing was described as "breathy," "squeaky," or "irregular," especially when the observers manipulated his body for experimental purposes. During the activity rating, one observer remarked, "He was markedly flushed . . . and his crying was about as hard as a baby can cry."

John's crying was often seen as a form of protest. For example, the mother noted that he cried when he was apparently not ready to accept his bottle (she explained, "He says, 'Don't rush me'"), or during his baths when a diaper rash on his sensitive skin may have made bathing of the genital area particularly uncomfortable. He was seen to cry vigorously during the experimental observations and sometimes to turn away from a bottle that he apparently did not want. This occurred before, during, and after a feeding, so that protest seemed to be more than a simple expression of hunger or lack of hunger. He objected several times to being laid supine, definitely preferring to be held in an upright position. As one observer stated, "Nobody could get away with holding John except in the position he preferred, because he would howl too loudly." At other times, the mother suggested that he cried to get attention (as during the early evening, when the family usually played with him) or because he was "angry." One observer described John as "resentful" of being handled when sleepy; the mother remarked, "When he gets to crying good, he always seems mad. . . . I don't know what he cries at." (This was a reference to his crying just after a feeding, possibly related to resistance to falling asleep, but this was not stated.)

John gazed directly at his mother for quite long periods of time (especially for so young an infant) and also focused on the observer for shorter periods of time, vocalizing vowel sounds that would have been more characteristic of an 8-week-old child. He was not yet able to follow moving people visually, and a marked strabismus was present at times. Frowning was also noted (as in response to bright lights, or accompanying delay in beginning to suck, or even sometimes during apparently contented sucking, which the mother related to the intensity of his involvement). She remarked, "That's his daddy all over. When he is doing something, he frowns like that."

At the end of the experiment, he relaxed comfortably in the observer's arms, smiling broadly, but without vocalizing as he had when the mother was in direct contact or within his immediate visual focus. In a few moments, his face puckered, and he would probably have cried had the mother not taken him.

The observer summarized the observation by the following statement: "He did not show a wide range of behavior during the afternoon, but everything he did was done with the utmost vigor—sleeping, nursing, crying, vocalizing. Thus, his behavior had an all-or-none quality to it, and few halfway states were seen."

Psychological tests, administered at home, clearly showed that John's development was at that time proceeding at a better-than-average pace. Motor and adaptive performances were equivalent to that of a child of 8— weeks, language to that of an 8 weeks child, and personal-social development to that of a 4+ weeks child.

John's impressive neonatal health and sturdiness were prized by his parents, who especially welcomed the birth of a son 4 years after the birth of a daughter. This was clearly evident in the warm, tender way in which the mother handled the baby, in her efforts to make him comfortable, in her pleasure at his development, and in her tolerance for his occasional irritable demands on her. She was sensitive to his needs, but also encouraged a good deal of independence on his part; for example, she gave him less physical support than some mothers did, and was proud that he could "feed himself" (i.e., that he took bottles at night and early morning in a propped position).

Despite this generally positive relationship between mother and baby, there were some potentially disturbing factors in the mother's mild doubts and anxieties, as well as an indication of perceptual distortions in relation to her own needs to be an independent, competent person. For example, it was surprising that she commented on a baby so obviously healthy and normal that she was glad he was not "feeble-minded," that she emphasized so strongly her wish that his eyes would turn brown like his father's, and that she hoped he would not be left-handed like her. Surprising, too, were her concerns that he not be tossed in the air lest he fall, that he not be placed in a sleeping bag lest he smother, that he be so overwrapped lest he be cold, and that he prepare himself to be "something better" than his father (i.e., that he obtain a better education and aspire to a more economically rewarding job). She made it clear that she felt adequate to use advice and help selectively; she did not rely on willing, available relatives for babysitting; she adopted a flexible feeding schedule, but rejected breast feeding as inconvenient and too time-consuming; she was unhurried, skillful, and alert to individual differences in her children, yet insisted that everything should be "regular and normal." She pointed out, for example, that she expected exact obedience and proper behavior on the part of both children. To obtain this, she was able to spank her daughter for pouting, and was proud that she could control her daughter's behavior with a simple word or gesture.

The mother's need to be independent probably was rooted in her own experience of a somewhat economically deprived life in childhood, her inability to acquire an education to prepare her for the professional career she would have enjoyed, and her identification with a mother who rose from a deprived early life to an executive position in the business world. The stress she felt from her own father's job instability may have accentuated her feelings that "every woman should be able to support herself," and also may have induced her to push her husband toward better-paid, more responsible, and more secure employment.

In appearance, Mrs. C. was unusually attractive; her grooming was not only immaculate, but well suited to her coloring. She was described as "a very quick-witted woman, who frequently had a ready response to our questions or comments, which made it especially pleasant to talk to her." Verbally fluent, she was generally open and direct, though she tended to deny and avoid things that were unpleasant or might be disappointing. For example, she had refused to hope for a boy baby lest she be disappointed; although somewhat physically uncomfortable and fatigued during the interview, she denied or at least minimized this; although obviously very pleased with her son, she actually went out of her way to describe him as a rather average infant (perhaps to avoid boasting, or to reduce future disappointment should he prove to be less advanced than she wanted to believe). Although she apparently discussed child-rearing procedures with her friends and read some popular articles on the subject, she made it clear that she preferred to be independent—to do things in her own way, based on her own understanding. For instance, she remarked that she did not understand how the observers found so much to record. One sensed that whenever she lacked total understanding, she felt vaguely anxious.

Mrs. C.'s feelings about independence were also reflected in her dealings with John. For instance, she was mildly inconsistent insofar as she encouraged independence at many points, but other times appeared overprotective of him, as noted earlier. While she was very sensitive to the baby's needs, she was at times somewhat awkward, and on at least one occasion held him overtightly. Several observers remarked that despite her obvious affection for the child, she did not always seem "particularly maternal"; this was reflected partly in her desire to return to work and perhaps related to her own desire to be independent. One observer noted her considerable pride about being an independent person, as she spoke about the smoothness of her pregnancy, how well the delivery went, and the fact that she did not feel in great need of help following the baby's birth. At the same time, she had very little awareness of natural dependent needs, which in fact seemed to be threatening to her. Specifically, the observer felt she might find it somewhat difficult to allow her children and her husband to be dependent on her. She minimized whatever conflicts she experienced in relation to dependence by presenting herself and her husband as "good solid citizens who live a harmonious life," an evaluation the observers saw as very likely honest and realistic.

Altogether, Mrs. C. was a likeable person, affectionate and competent with the baby, and intellectually alert and comfortable with the observers. She was, however, a woman whose mild upward mobility probably pressed her affectively freer and perhaps less well-endowed husband, and one who perhaps herself experienced some conflict between her wish to be independent and her equally strong desire to be a good mother.

John's father was a tall, good-looking man, strongly masculine in appearance and manner. While friendly and warm, he shared his wife's aspirations in regard to staying independent of both families and encouraging male sturdiness and independence in his son. He was, however, apparently less concerned than she about bettering his own vocational status, and was more impulsive and outgoing. His wife remarked, for example, that he made friends with people of all stations, that he frequently brought even casual acquaintances home for dinner without planning in advance, and that he was likely to buy impulsively or to plan recreational activities on the spur of the moment. He sincerely enjoyed his child, willingly cared for all the baby's needs except for changing soiled diapers, and anticipated sharing many masculine activities with his son when he was older.

Along with this degree of parental warmth, support, and concern, John enjoyed considerable affection and attention from both sets of grandparents and several other relatives. These experiences undoubtedly contributed to his sense of self-worth in a good world. (At the same time, the strong positive feelings between John and his relatives undoubtedly increased the severe loss he suffered later when both pairs of grandparents were divorced. Furthermore, the loss was the more intense because he not only experienced personal loss, but empathically shared parental sorrows, particularly those of his mother.)

In the light of future development and behavior, the infancy data became especially meaningful. We saw, for example, a vivid child who was vigorously active, unusually sensitive to sensory stimulation, emotionally labile, and highly reactive to autonomic changes. He was a warm, loving baby, but one who was also able to protest. So far as infancy tests could determine, he was developing at a better-than-average pace, with native abilities and personal style suggesting a potentiality for openness to the world—a basis for self-respect and security in a comfortable relationship with the world that would generally be experienced positively.

On the other hand, the urgency of his responsiveness and his sensitivities left him vulnerable to being overwhelmed and frustrated if his later skills did not match his needs. Loss of central vision in the left eye, as well as subsequent temporary losses of hearing (discovered only later), were sources of stress insofar as they interfered with basic school learning and with speech development.

Interacting with John's temperament and native capacities were the positive and negative family traits that have been noted. While his family was loving and supportive, the parents were occasionally inconsistent; sometimes they overprotected him and at other times they encouraged his independence. Furthermore, the capable and loving mother's pressure to be independent and her inclination to push the father beyond his own vocational aims were potential strains, which were later actualized.

There was also a history of economic deprivation in the maternal family, resolved by the grandmother's efforts to become financially independent while the grandfather was reported to be somewhat unstable in his job efforts. This combination of factors suggested a model from female relatives of independence and capacity to rise to challenges, contrasted with some inadequacy and lack of ambition on the part of male relatives. In a sensitive child like John, one could foresee some conflicts in the dependency area arising from his own needs and skills and from the inconsistency of his mother's handling. Also possible were some conflicts in identification with males, who, though physically sturdy and affectionate, were less dominant and forceful in some respects than the female relatives. Later in this chapter, it becomes clear how vulnerabilities in his native equipment and inconsistencies in family demands, in the context of an essentially stable family, intertwined in the making of a resourceful and appealing, responsible, and reasonable individual, but also one with poorly integrated ego development.

There are several details to be added to the infancy picture so far described. John was relatively healthy in his first year of life, and his motor development appeared to be normal. According to the mother's report at the beginning of the preschool Coping Study, he sat alone at 7 months, crawled at 8 months, and walked alone at 11 months. Of unknown significance was the fact that he was at 6 months exposed to and quarantined for meningitis; so far as is known, he did not contract the disease. Also of unknown significance, but possibly contributing to the acceleration of dependency overtly displayed in his slow speech development, was the fact that his tongue was clipped at 9 months of age when he was said to be tonguetied.

A major change in John's life occurred when he was 9 months old: His mother went back to work full-time, leaving him initially to the care of a responsible neighbor. In terms of our general knowledge of infancy, this is considered a critical or vulnerable phase, when the baby is likely to react most severely to separation from the mother. For this child, this separation was probably a special source of stress that created difficulty in the resolution of dependency and in the related speech problems. (Speech development was somewhat slow and articulation indistinct. Single words were comprehensible only at about 2½ years of age, and he talked in sentences only at about 3 years of age.)

Still, John was regarded as an infant low in vulnerability, and his general health and development were within an average range. There were no major health problems; motor skills were average or better; he related comfortably both to family and to others; and there were no signs of unusual fearfulness. Bowel control was established at 14 months, and bladder control sometime between 18 and 24 months. Nocturnal control was established at approximately 3 years of age.

Vulnerability shifted in the second and third years of life, when John was exposed to almost continuous stress from a series of systemic infections and to the separation from his mother, who continued to be employed in a full-time job. Repeated ear infections, requiring many penicillin shots and several courses of antibiotics, followed a fall into a lake. Subsequently, the left eardrum was lanced twice and the right eardrum once. Temporary hearing loss was noted, but there was thought to be no permanent damage. Susceptibility to colds was marked, and these illnesses were accompanied by hoarseness and spasmodic croup. Infections in the left eye left permanent scar tissue. German measles at age 2 and a severe case of chicken pox at age 2½ were accompanied by high temperatures, but his recovery was rapid—a point important to note in connection with his resilience in dealing with numerous other stresses.

Despite these physical complications, John had been left in the hands of a series of babysitters from his 13th to his 24th month. From necessity, his mother remained home with the child for 1 month at that time and then returned to work until John was 28 months old. Then she quit work on the advice of a physician, in an effort to alleviate John's demanding, clinging behavior and his poor speech development, which was largely restricted to grunts clarified by vivid and active pantomime.

We might say that the sturdy but sensitive and reactive baby of 1 month had become more vulnerable as a result of multiple somatic troubles and their sequelae, including temporary hearing loss at the time when speech ordinarily emerges. It was likely that the series of illnesses contributed to some slowing down of his originally advanced motor coordination, as well as of his speech. These, together with the irritability that often accompanies and follows a series of illnesses, no doubt interfered with consolidation of autonomy at this crucial stage. Moreover, the repeated illnesses in themselves and the frustrations they involved presumably interfered with the delicate process of integration at this stage of complex emerging functions.

The Preschool Years

Observations of John at the Menninger Foundation

At age 3½, John pulled his chubby body upstairs with effortful hanging on the stair railing and lumbered into Dr. Murphy's "Sensory Toys" examining room without quite noticing what he was stepping on. Yet he was not unmindful of his environment, which he took in with a steady appraising gaze, settling on a big gun. Then his face beamed with delight as he let out an appreciative "Ooh!," after which he requested, as though help could be taken for granted, "Help me take this out. . . . How shoot it? . . . Oh, shoot bear!" (in reality, a musical dog). Taking aim, John joyfully fired and then ran to pick up the soft stuffed dog, which he cuddled lovingly as he continued to manipulate the gun. This sequence of behavior and the choice of both an aggressive and a soft toy, along with his pleasure in the intermingled sound of the banging of the gun and the tinkling melody from the dog, aptly expressed his outgoing and trusting attitudes toward his environment, as well as his orientation toward action and his emotional lability. These choices, along with other toy preferences for things that worked or that could be manipulated, suggested that action was more important than expressing ideas or fantasy. His actions were typically exploratory and realistic, assertive but never stubborn or hostile. From his brief initial indecisiveness, one sensed that he might, when exposed to too many emotionally arousing stimuli, have difficulty sorting out his perceptions and feelings. When this happened, his tendency to go into action following only vague or casual observations without full integration of details led to frustration, particularly when his infantile language development blocked the easy communication with people that his warmth and lively spirit demanded.

In the Miniature Life Toy situation, John could be definite in his choices, but his expressive moods varied "from uneasiness to a spontaneous lilt." Easily pleased with success, he could also be easily discouraged by obstacles, which he dealt with at some times through ready acceptance of support. At other times, John gave up or lost direction, resulting in scattered, disorganized, and aimless action. Lacking persistence, he was sometimes helpless and babyish or impatient, dealing with these feelings by ineffective trial and error. Sometimes he forced or banged parts of toys when his efforts failed. Though highly alert to visual and auditory qualities of things, and to nuances of feelings in people, he did not look carefully and his vagueness sometimes led to bewilderment. Capable of reciprocal cooperation, he was socially amiable and ready to yield to adult protest.

When he was blocked or anxious, prominent emotional flooding (suggested by his flushed face, shallow rapid breathing, and frequent need for urination) interfered with sustained effort toward a goal, and frustration rose when his natural responsiveness was unmatched by easy verbal communication. Perhaps, too, anxiety arising from difficulties in integrating vigorous, active, and masculine identification with "his feeling for soft values" (as seen in his love for soft cuddly animals) interfered with full discharge of defensive aggressive impulses.

Altogether, John was seen at this stage as a warm, loving, and lovable human being, but one whose ebullience could fluctuate with periods of discouragement and disappointment, which were surprising in one so vigorous and reactive. These variations were partly understandable in the light of some fluidity of responsiveness, a reflection of some similar patterns seen in the father, and his own growing awareness of conflict between a need to interact and limited perception and skill. In this, the congenital loss of central vision in his left eye, repeated infections of both eyes and ears with some temporary hearing loss, extensive articulatory problems (doubtless aggravated by the latter), and some sense of deprivation lingering from the mother's absence at work all took a toll. These problems became more prominent after his entrance into school, where his sensory deficits created learning difficulties associated with increasing frustrations and exacerbation of conflicts concerning dependency. As will become clear later, however, John met these problems, and some others involving stability of the larger family group, with amazing resilience. This was fostered by his high degree of personal self-awareness and by his perspective and reasonableness in viewing his own resources and limitations, and his capacity to cope quite constructively with the exigencies of his life.

In the structured test (administered by the author) at the preschool stage, John dealt with mild apprehension of the new situation by ingeniously delaying departure from his mother and by making many potentially acceptable requests, terminating these only when she agreed to accompany him. Once assured of her presence, he became so independently involved in his activities that his mother was soon able to leave. With considerable interest, he inspected and explored test equipment and the room, moving about vigorously and actively, but rarely maintaining his interest in any one thing for long. Fine motor performances were handled somewhat awkwardly, often on a trial-and-error basis, and he refused to persist with test demands (such as paper cutting or drawing) that he found difficult or frustrating.

The intensity of John's interests and his desire to communicate were hampered by his motor clumsiness and his poor speech, leading to frequent emotional frustration and physical exhaustion. However, he had a proprietary air toward things he considered his (as when he said of a puzzle he assembled, "Don't break my picture"). It was easy to enlist his renewed efforts just because he seemed to want to please the examiner. For example, after once leaving the room and indicating his distaste for the test, he looked back over his shoulder, gaily calling out, "Hi." Once he said, "I can't . . . because I don't want to," an assessment which was at least partially correct, though it may also have served to deny the possibility that he might also fail.

In this situation, John emerged as a direct, lively, and vigorous child who expressed his wishes strongly without ill-feeling. With things, he was often impatient, careless, or rough, but never deliberately destructive; with people, he was forthright and emotionally expressive (enthusiastic, affectionate, disgusted, disappointed, irritated), but never hostile or indifferent. Perhaps a part of his resilience stemmed from the direct release of feelings without lingering resentment. Yet, from another point of view, the lability of his expression of feelings still left a residue of undischarged aggressive feelings, which emerged under stress in a form of impatience or disappointment. In this sense, he was both a highly expressive child and one whose sense of family loyalty and need for personal integrity sometimes imposed restrictions on his communication, thus laying a groundwork for conflict between his need to respond to and his need to develop differentiation from, a world that was both gratifying and frustrating.

Typically, John dealt with difficulty or failure by leaving the field; by removing or scattering offending material so as to eliminate it from direct focus; by delaying testing with reasonable requests, or with apparent interest in playing with test equipment; or by simply refusing to persist. He could be encouraged to try again, but these efforts rarely proved successful in the preschool years. Several times, when his mother restrained him from leaving the room, or offered him help that he had not demanded, he flushed, flailed his limbs, and protested noisily. John's activity, his impatience, and his short attention span suggested that test scores were a minimal estimate of his potential ability—a prediction borne out later by higher retest scores (see pp. 126, 130). At age 3½, a mental age of 3 years, 3 months and an IQ of 93 on Form L of the revised Stanford–Binet appeared to reflect a functioning level of low average quality, in which both sensory deficits and some emotional immaturity were deterrents to maximal display of cognitive resources.

A psychiatric evaluation by Dr. Toussieng when John was aged 3 years, 10 months was in essential agreement with the findings of the Miniature Life Toy play session and the structured test examination, though it focused more directly on some aspects of his immaturity and fearfulness and raised a question about organic brain involvement.

In the one-to-one relationship with a male adult, John was initially more hesitant and slower to become involved. His play tended to be monotonous and repetitive, without much sustained fantasy. He became increasingly aggressive to the point of physical exhaustion; still, there was no destructive behavior, and it became apparent that too direct expression of aggression was frightening to him. To avoid being tempted into expressing aggression, John appeared "to keep himself a baby and to see to it that he would not grow up too quickly if at all." Yet his play demonstrated many competitive feelings with adult male figures—once so strong that they broke through in direct physical attack. From these observations, the psychiatrist felt that John was "a rather immature boy who appeared to be fighting desperately with strong aggressive and competitive impulses that were not acceptable to him," although controls were not effective enough to prevent these impulses from breaking through at times. That he was making efforts to resolve these struggles through regression was suggested by his infantile behavior, coordinative awkwardness, lack of cerebral dominance, dysarthric speech difficulties, restlessness, and short attention span. On the other hand, these phenomena also raised a question about possible organic brain impairment.

During a Children's Apperception Test (CAT) examination administered in the same period, John's overt behavior reinforced our concerns about organic instability and again highlighted his immaturity in certain areas, with conflicts centering around dependency. The former was suggested by several aspects of his behavior, and the latter by his responses to the test.

For example, the examiner noted a limp, loose-jointed gait initially, with a readiness to trip or slip. There was also a kind of generalized excitement, which sometimes resulted in impulsive, jerky, and somewhat uncontrolled hand movements; John pounced on test materials with the fingers spread tensely apart. This was less notable later in the session, and postural adjustments were then made relatively flexibly and comfortably. Other indices of possible organic instability with a probable overlay of anxiety included rapid, shallow breathing, a frequent need for urination, and deviations in voice quality and manner of articulation. His voice was hoarse, strained, and tight; articulation and speech forms were very immature; phrasing and grammatical construction were awkward, and there were misidentifications and problems in word finding. These problems appeared to be related to poverty of vocabulary, as well as to a tendency to concretize for lack of clear conceptualization. Nearly continuous sucking and chewing on his fingers and clothing furthered the impression of immaturity and/or anxiety.

There was no resistance to leaving his mother at this time, perhaps partly because she was busy with packing (preparatory to moving out of town) and encouraged his independence. In the test itself, however, he seemed dependent on the examiner, of whom he asked many insistent questions. There was some delay in responding, but this seemed to stem from inability to handle or lack of clarity about test demands, as much as or more than from emotional resistance. He expressed distaste for the use of the microphone, which he objected to having near him. Later, however, he urgently wanted to hear the playback, only reluctantly allowing himself to be put off. Still later, he complained of being tired and insisted, "We are srew [through] weadin' [reading] dat [that] one." Toward the end of the test, he seemed to be trying to make his responses as brief as possible, evidently in an effort to be finished with demands that he found difficult and uninteresting. Increasingly, as the session proceeded, he seemed aware of his own expressive difficulties—perhaps experiencing the examiner's frequent failure to understand him as a form of criticism, which he had also experienced earlier from his parents.

Despite the generalized excitability and the strain under which he worked, and despite his poor speech and his tendency toward motor dyscontrol (perhaps reflecting organic instability or some pervasive tension accentuated by anxiety about the impending family move), John was friendly, cooperative, and talkative. He tried to fill in gaps in his vocabulary or conceptualization by identifying the pictured animals in terms of colors, movement, or function. Sometimes when he was confused, he offered several alternative meanings, leaving it to the examiner to determine the most appropriate. He was very definite in stating his preference as to how and when the microphone should be used, but he was also ready to defer to adult demands for delay or control; it was almost as though he welcomed such external control, which then would presumably clarify his own thinking. At times, he tried to avoid or terminate the test, but this seemed to reflect genuine confusion and discouragement rather than any negativism in interacting with an adult.

John's CAT responses seemed to imply a comfortable relationship with both parents, whom he saw as sharing his pleasures and including him in their activities. On the other hand, the father figure was viewed as a potential competitor and punisher, though the punishment was in terms of firmness rather than unreasonableness or hostility. Adult masculine figures were projected as strong, brave, and loving, but also as so powerful as to make the child feel weak and helpless by comparison. When the CAT cards raised issues of nighttime fearfulness, his speech became particularly immature, as though staying babyish was a useful maneuver to elicit protection. His habit of concretely describing single objects and of placing the examiner in the position of making the choice between alternative responses also had the quality of relating dependently. At other times, he could be very definite in expressing his wants.

Altogether, one had the impression in the CAT of a little boy who enjoyed people and welcomed new experiences, which, though generally pleasant, could also be frightening at times. Despite a rather energetic involvement in life, he was also aware of weaknesses and limitations; he dealt with these primarily by remaining a baby, thereby reducing both his own expectations and those of others.

The pediatrician who examined John at this time noted that he was particularly susceptible to respiratory and skin infections. Frequent colds, complicated by ear and eye infections, required repeated medication with penicillin and sulfanilamides; unusually strong reaction to heat and insect bites suggested marked skin sensitivity. Frequent need for urination, as well as increased pulse rate, elevated blood pressure, and systolic murmur under the stress of a physical examination (and in the excitement of play), suggested sensitivity in the cardiovascular system and probably also high autonomic reactivity. All of this implied considerable somatic reactivity in several zones, and a possible foundation for emotional lability interacting with this.

John at Home

John's behavior at home was quite consistent with the observations made during this series of tests. His warmth, emotional lability, high activity level, and strongly positive sense of self were all documented by the mother's natural and insightful reports. Her understanding was based on sincere affection, as well as on a realistic awareness of his limitations. For example, she described him as an active, vigorous child who ate heartily and had no time for naps (though he was always ready for bed at nighttime); he was "always going out to find the world," was friendly with old and young, was eternally inquisitive, and grew impatient with restrictions or delays unless they were carefully explained to him. Backyard fences and high shelves only offered challenges; he could not be kept in his own yard; on shopping trips, he resented delays when adults stopped to talk; in church and other public places, he could not be shushed, and his mother frequently felt obliged to remove him to avoid embarrassment. She reported that "if he decides he wants something, he goes right after it," and he can not accept "no" without "a battle between us." With peers, he was overbearing, argumentative, and often unwilling to take turns. He liked to play with his older sister and her friends, but he was unable to play for long periods because he interfered with their planned activities and showed little respect for their toys. Rebuffed by peers or his sister, he sometimes turned to imaginary playmates and followed his paternal grandmother's lead in talking to robins. He also shared with her a tremendous love for all growing and living things and a great curiosity about the world around him. Like his paternal grandfather, he enjoyed music and liked to sing. Altogether, his life was busy, often satisfying, but sometimes also deeply frustrating. In a sense, he was seeking stimulation from many sources, which led to richness of living, but also perhaps contributed to confusion at times.

His high activity level was rarely controlled by words; sometimes his mother spanked him or confined him to a chair. Of the two punishments, the latter was less successful, since it required constant supervision by the mother and was less well suited to the child's rapidly rising and dissipating feelings.

Sometimes after a particularly difficult day, both mother and child welcomed the father's homecoming—the mother, because the father (whom she considered more lenient) seemed better able to control John; the child, because he respected the father's definite limits, in the context of his warmth. Altogether, one saw a happy family with strong feelings; affection was frequently openly displayed, as was also disapproval. In this interaction, John's feelings were sometimes hurt, and his mother was sometimes nervous, but negative feelings were less frequent than were positive ones, and ill feelings were never of long duration. John respected and loved his parents; they respected and loved him. If the intensity of his need to be active and his occasional impatience sometimes got him into trouble, he was soon resiliently responsive again. In the mother's eyes, he was never "deliberately naughty," though he was sometimes careless and frequently irritating to her because of his vigorous insistence on freedom to move about and to explore areas and objects that she sometimes regarded as potentially dangerous. He was probably often frustrated by the conflict between his urgent need to interact and his mother's restrictions, or between his own outgoing, friendly nature and his difficulties in verbal communication or in seeing and hearing clearly. (The nature and degree of these conflicts were not recognized until some time later.)

In effect, John at this time was a vivid, active, warm, empathic, lovable and loved child, but also one whose lack of sensory sharpness and motoric smoothness interfered with the determined urgency of his need to see and interact with his world. Furthermore, he was, though distinctly charming and appealing, also a child whose energetic activity and emotional lability made him difficult to contain and something of an emotional strain on his mother. Thus, he was vulnerable to frustration from his own limitations and from the pressures of somewhat ineffective inner controls, as well as those necessarily imposed by his mother. Though naturally independent, he was by own limitations forced to be dependent in relating to a mother who by her own inclinations would have favored his independence.

In this complex of conflicts, John's rapid physical recovery from his illnesses, his inclination to view the world positively, and his mother's usually untiring patience and belief in him were bases for resilience. In the supportive preschool environment, his tendencies to regress and to deny were tolerated and even fostered at times, so that the frustrations he met, though sometimes quite intense, were only briefly overwhelming. With new pressures encountered at school (including more direct comparison with his academically more able older sister), as well as continuing physical problems and some family changes, he faced new stresses and experienced more self-doubt, but again he managed to handle all of this with considerable strength and resourcefulness.

John in the Latency Years

Early Latency

The family's move to another community involved certain new pressures; these were reflected in both mother and child and in the interaction between them. (The family visited John's grandparents in Topeka almost every year and cooperated with continued tests and interviews each time.) Mrs. C. told us she was sometimes exasperated with John when he failed to conform to her standards of neatness; he was also so continuously active as to be physically exhausting to his mother. In this context she felt somewhat guilty that she could not easily contain her impatience or his provocativeness. She also felt resentful and discouraged about his slow progress and was deeply concerned about his physical condition and his resistance to going to kindergarten in the new town. Though her attitudes were tempered by admiration for his "determination" as well as for his warm responsiveness to people, her deepened discouragement at this time was probably intensified by the physical strain of a miscarriage just prior to the move, and by her worries about her husband's new job and her part in pushing him to leave work he had preferred.

The cumulative effects of physical and emotional strains, as well as the mother's latent concerns about John's normality, were further increased by a series of problems in relation to John's health and school adjustment in kindergarten and the primary grades. For example, a tonsillectomy and an adenoidectomy at age 4½ were unsuccessful, and another operation was performed when John was 5½ years old. In kindergarten, where he was the youngest and least mature child in his class, expectable difficulties were magnified by frequent absences because of illness. Auditory impairments made it impossible for John to keep up with his class. He reacted by returning home several times each week, forcing the mother to take him back to school against his vehement protest. John still suffered from recurrent infections; he contracted measles, complicated with a very high fever and followed by a 15-pound weight loss. At about the same time, the father was acutely ill. Finally, it was definitely determined that John had a loss of central vision in the left eye, and he acquired glasses. (Glasses were required "to keep the eye in position," thereby lessening strain on the right eye, which despite repeated infections was not permanently damaged.)

Along with these strains, John experienced stress from beginning speech classes, from receiving radium treatments in both ears, and from acquiring competition in the form of a new and healthy baby sister. The radium treatments, in which long wires were run through the nose to apply local anesthesia and to insert the radium, were clearly stressful in several ways. Besides being frightening to so young a child, these treatments required him to lie motionless for 12 minutes—a situation that must have been agonizing for this active child. Furthermore, the administration of the anesthesia was painful, though the application of the radium was not painful. About all this, however, John was brave and uncomplaining, never so much as whimpering. There was little information provided about the speech classes, but one might surmise that concentration on this weak area would have been stressful to a child so eager to communicate. Finally, John was overtly loving toward and interested in the new baby sister, but it seemed probable that he suffered some feelings of being displaced as the baby in the family.

Giving as her reason the fact that John was the youngest in his class, the mother for one period considered withdrawing him from school, but this was not done due to the father's objection. At one time, she asked an examiner whether John was retarded; this recalled her early remark to the effect that she was glad that he was not feeble-minded—a feeling perhaps related to her contact with some handicapped children at a local institution.

Toward the end of the first grade, there were some signs of improvement both in John's speech and in his attitude towards school. However, his marks continued to be poor in the second grade, and John's loud verbal arguments with his older, probably brighter, and certainly more academically accomplished sister increased. Along with this, there were by then definite behavioral hints that John resented being displaced as the baby by the little sister. For example, he often demanded immediate attention from the mother (e.g., he would not tolerate waiting for lunch) and was unusually stubborn in making persistent requests even when the request was impossible in the mother's eyes (e.g., playing outdoors in his new clothes). These differences invariably ended in spankings, followed by tears, temporary retreats to his own room, and finally reparations on John's part. Clearly, these experiences were intense and disconcerting to both mother and child. For the child, they were frustrating and disappointing; for the mother, they were irritating and probably guilt-laden.

Nor were peer relations less intense. Though John preferred to have company rather than to play alone, he was likely to disagree with plans, to shout, and to punch vigorously enough that parents felt forced to stop fights before John hurt someone. The neighborhood children were, in Mrs. C.'s eyes, not properly trained. Despite Mrs. C.'s own experience of frustration with John's lack of control at times, she attributed differences in peer relationships almost entirely to the other children, and this projection of blame on her part resulted in strained relationships with neighbors. She was also angry at the neighbors' description of John as "belligerent and immature." In a sense, her anger probably was protective of John, but also was a reluctant admission that she too experienced him in these terms.

In another context, when Mrs. C. described John's new fearfulness of the dark, she exclaimed, "Perhaps most of John's troubles are his mother"; this suggested a sense of guilt, but one that was selectively applied. Thus, there were intermingled feelings of discouragement, defeat, sense of guilt, projection, and perhaps also some displacement of feelings about her husband's inadequacy. Nonetheless, these feelings were at least partly balanced by positive feelings of admiration for the warmth and consideration of both husband and son, who often just short of the mother's breaking point demonstrated their warm affection for her. In effect, the mother's feelings were intense, were usually expressed directly, and were not allowed to fester. This suited John's own reaction patterns insofar as it offered immediate release, followed by a time for making up. Thus, despite repeated frustrations, John was able to try again and to seek new reassurances, behavior which must have been experienced as satisfying, since he never entirely lost his viewpoint that the world and his family were basically good.

Following this series of misfortunes and raw emotions, there was a period of greater stability, during which John showed numerous signs of maturing. His warmth and empathy continued undimmed. His health, though still precarious, was better understood, as were the sources of his early school difficulties. Behaviorally, he was more serious and often engagingly earnest in his efforts to master basic school subjects; he was also less distractible and more likely to persist in difficult tasks. His persistence was noted, too, in his laborious efforts to master bicycle riding, an experience that included numerous falls without complaint on John's part; though never becoming entirely proficient in riding his bicycle, John learned well enough to find this activity

pleasurable. His speech improved to the point of becoming more comprehensible, though he still spoke in husky, slurred tones, made a
number of articulatory substitutions, and often fumbled for words to
express his rich perceptions and his love for people and animals. In this,
his thinking often appeared ingenious and even somewhat poetic: For
instance, when failing to recall the names of the four seasons, he
explained that they were "the going-fishing season, the bike-riding
season, the ice-fishing season, and the walking-down-the-valley season."

Both gross and fine motor skills improved, though there was some
lack of control of the body when feelings were high. Laterality was
definitely established to the right, but drawings were primitive and
disproportionate in size. His writing was a slow, laborious process with
scrawled, large, inaccurately formed numbers and letters, made only by
bending very close to the page and holding the pencil in a cramped,
awkward position.

Difficulties in focusing on small visual details handicapped John in
learning to read and to spell—processes in which there were directional
confusions, reflected in poorly established left–right orientation and in
the formation of similar letters, such as "B" and "D" or "U" and "N."
Nor was he better equipped to learn phonics, since his auditory discrimination was poor. These difficulties interfered, too, with his learning
arithmetic, since he could neither easily make the numbers nor clearly
see written examples. Furthermore, rote memory was somewhat below
average, perhaps partly as a result of the pressure and discouragement
he felt when he was asked to attempt such unrewarding and difficult
tasks as these school subjects. On the other hand, meaningful related
facts about people were well retained.

His IQ on the Stanford–Binet rose to 106, a 13-point increase over
the score he obtained at age 3½. This resulted partly from the care
he took to delay and to handle motor tasks carefully; however, with
increasing difficulty, his performance showed little planning or organization and was likely to be impulsive. He had difficulty discovering or
applying organizing principles for himself, whether the task was one of
motor assembly or verbal abstraction, but his knowledge of the natural
world and of human relationships was superior. It was also clear that he
could learn associated facts quite well when he was given a good deal of
support and encouragement.

His most prominent difficulties lay in abstracting, generalizing, or
integrating, so that much of his thinking appeared to be primitive and
concrete. These difficulties, seen in conjunction with his awkwardness
in motor execution of written symbols and his lack of sensory clarity,
were undoubtedly major factors in his slow acquisition of both speech
and basic school subjects.

Furthermore, all these aspects of his behavior, along with the impulsivity already noted, suggested to the psychiatrist "the possible presence of organic brain damage . . . however, there is nothing to indicate a specific localized lesion." This opinion was shared by our neurologist, who found "mild scarring and dulling of the eardrums bilaterally" without serious auditory impairment. Additional findings included "divergent strabismus of the left eye," scarring of the left cornea, "some type of deformity of the optic nerve head," and "some change in the pattern of blood vessels on the medial side," although gross visual fields were intact. Gait and coordination were regarded as normal, though ungraceful. Fine coordination was adequate, though slow and less skillful than average. There was "no evidence of any fixed or focal disorders on the EEG recordings." A diagnosis was made as follows: "Developmental aphasia, predominantly motor type, improving . . . [without] indication of acquired brain damage. . . . This boy's difficulties with words appear to be on the level of word finding and word production, with either relatively little or no difficulty in the symbolic or understanding level."

In these, then, there were numerous realistic problems in John's physical development, complicated by intensification of mother–child conflict and by a series of environmental pressures. Yet there were always some positive factors that apparently contributed to John's resilience and resistance to defeat. His mother recognized John's problems with impulsiveness, perceptual deficits, retardation in speech, and possibly his weaknesses in organization and integration. She provided him with a good deal of support, but she herself was often pressed nearly to the breaking point and was very discouraged, angry, and guilty. Her discouragement was related to the piling up of misfortunes; her anger and guilt were related to the fact that she felt unable to control her own feelings or the impact of events on family behavior. Complicating this picture was the mother's disagreement with the father about his vocational future and in relation to some aspects of the child's handling. Furthermore, she valued her own independence and admired independence and determination in her son. However, her needs and anxieties contributed to some overprotectiveness of the children, (granting the realistic needs for protection) without fully taking into account John's own difficulties as these became more obvious in the school learning situation. In turn, John's awareness of parental clashing in a family so capable of great warmth and affection doubtless presented him with integrative difficulties, and made it necessary for him to "stay little" and to avoid clashes with adults.

On the other hand, John's great warmth toward people, his expectation of help, his persistence when he experienced encouragement and support from adults, and his eagerness to communicate and to learn were assets ready to be mobilized by sympathetic teachers or parents. John's awareness of his own difficulties, or those that he might encounter, and his willingness to take the initiative in making reparations after conflicts with his family contributed to his resilience. He never really lost trust in himself despite the numerous frustrations he met. Nor was his faith in his family and other people destroyed, despite the many conflictful interchanges with his harassed and frequently irritated but also loving mother. In this, he was undoubtedly helped by the steady affection and firmness of his father; by the background of a relatively pleasant and comfortable early infancy; and by the fact that his health, though still a matter of concern, was gradually better understood and controlled. Other factors that prevented despair were his capacity to discharge some aggression and to make amends. Though his emotions could certainly have been regarded as labile, they were discharged and therefore allowed him to begin anew. Certainly often in physical pain, often frustrated and discouraged, he was yet able to protest and to defend his own integrity and privacy, to turn away at times, to lose himself in his own fantasy, to act dependently at times and to move ahead autonomously at others, to expect and seek help, and to find pleasure in what he could accomplish. His overall coping patterns could be said to be ingenious, flexible, positive, and generally realistic. He was moved ahead because he never became entirely defeated, nor did he lose his self-respect or his urge to master. Despite his impulsivity, (foreseen at 4 weeks of age and probably increased by his autonomic reactivity and his largely acquired organic instability) he was learning to delay and to persist, to deal with frustration, and to harness his energies, eagerness, and determination in a struggle that, though subject to setbacks at times, was directed toward growth. In all this, his personal charm, warmth, and understanding of people made him appealing and aroused the sympathetic support of all who knew him.

Later Latency

In the later latency years, the gains and growth already reviewed continued as John's personal health improved and as family life stabilized. This was observed both in a visit by Dr. Murphy to the family home during John's 9th year and during tests made 6 months later by Dr. Moriarty at a time when the parents were visiting the Topeka grandparents. Interviews by Dr. Murphy with both parents testified to a wide range of interests and activities in which John engaged with a good deal of loving warmth, as well as to rough-and-tumble aggressive motor release. This was illustrated in John's play with his new dog, who was "his baby, his pal, his fantasy companion, his roughhousing play-mate, everything that a dog could be for a little boy."

Both parents actively participated in and encouraged John to enjoy indoor activities such as checkers and experiments with a chemistry set, and outdoor activities such as boating, swimming, camping, and organized Boy Scout activities. The mother served as Scout troop's den mother for a period of time. The father took time to go hunting and fishing with his son and to help him learn to handle guns, model trains, and his bicycle effectively. In this, the father's natural un-self-conscious warmth for John contributed to a good deal of shared pleasure and to John's growing sense of confidence, increased attention span, and willingness to use offered opportunities for new experiences in a way that both made use of parental support and allowed him to maintain his own autonomy. Along with this, the family shared a number of church activities; grace was said at meals, and John took his turn in leading this ritual.

For her part, the mother was consciously trying to be "more casual," to reduce the tension over the father's job, to settle down in the new community, and to provide an atmosphere that would foster John's security and progress. She found this easier to do because she tremendously enjoyed the summer camping, found a number of satisfying personal relationships in the winter, and above all was less worried about John's physical health. (For 2 years, he had rarely been ill.)

In school, John made some gains with the help of a sympathetic third-grade teacher. In the fourth grade, he was again under pressure when the "platoon system" required him to move from room to room with different teachers for different activities. This was reflected in his forgetting materials and assignments, and in some resentment that he was never quite finished when the periods ended. He was able to accomplish average or nearly average work, however, and liked all of his teachers except one art teacher, who had ridiculed his work in front of the class. The mother's conferences with the teacher and the principal regarding his visual difficulty eliminated further ridicule, but John continued to dislike the class. Interestingly enough, the mother had not focused before this on John's visual difficulties, because she did not wish his teachers to consider him "defective."

Six months later, when the family was visiting the grandparents, both interviews with the mother and several sessions with John validated the impression that the family as a whole was attempting to deal positively with problems in a direct, active, and clear-headed manner. The help and support of both parents and of his teachers, along with John's own drive for autonomy and his deep and varied interests in people, his pet, his school, and play activities, were all part of John's observed progress. Continued difficulties with arithmetic and the one unpleasant experience in the art class suggested that school could still present problems, but he accumulation of successful and gratifying experiences offered a positive background on which to build.

Early in these sessions (which took place when John was 9 years, 8 months old), it became apparent that the real reason for the Topeka visit was the parents' desire to offer support and help to the paternal grandmother, who was currently seeking a divorce. In regard to this, John was somewhat evasive, though he expressed strong sympathetic and protective feelings toward the grandmother and a wistful hope that he could still see his beloved grandfather. Beyond this, he made it clear that the divorce was a "private matter" he did not wish to discuss.

He indicated at this time that he accepted facts—the divorce, as well as his own sensory limitations and academic problems—fairly philosophically, with the faith that the world was really a good place and the trust that things would generally turn out all right. For example, in regard to limitations in his own skills, he remarked, "I feel bad when I first do it [i.e., make errors], but then I get over it. I just do my best." Furthermore, he was convinced that although his mother could sometimes be quite demanding and harshly critical, she was always ready to help him when he needed reassurance or specific concrete suggestions.

He saw his father as less harsh in discipline, as one who helped him master typical male activities, but who was less available than the mother. As an unconscious level, there were some indications that the father's masculine vigor was mildly threatening to John; however, there was on the whole "apparently a relatively good balance between the past and acceptance of things that have to be, and an active orientation toward mastery. . . . He seemed to have accepted his sex role and to have established a fairly good male identification."

Will all observers, John was friendly and pleasant, though perhaps more serious and constrained than he had seemed in his early years. He was courteous and attentive; he was still mildly tense in examinations, but distinctly proud of his improved speech and of his efforts to look ahead and to learn. His Wechsler Intelligence Scale for Children (WISC) IQ placed him in the high average range, still reflecting good general knowledge but with some vagueness in integrative processes and occasional difficulties in verbal communication.

A year later, on another visit to Topeka at 10 years, 7 months of age, John's full-scale WISC IQ was 120—27 points higher than his preschool Stanford–Binet IQ of 93. His performance was now less variable in the separate tests, and his responses in general were better organized and more detailed. There were, however, still some residual signs of looseness and confusion in thinking. Word-finding problems were by this time minimal, appearing more often as hesitancies or delays in speaking than as substitutions or rewording.

Toward the examiner, he was gracious and friendly, but less spontaneous and enthusiastic than he had been as a younger child. It was as though he were consciously trying to appear to be grown-up and casual. He considered each new demand carefully, apparently bending every effort to be precisely accurate. This probably made his overall performance more effective, though it also suggested a laboriousness that no doubt reflected some tension from his great effort to be controlled and focused.

At age 11½, when John was next seen in Topeka, Dr. Toussieng felt that the obsessiveness of John's thinking sometimes made him confused and uncomfortable, though vigorous abandonment to activity and a deep enjoyment of life somewhat mitigated this impression. At this time, John seemed to be enjoying fairly comfortable positive relationships with his family and with peers. His trust in the world was still predominant, and his keen awareness of some limitations in himself and his world were matched by vigorous efforts to master whatever problems he faced. His grades were consistently average, and he found new satisfactions in school, particularly in a science class with a male teacher who encouraged experimentation. These gains were probably related to improved general health, though they also reflected increasing family stability. Following some special training in connection with his job, the father seemed to be happier with his work and also had more time to spend with the family. This reduced interparental friction, which perhaps also diminished after some discussion with the family minister. Another divorce—this time of John's maternal grandparents—was upsetting, not only because of his own feelings but also because of his empathy for his mother's feelings. However, this threat to the security of the larger family group seemed to increase the cohesiveness of the immediate family. In a sense, this second divorce of grandparents focused the involvement of John and his parents on their own immediate family, and increased their feelings that they had finally become completely settled in the new town to which they had moved when John was 4 years old.

John in the Prepuberty Years

Early in John's 12th year, when he was a seventh-grader, his mother was interviewed during a period when she spent 5 weeks in Topeka in order to attend to some pressing family business. At that time, she was certainly more positive about John than she had been in the early latency years, though she was frank in expressing some negative feelings at times. She described him as forthright and open, sometimes impulsive, but often quite determined and persistent. She thought of him as a child who could reach out for whatever he needed, or protest against or reject things he disliked—a picture much like the impressions examiners had of him as an infant. She remarked, "John is still impulsive about some things. . . . He still has to run"; apparently, however, he was much better able to accept prohibitions than he had been earlier. At 7 years, "He was so demanding as far as time was concerned, and I just felt that I didn't dare take my thoughts away from him for a minute." At 12 years, he was direct and forthright in his requests and expected no deceit from others. This was true in regard both to doing something he wanted and to expressing opinions. "Sometimes he and his father don't agree on something and . . . oh, John will stand, and the tears will be running down his face, and he'll say, 'Now, you're going to have to listen to my side of it, Dad.'"

She felt too, that "John forces him [his father] into his role of father a lot more than the other children." In this regard, she mentioned John's urgent requests each spring and fall to go hunting, fishing, or on overnight camping trips with his father. Usually, the father agreed and each trip was enjoyed by both father and son, though perhaps by the son more so than the father, who sometimes found John's energy fatiguing. The mother admitted, too, that standards of neatness and cleanliness on the male campouts were less than those she would have required. She felt that those trips increased closeness between father and son, and she also expressed the opinion that her present absence of 5 weeks was bringing the two closer, as they were forced to do so many things together.

John's hearty enthusiasm and vigorous participation characterized everything in which he was interested, and his interests covered a wide range, though some persisted much longer than others. For example, he continued to love nature and the outdoors; in his mother's words, "He sort of clings to nature and animals, still." He shared with his family great pleasure in summer camping, where he enjoyed hunting, fishing, swimming, and boating, and in winter he went tobogganing, skiing, and ice fishing.

John loved animals of all kinds, but was no longer allowed to have a dog of his own because he was found to be allergic to fur. It was also necessary for him to handle game as little as possible because his eyes reddened and easily became infected. In relation to this, Mrs. C. reminded the interviewer that John had only peripheral vision in the left eye; apparently, he saw only some light with the left eye, and forms were vague. This interfered with the playing of team sports to some degree: He liked to play football and baseball informally, but was not good enough to play on a team. Mrs. C. felt that John probably would not have been a team member in any event, because he was "clumsy as a cow" and would also have objected to the steady routine of concentrated practice. On the other hand, she mentioned that he was planning to take guitar lessons and hoped to sing in the junior choir at church. Whether these interests would be lasting was not known.

Other interests included coin collecting, which John studied seriously, making purchases only after carefully going over coin catalogues. Intermittently, he liked to bowl and play pool.

Though John was quite interested in girls during the sixth grade, he said little about girls in the seventh grade and did not date regularly. The mother felt that he had reacted strongly to the pregnancy of one of his classmates and interpreted his silence in this way: "He's thinking this over. This is a new part of life that he never was familiar with."

He was beginning to think about his future, particularly as he heard his older sister's friends discuss college and service requirements. He was definite that he wanted to join the Navy. Afterwards, college was a possibility, as he thought he might like to be a veterinarian; however, he was also intrigued with the idea of farming, perhaps patterned after the somewhat primitive existence of a bachelor great-uncle who took great pride in caring for pure-blooded animals. Perhaps, too, he saw such an existence as avoiding the pressures and restraints of family life, as well as the possible disappointments in marriage, which he had seen in the divorces of both sets of grandparents. In any event, he earnestly told his mother that he hoped she and his father would never divorce, and he did not commit himself to a prospect of marriage. For the present, he was content to defer these decisions, to enjoy those activities that allowed him to be active, to be outdoors, and to move along at a pace he could determine (i.e., without requirements to defer to rules and regulations of team members).

He was now concentrating on school, which seemed to be a positive and rather exciting experience. His mother remarked, "He seems to be getting along much better than he ever did . . . and seems to understand what he is learning." She reported that his grades were mostly C's with a few B's and that there were "no real problems," though spelling continued to be difficult for him. He liked all of his teachers and all subjects except art, but this he took philosophically as part of his education.

When John himself was seen 3 months later, it seemed clear that the mother's appreciation of him included a balance between awareness of his limitations and admiration for his strengths. Furthermore, the balance between honest affection and decisive discipline kept paths of communication open between the two, so that it was possible for the mother to encourage his independence, to give him support, and to set limits for him without damaging or distorting the relationship. In this atmosphere, John was able to express anger and criticism and to seek an independent identity without losing the love of his mother. In the process of growing up, he could be frank in expressing opinions openly and fearlessly, and could also sometimes be boyishly aggressive, impulsive, or moody without sacrificing his capacity for giving and receiving warmth. In this, one was reminded of his preschool play with the musical dog and the gun, when the potentialities of each were realized and enjoyed. Along with this, there was also an appreciation of reality as neither ideal nor perfect, sometimes depressing and difficult, often serious, but also funny. Thus, John could say, "I grew up last year when we had all this trouble" (in relation to the bitterness and instability in the maternal grandmother during and following her divorce, which still created intensely unpleasant interactions between family members), but he could also laugh when appropriate, even about serious things like religion. As his mother commented, "He's going to be able to be happy in his life no matter what happens. . . . I mean, he is going to be able to take life as it comes and still have this wonderful-to-be-alive feeling."

Much of John's strength appeared also to come from the father's stability and perspective, geniality toward others, and pride in his own family. Despite the lack of challenge in his work, he was able to provide comfortably for his family, as well as to arrange a schedule that would allow time to teach John skills. For example, he encouraged John to try the boat at full throttle, to seek out ways of earning his own money, and to plan ahead for a realistic future. He was able to admit that he might be more reckless than John, but he fully sympathized with his son's caution and was proud of his sensible stance, which allowed him to find adventure without danger. He could admit that he did on occasion lose his temper without feeling guilty, and could appreciate his wife's occasional exasperation with John without lessening support for his wife or losing his son's respect. In essence, both parents were united in providing family closeness and in setting an example of a positive and constructive approach toward whatever life held for them.

John's own capacity to take life as it comes, to enjoy what was available, and to deal with problems realistically but with humor was reflected in the projective tests given by Dr. Moriarty at this time. Overtly somewhat tense and somber (presumably in relation to pressures in the relationship to the grandmother and in response to a serious injury of another family member), John involved himself gradually, as though he chose to stay in control of his feelings and of the extent to which he would communicate. Yet he was not totally distant or unresponsive. Though somewhat troubled by shading, color, and vagueness in the Rorschach cards, he was always able to give good responses following some loss of perspective. He did this first by putting distance between himself and his perceptions and by keeping to concrete details, followed by making original additions that suggested a sensitivity to the beauty of the world. If his perceptual style was at times lacking in integration, it was also effective in holding stimulation to those details he could handle and at a tempo he could manage. Then, when he was ready, he could move on to more organized and more original perceptions. Sometimes immature and occasionally impulsive, he was likely to restrict his functioning in ways that had clinical overtones of obsessiveness, distancing, and withdrawal; ultimately, however, reality testing and a remarkable capacity to stay with the difficulty until he reached his goals kept him from being overwhelmed. One might speculate that it was by similar techniques of controlling the amount and intensity of stimulation and of moving at his own pace that he learned to read and write in the face of odds that might have been overwhelming to a child with less determination, less personal integrity, and less optimism.

John's preferences for a series of picture postcards of works of art, landscapes, and architecture gave further support to these speculations. John's range of interests in this informal task was broad, but he always chose the uncluttered and the clear-cut. He liked bright, colorful pictures where meaning was determined by firm lines and form, and scenes in which warmth and humor in human relationships were depicted. Often he selected familiar paintings like *The Last Supper*, but he also was attracted to scenes portraying experiences that were new and exciting, such as Picasso's *Bullfight*. Still life was not attractive to him, especially if the scene struck him as "fuzzy." This was perhaps a rejection of the discrepancy between his urgency to see clearly and the limitations that had been imposed by his visual problems. He preferred pictures of animals, especially if he saw human attributes such as "courage" in a metal bird or "comedy" in the stance of a horse. He rejected sculptures that appeared broken, impaired, or incomplete, landscapes that seemed to him to be overcommercialized or looked like "a fraud," or scenes where people were crowded together. Altogether, his preferences and rejections reflected his own need for completeness and warmth, his basic honesty, his love of natural beauty, and his requirements for vigorous interaction with a simple, unhurried, and sympathetic environment. His rejection of the impaired and the vague suggested his deep sensitivity to his own sensory limitations, and perhaps also his search for identity.

John at Puberty

Approximately a year later, when John was 13 years, 7 months old, he was again interviewed in Topeka, and a variety of speech, hearing, and neuropsychological tests were made.

In the speech and hearing sessions with an unfamiliar male examiner, Dr. Clyde Rousey, John was somewhat uncommunicative and unspontaneous, though entirely cooperative. Findings suggested "some neurological dysfunction," probably "localizable in the right hemisphere . . . with a possibility of some cerebellar dysfunction." There was also evidence of some constriction of feelings in his hoarse voice and restricted pitch range, and of persistent anxiety in the sharp whistle accompanying the production of sibilant sounds. To this unfamiliar examiner, these findings raised questions about the meaning of John's apparent underachievement in school and the extent to which his thinking was subject to disorganization. I reserve discussion of these speculations until after I have presented other data obtained at this time and a year later.

An extensive battery of neuropsychological tests, by contrast, gave "no evidence of impairment of higher brain function" in a child whose IQ was in the bright normal range. John's WISC verbal IQ at that time was 113, his performance IQ was 111, and his full-scale IQ was 113.

During these tests, given by Dr. Moriarty, observations made by a familiar woman examiner (Dr. Murphy) who later interviewed John privately suggested the presence of open but subtle affect exchange, with an undercurrent of anxiety and a persistent need for overt motor discharge. However, there was a high degree of persistence, a capacity to sustain effort and control impulses, along with a distinct capacity to find amusing both his own reactions and friendly gestures from the examiner. The observer saw him as an irresistibly good-natured child, unspoiled and un-self-conscious in his warm, genuine responsiveness to people. In this situation, his observed behavior was characterized by "a considerable capacity for modulated acceptable discharge of tension, open affect, and freedom from repressive tendencies which might have contributed to the accumulation of undischarged tension." Also assets in coping with the pressures he faced were good reality testing and recognition of what he could or could not do, along with freedom from unrealistic aspiration level, resilience in recovery of his self-esteem, and capacity to tackle each new task with renewed interest even after a discouraging failure.

In Dr. Murphy's interview, John's soft voice and his seriousness of manner communicated undertones of depression or disappointment, as well as boredom. It seemed possible that these feelings were related to a sense of inadequacy in the recent tests and in school, and perhaps also to the fact that the family were not planning to spend the summer in the woodland cabin where they had stayed for many years, and which had earlier been one of his major satisfactions.

Nonetheless, John talked willingly and revealed a number of interesting attitudes about his teenage life. He made it clear that in some ways he was a typical teenager, yet in other ways he differed from his age group. Like other teenagers, he wanted his opinions to be taken seriously and resented his father's disciplinary reactions to "talking back," which John experienced as "taking a stand." Apparently, "go-arounds with Dad" were somewhat stressful for both parties. He felt that his mother was more willing to listen and that he could "talk Mom into it." He identified himself with his teenage peers to the extent of excusing mild mischief on the basis that it was not really hostile, but simply fun-loving or adventure-seeking experimentation with new grownup modes of behavior. He did admit, though, that most teenagers do not stop to think of consequences.

Also like many teenagers, he felt that the teen years are "a tough time" because "you can't do anything—you can't drive a car; you can't get a job . . ." and there are not enough recreational outlets.

He differed from many teenagers in not identifying with group or gang activities. Instead, he chose a few close boyfriends and one girl-friend. He was unusually clear-cut about avoiding "doing things one shouldn't do," especially when sexual activities were concerned.

All in all, John seemed to be generally helpful, tolerant, and under-standing of people, and he used solid good judgment in relation to his own behavior. He liked people and sought their friendships, but he did this selectively: avoiding large groups, which might have loosened his impulse control and subjected him to threatening stimulation. Friction with his parents was moderate for his age, largely because it was balanced by a good deal of mutual love and respect, an advantage he had enjoyed since early childhood.

A later series of tests and interviews in Topeka when John was aged 14 years, 7 months, and at a time when he was under considerable pressure, offered some clarification of already known aspects of his life and raised some important questions about ego integration and the stability of impulse control. After presenting these data, I describe the nature of the stresses he faced, and then attempt to assess the balance between strengths and weaknesses in the light of earlier and ongoing development, as well as probable future adjustment. An important aspect of such an assessment is the apparent divergence between several observers' experiencing of John's reactivity and his style of dealing with stress in the face of different demands and in the context of different interpersonal interchanges.

With an unfamiliar male psychologist who focused on assessing John's perceptual style, John appeared to be anxious and maintained a rather strained reserve, with some release of tension in motor activity. This observer experienced in John chronic angry feelings, apparently handled by "avoidant withdrawal and acting out as means of partial control," and raised the question as to whether there was in some situations "danger of sudden outbursts of motoric expressions of anger." In a Photo Sorting Test, consisting of 36 pictures of people of widely varying ages and activities, this observer saw John as avoiding real participation by giving superficial classifications focusing on limited aspects of the stance or activity of the persons depicted. This was the more impressive in the light of more open reactions to feeling states in a test some 5 years earlier. The observer concluded that John "must be somewhat more tightly but imperfectly controlled" in the puberty years, and was probably "carrying a rather heavy burden of feeling states which he had very inadequate means of expressing," especially since he was overtly polite, pleasant, and cooperative.

The speculation of possible disorganization in thinking, along with some awareness of his own tenuous impulse control, was also made by Dr. Rousey on the basis of John's continued articulatory substitutions, his restricted pitch, a prominent whistle in sibilant sounds, difficulties in auditory discrimination (without evidence of organic impairment), and faulty diadochokinetic rates (suggesting at least diffuse neurological impairment or instability).

In the neuropsychological tests, John was tense, somewhat uninvolved, mildly resistant, and rather intolerant of frustration. WISC scores were relatively unchanged (verbal IQ, 114; performance IQ, 107; full-scale IQ, 112). Neuropsychological tests fluctuated within a small range, with some tests handled better than they had been the preceding year, others more poorly. He was somewhat slower in some motor performances, and there was a faint suggestion of somewhat poorer organization in thinking, but no definite indication of neurological impairment as reflected by cognitive–perceptual tests. The Wide Range Achievement Tests in relation to current grade placement showed about 1 year's retardation in reading and 3 years' retardation in spelling, whereas arithmetic exceeded group placement by a year and a half. The neuropsychologist felt that the possible presence of brain dysfunction, not then measurable by tests, might make him more vulnerable to aging changes in later years.

An account of the stress to which John had been exposed was gained from an interview with his father, who, despite the stability ordinarily observed in him, admitted being "all shook up" over a very disturbing verbal browbeating from the paternal grandmother in John's presence the preceding evening. The bitterness and emotional intensity of the grandmother's diatribes and his father's reaction must have been seriously upsetting to John, who later told the psychiatrist that his most serious "emotional problem was the griping and bickering between his paternal grandparents, especially since they had in his early years been so loved and admired. With the fresh memory of this shocking experience the evening before, combined with the pressures

John always felt in tackling verbal or sensory tasks with new or relatively unfamiliar people, it was not surprising that he functioned in a
somewhat unorganized manner. Nor was it surprising that he withdrew from new and untried contacts, since his most trusted relationships (with his father and grandmother) had been so recently threatened. Beyond this, we knew from previous behavioral samples that
John was likely to withdraw initially from overwhelming stimulation or
to reduce the area of stimulation to manageable proportions. And in
addition, we knew from observations of other normal puberty-age
subjects that reserve and constriction appeared to be common reactions
at this stage.

Considering the personal threats to this sensitive boy who had so
recently had an experience that might have been severely traumatic
even to a less empathic individual, John's "avoidant withdrawal" in tests
at this time may have been highly appropriate and strategically ego-
syntonic. Such an interpretation seemed the more reasonable when we
reviewed the more positive way in which the psychiatrist experienced
John, as well as the evidence furnished by John and his father of
improved functioning in many areas of the boy's life.

For example, both John and his father independently testified that
he had moved from a close association with a few friends into a larger
group, where he enjoyed a variety of contacts, and that in many respects he led a remarkably full, rich life in which he was neither in a
hurry to grow up nor nostalgic about the past. In assessing his duties
and chores, John could be forthright in expressing some resentment
that his mother's job forced him to stay home to care for his younger
sister ("It would be a lot easier if my mom wasn't working"), and he
could selectively see disadvantages as well as advantages in the regular
paper route he carried. For instance, he disliked the early rising and the
fatigue of trudging through the snow on a cold morning; on the other
hand, he relished the idea of earning money, gloried in the cool fresh air
and the freedom of being alone in the quiet early morning, and looked
forward to his daily friendly contacts with neighborhood dogs.

On the whole, he dealt with frustrations and difficulties (as in
school) by philosophical feelings that "You've got to take it." As he saw
it, schooling was a necessity for a future that would be secure, economically rewarding, and interesting. In this regard, John toyed with the
idea of going into forestry or engineering, but he vastly preferred his
long-time aspiration to be a veterinarian with his own hospital. He
fantasied that the hospital would be situated on a ranch, which would
not only provide additional income, but give him the space he needed
and the opportunity to enjoy nature in a simple and uncommercialized
setting. Nor was this projected future only a pipe dream, because John
was fully aware that the initial financial outlay would be considerable,

and that it could be accomplished only by careful planning. He had taken into account, too, the probable need to defer marriage and the possible interference of his allergies to fur (a discomfort that, though decreasing, was still a problem).

In other words, John seemed to have some doubts and reservations about his ability to realize his goals, but he was ready to make the most of whatever happened; to accept some defeats with renewed efforts in areas where he could be successful; and, above all, to make the best of disappointments without floundering in his own miseries. He said of his average grades, for example, "I'm not going to gripe about them. Of course, I don't gripe anyway. If I get it, I get it." In this, too, was the feeling that if he himself recognized his efforts to do his best, then others' criticism was less stinging ("I wasn't worried about it because I know I tried").

John's sensible practical judgment was seen, too, in his discussion of his relationship with his parents, of whom he said, "They aren't strict. I think they are fairly reasonable. At times, I don't think so, naturally, but I think they're fairly reasonable. I don't particularly care for all the chores I've got at home, because I don't know many boys that have them, but I know other mothers that work, too." In turn, he sympathized with his mother's wish for a more attractive, stylish, and *convenient* home (as was also true of the father, despite his own greater emphasis on a *comfortable* home and adequate provision for the children's education). He could also recognize that his father's fast driving was not dangerous for a man with "fast reflexes," though he rejected this for himself.

Altogether, John in puberty seemed to be a boy with essentially good judgment and a rich sense of the pleasures and humor in life; though aware of difficulties and handicaps, he was neither depressed nor lacking in self-respect. Toward the family, friends, and acquaintances, he expressed a mature tolerance for differences in viewpoints and behavior, and had a good capacity to select for himself what he liked and to reject what he disapproved of. The resentments he had were not too great, and could be expressed, when he chose, to those in whom he wished to confide. If he sometimes withdrew, he seemed to do so with conscious awareness of his need to sort out his own feelings and to deal with them in ways that were not overwhelming. In the face of his sensory deficits, his own emotional lability and depth of feelings, the emotional pressures from the larger family, and the parents' strong reaction to these pressures, John was indeed remarkably resilient. Whether the controls he imposed and the further pressures of adolescence would be too great was clearly an open question, but the strength with which he had previously dealt with physical pain as a young child, his persistence in his struggle to learn academic subjects, and the overall warmth of his reaching out for others suggested continued positive development.

Synthesis and Summary

From many points of view, John was and continued to be an intriguing boy. Clinically, his development exemplified the need for care in assessing behavior at any one age level. That is, to avoid error, one must keep in perspective the changing, ongoing development in relation to inner and outer events and their impact on the child in his specific environment. Methodologically, it is important to focus on the demands of each new experience, weighing interpretations by each observer according to the structure imposed on each by his special interests. Theoretically, one can raise a number of speculations as to what factors commonly play into resilience; in turn, these can be clarified and in some measure understood.

Setting side by side the vulnerabilities and pressures and the positive factors in the environment and in John's own coping style, one can raise some questions and move toward some answers, but to say that these are more than speculative would be presumptuous.

Apparently active and intense from the time of his mother's first experience of intrauterine movement, John even as a neonate was a baby who was especially adept in communicating his needs and expressing his protests. As an infant, he seemed to experience actively, to react strongly, and to seize the world with intensity. As early as 4 weeks of age, he was described as a child of high activity level and high autonomic reactivity, and as one in whom "few halfway states were seen." At that time, his physical health and sturdiness, as well as his better-than-average development as indicated by psychological tests, were assets that developed favorably in a warm, loving family with an unusually competent mother and proud, vigorous father. However, even at that time, there were some indications of conflicts between the mother's needs for personal independence and her equally strong needs for family closeness. Important, too, were some observable inconsistencies in her way of encouraging his independence (e.g., "feeding himself") at the same time that she was deeply concerned lest he be injured or harmed in some way and therefore was somewhat overprotective. In other words, she was both sensitive to the baby's needs and bound by her own need for integrity as an individual.

Furthermore, John's vigor and intensity, while very appealing and a factor contributing to and supporting his openness to the world, his

self-respect, and his empathy, was also a source of vulnerability. Predic-
tively, vulnerability would have been expected to increase when his
urgency to interact was not matched by his integrative skills; this we
later saw to be the case. Beyond this, we saw some instability in the
larger family (later verified by the divorce of both sets of grandparents)
and some mild interparental friction, both of which were threatening to
this vivid, intense child. Nonetheless, the first year of life showed no
deviant experiences or behavior, beyond the fact that John's tongue
was clipped at 9 months of age.

During John's second year, he was stressed by frequent infections
localized in his ears, and also suffered a severe case of chicken pox with
accompanying high temperatures. Even more stressful was his mother's absence from the home in full-time employment. Equally impressive was the fact that the mother quit work in response to John's
clinging, demanding behavior and retarded speech development.

In the preschool years, the systemic infections continued, subject-
ing John not only to severe pain and frightening treatments, but also to
temporary lack of clarity in seeing and hearing. In a child who very
early wanted so intensely to see and hear clearly, and who later rejected
the vague or impaired in his projective tests, we cannot underestimate
the traumatic effect of these experiences. At the same time, we should
remember that despite John's capacity to protest, he could take the
accompanying pressures with unusual equanimity, never whimpering
when he understood that medication was given for his benefit. Here,
we saw a basis for his later acceptance of difficulty and his freedom
from a sense of defeat in the face of academic problems and emotional
strains from the larger family.

We should also recall that for a period the mother was harassed
almost to the breaking point, feeling anger toward neighbors who
complained of John's "belligerence" and guilt about her inability to
control his impulsiveness. Yet these natural reactions were at least
partially balanced by the stability and steady affection of the father,
who was more able to set limits and to tolerate John's discharge of
feelings.

After John's eighth year, his illnesses diminished, partly because
they were better understood and controlled. However, the pressures of
the move to the new town persisted, and subsequent instability in the
larger family relationships contributed ongoing stress. John reacted
both by expressing needs for independence and by enjoying a dependency that allowed him to put off growing up.

In subsequent years, we saw John as a warmly empathic child who
gradually learned to control his impulsivity through narrowing the
field of stimulation, focusing concretely on some details and leaving
others to the future. Perhaps as a part of this, he managed always to

live in the present, without nostalgia for the past or too much urgency to move into the future. Each demand was an entity in itself, and in this he gained a good deal of support from both parents, who were openly proud of his improvements and equally disappointed when he failed to meet their standards.

From a positive viewpoint, John enjoyed the warmth and love of relatively stable parents who always respected him for the warmth and determination they saw in him; this respect and love supported his identification with them. If they were at times harsh or overdemanding, they were also able to love and control, and always willing to accept the reparations he offered. The resentments present in John at puberty were mild, realistic, and unlikely to change the basically stable and close pattern of child–parent relationships. There is no question, however, that as John grew older he became overtly less impulsive and perhaps somewhat less outgoing in the presence of others. This was more notable in new situations with unfamiliar people, especially when test or interview demands focused on his less adequate areas of functioning.

It is important here to take into consideration the degree to which autonomic and neurological instability were involved in John's development. On this point, our records were not altogether clear-cut, though both the early observational material and the tests and behavioral demonstrations through John's growing years repeatedly confirmed impressions of emotional lability and high autonomic reactivity. Slow speech development, continued deviation in pitch, poor voice quality, and articulatory substitution, along with some awkwardness in motor coordination and a kind of concreteness in thinking, all supported an inference of neurological instability. However, aside from a diagnosis of developmental aphasia, motor type, in the latency years, and the suggestion in the speech evaluation of some diffuse impairment, this impression was never fully validated. At the same time, history of some emotional instability in the larger family, and at least temporary periods in which the mother's doubts and anxieties created tensions (if not grosser disorganizations), suggested the contributory role of emotional factors in reducing total integrative effectiveness in the child. For practical purposes, these organic and emotional factors could not be separated or differentiated clearly.

When we add to this a picture of a positive, reality-oriented coping style that tended to isolate, to deal with parts rather than wholes, and to stay with the specific and present, the emerging personality structure in this background becomes still more complex. We might well have seen more disorganization in an individual with less sense of well-being, less capacity to struggle, and less consistent support from his parents.

A relevant aspect of John's coping with stress at any one period was the nature of demands in relation to developmental stages—for instance, the apparent withdrawal and constriction at puberty in response to the examination of sensory defects. Since many teenagers do manifest some reserve at puberty, what was seen in John was not in itself considered excessive. The strain this conscious control placed on an essentially outgoing, reactive, and intense youngster is yet another point that probably awaits future development for final assessment.

At this point, in the light of what is known of John's strengths and weaknesses and of the many pressures he experienced, one can conclude that he was an amazingly resilient individual who in many respects maximized the resources he had. In this light, his integrative weaknesses were less impressive than the warmth with which he embraced the world, and the persistence with which he set about to establish himself as an individual in a world that, though difficult, was never overwhelming or defeating. Contributing to this was the basic stability of his parents; their belief in themselves and in him; their openness in expressing both positive and negative feelings; and, perhaps most important, his own energetic drive to master. In summary, it is easy to agree with his mother's statement at prepuberty: "He's going to be able to be happy in his life no matter what happens. . . . I mean, he is going to be able to take life as it comes, and still have this wonderful-to-be-alive feeling."

Resilience in Children at Risk   III

Although distressing, it is not surprising to learn of the failure to cope with misfortune (and, frequently, the development of major psychopathology) among persons otherwise vulnerable through such factors as increased genetic loading for major psychiatric disorder, temperamental characteristics such as increased impulsivity, or childhood environmental circumstances such as poverty. More remarkable is the capacity to maintain adjustment when confronted with increased vulnerability and adversity. Study of the development and maintenance of competence when confronted with misfortune provides important information regarding the course of human development and the determinants of continued resilience.

Building upon several decades of detailed study regarding the development of offspring of parents showing major psychopathology, the first three chapters in this section consider factors associated with the ability of these offspring at risk for such psychopathology to maintain resilience. Worland and his colleagues from the St. Louis Risk Research Project focus principally upon cognitive competence among offspring of psychotic parents, while Fisher and his colleagues report on psychosocial factors associated with continued resilience, particularly aspects of the relationship of parent and child that might lead to competence rather than to socialization into parental psychopathology. Aspects of the parent–child relationship leading to increased resilience in these otherwise vulnerable offspring are discussed by Musick and her colleagues; their chapter is based on a continuing study of children and their parents treated together in an intensive primary prevention project. These investigators focus on attributes of the mother that enable the child to maintain resilience, as well as upon such characteristics of the child as likeability.

Study of abuse and neglect of young children has also focused upon aspects of the parent–child relationship likely to lead to adverse outcomes in the child's development. Farber and Egeland focus upon vulnerability that is primarily due to adverse environment rather than to constitutional vulnerability. These investigators suggest that particular interventions may be helpful during the first year of the child's life in reversing effects that may adversely affect subsequent development. This recognition of the extent to which early adversity may be reversed raises more basic questions regarding determinants of resilience in young children.

Environmental adversity is also the focus of Felsman and Vaillant's report, which presents important findings from a continuing study of persons first identified by Sheldon and Eleanor Glueck more than four decades ago. Selecting a subgroup of this study population with the greatest environmental adversity in childhood, and focusing upon the persons' experience in their subsequent life history, Felsman and Vaillant focus on aspects of competence during childhood that are most directly related to successful adult outcome, particularly courage and determination persistently shown over periods of many years.

The advantage of this experiential perspective for studying the development of competence and resilience is also shown in Peck's detailed report on adults whose childhoods were marked by family instability, and whose attainment of personal reliability—the result of years of determined and persistent effort—came about only after periods of re-enacting the difficulties of their childhoods. Peck's discussion gives particular consideration both to the advantages and to the psychological costs of this effort at maintaining stability in the adult years.

6

Children at High Risk for Psychosis Growing Up Successfully

E. JAMES ANTHONY
Chestnut Lodge Hospital

A Serendipitous Finding

Prospective studies of children at high genetic risk for psychosis (schizophrenia or manic–depressive disorder) uncovered three subsamples, two of which had been anticipated and included in the research design. The third was discovered accidentally when new methods were applied to the investigations. The clinical bias at work among our research group insured that the main thrust of inquiry was directed toward sickness in its various psychotic and near-psychotic forms, and that the mentally adjusted half of the sample was more or less taken for granted. About half the children in this half of the sample (25% of the total group) were recognized as being free from significant psychiatric disorder, although they showed transient disturbances from time to time during their development; another subsample (15% of the total group) seemed relatively well adjusted and asymptomatic. It was felt that this type of distribution was predictable in response to any kind of stressful circumstance. That this half of the sample was growing up successfully did, however, arouse enough curiosity to induce us to investigate the basis for this, and the nonclinical investigators began to explore the competences and coping skills responsible for this resilience.

It was the third subsample (about 10% of the total group) that came as a surprise when the normal end of the spectrum of adjustment was explored with the new methodology. These children of psychotic parents were not simply escaping whatever genetic transmission destiny had in store for them, and not merely surviving the milieu of irrationality generated by psychotic parenting; they were apparently thriving under conditions that sophisticated observers judged to be highly detrimental to a child's psychosocial development and well-being. Unfavorable hereditary developmental potentials and environmental conditions were working together against these children, and still they thrived. On examining the living conditions of these families more circumspectly and even living in with them (Anthony, 1975b) my colleagues and I found that about a fourth could be described as "average, expectable environments"; about half could be labeled difficult and trying as a result of erratic parental behavior; and about a quarter could only be judged as deplorable. An experienced clinician like Bleuler (1978) spoke of such childhood conditions as often "appalling" and "horrible," and felt that the suffering induced was a direct consequence of the psychosis and psychotic personality disorder of the parents. He quotes one grown-up child of a psychotic parent who spoke of his experience: "When you've been through that . . . you can never really be happy; you can never laugh as others do; you always have to be ashamed of yourself and take care not to break down yourself" (p. 410). One can survive such a holocaust, but can one thrive in it? Can one flourish and prosper and create a superior mode of life?

In the first enthusiastic acknowledgment of the existence of this anomalous subgroup, the term "invulnerable" was applied to it. More specific designations such as "superphrenic" and "supercycloid" also came into use, with both subsumed under the generic "supernormal." "Invulnerability" struck many critics as mythological rather than scientific, and the less provocative term, "resilience," was increasingly adopted, even though its underpinnings were as much in doubt as "invulnerability."

If one thinks of this concept in a relative way, the notion of complete invulnerability is undoubtedly fictitious and part of human wishful thinking. The word "invulnerability," however, suggests a contradiction in terms unless one specifies its use in the context of a particular threat. Thus, a child may become immune from regular exposure to the psychotic process and still be vulnerable to other types of stress. Some children may become habituated to repeated threats (the so-called "inoculation" effect). Other children exposed to the same recurrent disturbances begin to find ways of mastering them, especially if there are successful models of coping immediately available. The resilient child is characterized by sound normal defenses, a wide range of coping skills, many available competences—constructive and even creative capacities that provide imaginative ways of dealing with frightening realities—and an inherent robustness that enables him to generate a psychoimmunity.

Although resilient children can generally be described as good copers, and although they all manifest a high degree of competence, their ways of coping and their types of competence may be very different.

Constructive and Creative Competence in the Service of Resilience

In constructive competence, there is a fairly practical, concrete, down-to-earth approach to tasks and problem solving. It implies a great deal of "doing," and its efficacy is judged by "things getting done." The individual who has acquired this type of competence is characteristically self-confident when carrying out a project and is able to organize the activity, plan the procedures, and persist in his efforts until he brings the matter to a successful conclusion. For the most part, he enjoys working independently, but he can also immerse himself harmoniously in a working group. Although he cherishes his autonomy, he knows when to ask for help and makes good use of it. In short, he copes well by himself or in conjunction with others.

In creative competence, the individual is no longer limited by the situation or the methods at hand. He can extend the dimensions of the task and invent means to carry the work further into the realm of exploration. He can move from the practical to the abstract and solve the problems "inside his head."

Constructive competence of the bread-and-butter variety helps to keep the wheels of reality rolling, whereas creative competence may take flight from reality and investigate, in novel ways, the less tangible but no less important facets of a problem.

In terms of theory, Piaget (1951) has furnished us with the framework especially pertinent to this topic of differential competence. Figure 6-1 presents a schematic epitome of Piaget's major developmental constructs, which basically have to do with the interactions of "assimilation" (or taking in of the situation from the outside) and "accommodation" (or adjustment to changes brought about by assimilation). When assimilation and accommodation are on equal terms, there is a state of equilibrium that allows cognition to develop without distractions from inner and outer worlds. There are situations (and there are individuals) where (or in whom) there is always a primacy of assimilation over accommodation, and there are also situations (and individuals) where accommodation is preponderant. Depending on the stage of development, whether sensory–motor, egocentric, or operational, the balance or imbalance of the two fundamental mental functions shapes and colors the interests, occupations, and activities of the child, who can therefore exhibit a wide array of competences at every developmental stage. The competence is associated with and appropriate to the stage, so that one can speak of a competent infant, a competent preschooler, or a competent school child. The individual does not outgrow the different phases, but incorporates them in the next period of develop-

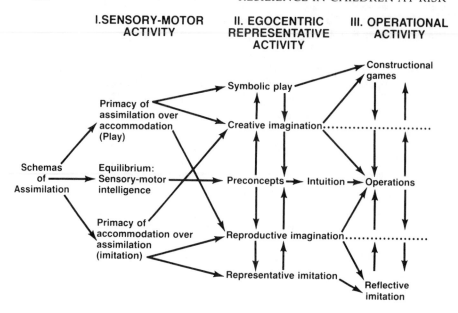

Figure 6-1. Schematic representation of Piaget's major developmental constructs. (From *Play, Dreams and Imitation in Childhood* by J. Piaget [C. Gattegno and F. Hodgson, Trans.], 1951, London: Heinemann. Reprinted by permission.)

ment. If, therefore, in addition to the developmental task, the child is confronted with environmental demands that are in excess of the psychosocial environment appropriate to his phase of development, he can make use of his acquired competences to deal with these exigencies. What may happen, however, because of inborn propensities or because of the abnormal pressures from the milieu, is that he may move toward imbalance or balance in his cognitive functioning.

If assimilation becomes the dominant mode, the child may no longer tackle reality head-on, but may resort to sensory–motor play, symbolic activity, fantasy, creative imagination, or games generated by him to "play out" his difficulties, and may use operational thinking to construct situations that can be staged dramatically. Thus, he is exercising his potential to become a writer, a playwright, a poet, or an artist. His life predicaments will tend to loom to the forefront of this activity, and the dramas enacted will often reflect his own personal problems. In this way, he can also bring his dreams and daydreams to life for presentation to an outside audience, but its interest would be subsidiary to his own.

A well-balanced cognitive competence will be reflected in an enhanced sensory–motor intelligence, followed later by the building up of preconcepts, intelligent hunches, concrete operational activities limited to the here and now, and ultimately a growing capacity for abstract thinking that allows for the elaboration of psychological, logical, mathematical, and philosophical systems. The child's conception of the world emerges along this developmental line, and eventually his creative products could reach an intellectual level high enough to alter an academic or technical field.

With the primacy of accommodation, the role of the caregiver and caretaker becomes crucial, since the processes of imitation and identification reduce free, spontaneous imaginative activity and enhance constructiveness based on adult models in the immediate environment. In the assimilative mode, self-perpetuating fantasy creates representations that are not reality-based; in the accommodative mode, the representations are largely reproductions derived from imitation. Under conditions of equilibrium, representations can abstract material from fantasy life while maintaining some degree of control over it, and can take from imitative life examples of models used by significant others.

With Piaget's paradigm in mind, one can obtain a developmental viewpoint of different competences in the making. For example, there is a constructive type based on learning from copies, with the degree of competence reflected in the accuracy of the representation, which would not be the individual's product so much as the reproduction of resources available around him. Second, there is a creative, imaginative competence that transforms reality in keeping with the more wish-fulfilling fantasies of the individual. Third, there is a creative conceptualization of the individual's environment pursued systematically through a wide range of logical operations.

If the environment is psychotically disordered, with gross distortions of reality prevailing at times, one type of child may deal competently with the overwhelming stressfulness by means of reproductive representations that permit various forms of constructive activity but keep close to the realities adjoining the psychotic unreality. A different type of child may substitute his own brand of unreality, based on his inner fantasy world, for the unpalatable and disturbing unrealities imposed by psychosis. A third child may make full use of his well-balanced cognitive competence, so that his representations take the form of making systems that comprehensively cover the areas of his concerns.

One has also to remember that these various activities are often taking place in juxtaposition to the adult's psychotic outpourings and that the reproductions, the systems, and the fantasies have their interactive counterparts in echo phenomena, delusional fantasies, and paranoid delusional systems.

Before illustrating these different responses, one needs to consider the bizarre psychotic constructions of the parent, because if the child is to function and develop successfully, he needs to use his whole range of competences to counteract the strange substitutes for reality put forward, sometimes very convincingly, by the psychotic parent.

A brief vignette illustrates the interactions involved. Segal and Yahraes (1978) comment on a case from the St. Louis sample that I have reported:

> Anthony tells of a woman, suffering from schizophrenia of the paranoid type, who insisted on eating at restaurants because she thought someone was poisoning the food at home. Her 12-year-old daughter adopted the same phobic attitude. Another daughter, 10 years old, would eat at home when the father was there; he was normal. Otherwise, she would go along to a restaurant. But a seven-year-old son always ate at home, and when the psychiatrist asked how he could do so, the boy simply shrugged and said, "Well, I'm not dead yet." The older girl eventually developed an illness like her mother's. The younger went to college and did reasonably well. The boy—the invulnerable—performed brilliantly all through school and afterward. His mother's illness apparently had given him both a tremendous need and a tremendous ability to overcome all sorts of problems. (p. 284)

The older girl was shy, seclusive, and oversensitive, given to somewhat peculiar fantasies and therefore extremely vulnerable to her mother's delusional idea. The second girl was imitative: When she was with her mother, she felt, thought, and acted like her mother, and when she was with her father, she did the same with him. She did not become overinvolved with either, and so could hold her own without succumbing to the ideas presented by the mother. At college, she formed an attachment to a teacher and incorporated a great deal of her ideas and values. The boy's response was autonomous. He was cognitively well balanced, and thought clearly and logically. His pragmatism was in sharp contrast to the "what-if" reactions of his sisters. Later he began to systematize his ideas concerning schizophrenia and developed into an outstandingly creative person, a true "superphrenic" whose remarkable capacities allowed him to master the corrosive presence of the severe mental illness to which he was exposed.

The mother's delusional ideas, however, were not simple ad hoc products, but part of the fabric of her life. The poisoner in the house that she suspected was her widower father, who had come to live with them and with whom her relationship since childhood had been tempestuously ambivalent. She had always loved him, hated him, and feared him. On a primitive oral level, there were fantasied concerns that he might want to put something "bad" into her mouth and thus harm her, however much she might wish it. As an adolescent, she had to leave home because she was tormented by fellatio fantasies about him. When her mother died, she invited him to come and live with them, even though she had taken flight from him before.

In many instances, the delusional ideas of the parent are presented very seductively and are difficult to resist. For profound unconscious reasons, the parent has a high degree of investment in these particular notions and may even make credence a test of love: "Love me, love my delusion." Many of these psychotic systems represent highly creative efforts, although they are so idiosyncratic that strangers do not find them appealing and may simply dismiss them as nonsense.

Ferenczi (1913) pointed out what a hard fight the achievement of reality testing is for the young child and how influential the adult in the child's environment can be in helping or hindering this crucial development. Even in the most average environment, transient setbacks can be brought about in imaginative children by the fairy tales told to them by adults in search of their own lost childhood omnipotence. These are what the child has to grapple with to achieve a reality orientation: "How overwhelming it must be for a child to be constantly confronted by the delusional fantasies of a highly significant person whose love he wishes to preserve beyond the calls of reality" (Anthony, 1971, p. 265). When the magical/phenomenistic system of the nursery school child comes into close contact with the psychotic system of the mother, the two can powerfully reinforce each other. Piaget (1926) compared the child's imaginative productivity at this time to the notions of delusional psychotics, especially in the early stages of the illness, when reasoning is based on fantasy, when every probability can become a certainty, when ideas are meshed together on the grounds of juxtaposition, and when symbolic functioning is constantly inspected for hidden meanings. Fantasy becomes a fact and facts become fantasies, and all is absolute.

Lidz, Fleck, and Cornelison (1965) also wondered at the abnormal pressures at work in the "subculture of psychosis." The wishful perceptions of events can result in

> a strange family atmosphere into which the children must fit themselves and suit this dominant need or feel unwanted. Often children must obliterate their own needs to support the defenses of the parent whom they need. They live in a Procrustean environment, in which events are distorted to fit the mold. The world, as the child should come to perceive or feel it, is denied. Their conceptualizations of the environment are neither instrumental in affording consistent understanding and mastery of events, feelings, or persons, nor in line with what persons in other families experience. Facts are constantly being altered to suit emotionally determined needs. The acceptance of mutually contradictory experiences requires paralogical thinking. *The environment affords training in irrationality.* (p. 180, my italics)

The child has to cope with the powerful ideas brought into the household by the psychotic creativity of the parent, and his ability to resist them may be limited by the resonances set up in his own mind. One needs to look at psychotic creativity in terms of its dyadic repercussions in the offspring.

Psychotic Creativity

It comes as a surprise today to read that Lombroso (1891), at the end of the 19th century, felt that genius could be the expression of a "degenerative psychosis." According to him, psychotics were people who "almost reached" brilliant ideas and discoveries, but the end points were thwarted by distortion and degradation. He also referred to "near"-psychotics or "mattoids," who were eccentric and unconventional in their ways but remarkably proficient in literary, artistic, and scientific activities, although they still had a certain "sick" quality about them.

Jung (1907) noted the congruence that exists between the symbolic processes in schizophrenic thought and in the magical/archaic thinking of primitives and small children. When it comes to abstract expression, it is difficult to distinguish between artistically gifted schizophrenics and abstract artists, and the suggestion has been made that both are engaged in making use of creative means to discover underlying segments of their egos that contrast with the chaotic nature of their conscious egos. In the process of "discovering the ego," there are two contradictory forces at work: In one, there is a retreat to a schizophrenic way of life and an autistic rejection of the environment; in the other, there is a deep longing for contact and communion and a push toward such mergings.

These contradictory thrusts become understandable within the framework of Piaget's schema as described earlier. The equilibrating process involves the harmonizing of ingoing assimilations and outgoing accommodations, but when imbalance occurs, either an undisciplined, autistic cognitive mode may result or the individual may lapse into echo behavior, imitating whatever models are presented to him.

The schema brings into continuity normality and abnormality, childhood and adolescence, modernism and primitivism within the same frame, so that, depending on the degree of equilibrium, the individual may display different amounts of magic/phenomenism, operational thinking, and mirroring reactions. The ratio of assimilation to accommodation will thus determine the turning away from or turning toward reality, with gradations between the two.

If one accepts this continuum, the "existence of latent schizophrenic life in normal individuals" (Bleuler, 1978, p. 484) no longer appears self-contradictory, particularly in the offspring of schizophrenic parents. If such is the case, one would expect continuous resonances between the latent and manifest propensities as evident in creative products. The creative fantasies of the child may thus interact with the delusional fantasies of the parent, especially in cases of *folie à deux*. Here the creativity of both parent and child becomes "sick," and this is likely to take place when the child is dependent, submissive, and suggestible. The following case illustration (Anthony, 1971) highlights the interactive element:

> A little girl aged five, living alone with her widowed mother, told her that she had seen a scarecrow in a field adjacent to their home. It waved to her and whistled. She heard it say that it would come and get her. The mother became perturbed and said that, when she was small, scarecrows sometimes got free and came into the house and that when they did, you could usually expect a death to take place. The mother warned her to be careful and to keep away from that side of the field. The next day, the child came running into the house screaming that the scarecrow was coming after her and that it was going to kill her mother. The mother immediately rushed out with a broom, and the neighbors heard her shouting that she was not going to let any devil get into her house. That night the child had a severe night terror and screamed that the scarecrow was in the room and sitting on her chest. The mother put on the light, barricaded the door with a heavy chair and took close hold of the child who continued screaming. The next morning, the mother told her neighbor that "they" were not going to get her or her child and that she knew what they were up to. She and the child now slept in the basement, both in a state of great apprehension, and the mother began to have nightmares. She explained to the child that the "scarecrow people" were devising all sort of tricks, such as dreams, to get into the house and kill the occupants. According to the mother, it was the child that they were after and according to the child, it was the mother. Four days later, the police broke in and found the pair virtually starving and panic-stricken. The mother was hospitalized with the diagnosis of schizophrenia and the child placed in a residential home. For about four weeks, the child continued to interpret events in her environment in terms of the "scarecrow people," but then gradually subsided and eventually disappeared. (p. 256)

In a follow-up, 5 years later, the girl was living with an aunt who had custody of the child. She was doing well at school and was considered to be a gifted child with a special talent for imaginative compositions. However, she did not have any close friends because of her seclusive nature. Her nightmares persisted. The clinician labeled her "schizoid," and suggested that she might be at high risk for schizophrenia. At a further follow-up when she was in the 10th grade, she was clearly an unusual girl, sometimes mixing well with her peers, but often withdrawing into her own private world about which she wrote little stories, illustrated with free-hand drawings. These were clearly promising productions, and she seemed to thrive on the praise that she was given. But her nightmares continued.

It was noted that both mother and child showed the same high capacity for fantasy, and both were subject to the terrifying dreams. Both slipped very quickly into a world of unreality, but whereas the mother remained chronically unrealistic, the girl bounced back and made increasingly creative use of her fantasy life. Hartmann (1984) has, in his sleep studies, arrived at similar conclusions:

> Our studies also suggest that those who have continuing nightmares, or other signs of thin boundaries in childhood, may be vulnerable to developing schizophrenia. If we can identify these at-risk people, we may be able to help them—in structuring reality, in developing a particular artistic talent, in bearing pain without losing touch with reality. . . . [T]hin boundaries can be valuable and useful characteristics if associated with the right combination of intelligence, talent in some particular direction, and interpersonal support. Having thin boundaries can be an advantage in allowing insight into one's own mental content and mental processes, and presumably those of others, making one a better writer, painter, teacher, therapist, negotiator. Scientific, as well as artistic creativity, requires "regression in the service of the ego" implying an ability to regress to a point where different realms of thought are merged, to temporarily ignore boundaries in order to put things together in a new way. This regression may be easier for people with a tendency to thin boundaries. On the other hand, keeping regression in the service of the ego may be more difficult for them than it is for others. (pp. 168–169)

The girl in the case described above clearly had "thin boundaries" that facilitated a free psychological exchange between her and her mother. They seemed to be equally susceptible to the outside "persecutors," but it was difficult to determine whose morbid imagery was contaminating whom. The girl's proneness to nightmares rendered her, according to Hartmann, disposed to both mental disorder and creative capacity.

Elsewhere (in Chapter 1, this volume), while agreeing that children can be captivated by vivid delusional fantasy to the point of creating similar productions themselves, I have also argued that the creative fantasy can provide the child with an extraordinary capacity to cope with incipient or threatening mental illness in himself. The child can, therefore, respond fantastically to emerging mental disorder in himself in an attempt to prevent it, as well as to the emerging mental disorder in the parent. A good deal depends on the child's ego strength as to which way his creativity carries him: If he is ego-resilient, it will lead to acknowledged works of art and composition, and if he is ego-vulnerable, it will give rise to delusional ideation (Barron, 1963). It is difficult to separate the creative person from the creative process that he undergoes in order to generate a creative product, but in general it would seem that if the person is "sick," the process is more likely to be morbid and the product clinically deviant. There is some suggestion, also, that divergent thinking is more likely to be associated with "sick" creativity; however, such a claim has limited value, since it is in divergent thinking that one finds the most obvious indications of creativity in general (Guilford, 1957).

Another crucial factor involves the "distance" that the child can put between himself and the delusional fantasies of the parents, and this is a function of both age and representational competence. It takes a degree of dispassion to transform frightening and bizarre delusions into manageable facts, fantasies, or fictions. If the child is unable to put distance between himself and the psychotic outpourings, the transformations may prove beyond his capability and may sap rather than enhance his resilience. His problem is whether he can distinguish between the parental version of reality and the consensual account of others; there may be frequent conflicts between the two presentations, with the delusional one being far more seductive and harder to resist (Anthony, 1968). Moreover, when the child is incorporated into the delusional system itself, as a persecuting or victimized character, and is abusively treated as a consequence, he may be quite unable to make an objective and realistic appraisal of his predicament. Bleuler (1978) has reminded us that some psychotics can make very good parents, and that some children can see beyond the gross disturbing pathology and appreciate these parental qualities. There may be "some" children who can make this differentiation, which even clinicians find difficult to make, but this may depend on the extent to which the nature of the parent's psychosis permits the child to step outside the situation and not be drawn into a maelstrom of feelings. It may happen with parents who are profoundly withdrawn and inaccessible, of the type I have referred to elsewhere (Anthony, 1975) as "noninvolving." However, a disorganizing, chaotic, and intensely paranoid parent may so undermine the child's sense of security and safety that he is often quite unable to draw any kind of sustenance or benefit from the contact. This is the involving type of psychosis as seen from the viewpoint of the child.

Yet, it is not without sound basis that Lidz et al. (1965) have spoken of a "training in irrationality" for children whose sense of reality is still not firmly structured and who respond to paralogical ways of thinking and communicating as if to the facts of life, since their own developmental mode is concordant with it. They, too, are accustomed to autistic reverie and are not too distant from primary-process thinking. But the overriding fact is that they are dependent, uncertain of their own bearings, and thus extremely vulnerable to the parent's interpretation of reality.

Minkowski (1927) and his wife and coworker Minkowska (1925)

made an interesting differentiation between "rich" and "poor" autism in schizophrenics. In the "rich" variety, the inner life resembles colorful dreams, but in the "poor" sort, it is characterized by rigid systematization; by a search for symmetry with an all-inclusive mathematical formulation; and by an imagery that runs out on infinite rails, cannot be influenced in any way, and is suffused with a cold, impersonal timelessness. As Minkowska put it, "The life of the imagination supersedes reality, and thought supersedes experience" (quoted in Bleuler, 1978, p. 492). The reason why the schizophrenic deals incompetently with reality and experience is that he cannot view them in a consistent, coherent, natural sequential order (Binswanger, 1959). As a result, holes develop in his total experience, and in turn this brings about a cleavage in the act of living. What he lacks are adequate solutions to the dilemmas that constantly confront him, and it is this incoherence that he presents to his children.

Even if the child is dazzled by the profusion of fantasy in the "rich" autistic, he may still be struck by the incompetence and lack of basic coping skills of the parent. Unfortunately, he cannot but identify with this inadequate model that leaves him vulnerable to life's ordinary processes, unless he is able to develop ways and means of his own to meet these demands in addition to the extraordinary ones imposed by the parent. In some ways, the schizophrenic recreates a new kind of world for his child that cannot be correlated with actual experience. As Ey (1959) put it, "Schizophrenia is tantamount to the building of a world based on the principle of strangeness" (p. 147). What the child of the schizophrenic longs for is the familiar and the commonplace. At times, he can almost feel his parent trying to make him different from other children, and like every child, he wants to feel, to behave, and to think like his peers. Because the schizophrenic lacks organization and structure in his thinking, he may struggle to establish some pseudo-order by the process of symmetrization and the establishment of symmetrical relationships, and in this way may try to harmonize his inner and outer life. One often sees evidence of this in compulsively repetitious statements from the offspring of schizophrenics: "I love my mom; my mom loves me." This allows some degree of equilibrium to be achieved.

The Different Faces of Competence in Children of Psychotic Parents

The competence of the children of psychotics is directed toward breaking the stranglehold that the parents have on them and rising above the "horrible," to quote Bleuler (1978), milieu that hampers their development. They constantly interact with delusional fantasies, murderous abuse, incestuous attacks, and gross neglect; within this malevolent setting, they need to develop strategies that can buffer them and, at the same time, give them a chance to generate coping skills. Within the framework furnished by Piaget, the three types of competent responses can be illustrated from various sources.

Constructive Competence: The Case of Vreni

Vreni (described by Bleuler, 1984) was a 14-year-old Swiss girl who stayed at home to take care of younger brothers and sisters and her alcoholic father, who suffered from a vascular disease and was frequently promiscuous. Her mother was a patient at the Burghölzli and suffered from a syndrome that left her emotionally flat and quite indifferent to her family. When Bleuler first encountered her, she was taking a large bag of washing to her mother; he informed her that the hospital took care of this for the patients. She said that she understood this, but that her mother was pleased when she did her washing. He found out that she was not attending school, which in Switzerland was "almost a miracle." At the time that she was 2 years old, the misery had started. As the mother withdrew more and more, the father became increasingly irresponsible and both mentally and physically ill. When the mother was hospitalized, Vreni stayed at home to look after the family. A welfare worker visited the home and brought back "sensational news": The household was kept in perfect order by Vreni; the smaller children were healthy, happy, well fed, and well dressed; they went regularly to school, and their teachers had no complaint about their behavior. Bleuler tried to help Vreni, but she did not need help—she did everything herself and never asked for anything from anyone. However, she did wish to become a nurse, and Bleuler arranged for a private teacher for her. She worked hard and was accepted in a nursing school, but then she decided against this because she felt it was her duty to continue the care of the family, and this she did. At the age of 22 she married and had two healthy children. She was altogether a very healthy and happy wife and mother, in spite of a childhood that had become so threatening soon after infancy. Bleuler describes her thus:

> She is certainly not a "superkid." Her IQ is average, she lacks particular interest or talents, and she was not fitted in any particular way. *One could point to the fact that the living conditions of the child only began to deteriorate after babyhood.* From her case history we are tempted to say that life gave her a rare chance in her childhood: the chance just to do what she liked to do and what she was able to do. She loved and still loves children; she was proud to care better for her sick father and for the other children than her mother had; and she was able to take over her mother's duties with a good heart and a practical skill. (p. 541; italics added)

Bleuler suggests that such stressful childhood experiences may not inevitably and inexorably lead to an abnormal adult outcome if a child can develop a sense of purpose and a satisfying life task appropriate to his nature. In the context of this chapter, one would say that Vreni's comparative invulnerability stemmed from an increasing constructive competence that made her indispensable to the family as a whole, and, at the same time, let her cope successfully with significant mental disorder in both parents. One sees in Vreni both the compassionate and dispassionate features characteristic of invulnerable children. In terms of the Piaget model, she was totally in the accommodative mode; her competence stemmed from imitative and identificatory sources. She wanted to be a mother like her mother, but was a far more successful one and worked hard at it. She was even proud that she did better (and possibly unconsciously pleased but guilty at having taken her mother's place). From being a highly successful surrogate caretaker, she wanted to train to become a nurse and look after other people, but then decided to create her own home and to provide very successful caretaking for her own children. She was *not* a "superkid," but she was a good coper, competent, self-assured, confident, and well defended against the on-slaughts of parental mental disorder.

Creative Competence: Assimilative Mode

The case of Hans Christian Andersen (see Andersen, 1847), mentioned in Chapter 1 of this volume, is striking enough to merit repetition in this different context. Andersen felt that he had been "a case" ever since he was small, and his sense of vulnerability stayed with him all through his life as he hovered constantly on the edge of psychosis. His depressions became severer and more frequent as he got older. "Bear with me," he wrote to a friend. "You know I have a screw loose." His grandfather, with whom he was closely identified, was a wild-eyed old man who made artistically carved figures of birds, beasts, and gro-t sque-headed men and peddled these figures in the countryside, and who sometimes walked down the street decked with flowers and wearing a paper hat, singing strangely as he went. Inevitably there was a jeering mob of urchins at his heels. Lombroso (1891) would have labeled him a "mattoid," but he eventually became psychotic. Andersen could never rid himself of the fear that one day he would end up like his grandfather. "I knew I was of his flesh and blood," he would say, and study himself in the glass where he seemed to detect a close resemblance. His father was also a solitary man who spent a lot of time with his son, but his mental faculties gradually declined, and he too soon became psychotically delusional.

People were aware of Hans's combination of extreme vulnerability with resilience. He was described as "a sensitive plant *but able to unfold and withstand the most inclement weather*" (Andersen, 1847). From very early on, his extraordinary competence showed itself in his gift for creative fantasy, his high intelligence, his eagerness, his enthusiasm, and his extraordinary persistence in the face of setbacks. He was always determined to see things through to the end. His wit and humor enchanted his friends, and he was able to laugh and poke fun at himself. He himself thought that he thrived for various reasons: because he had an extraordinary capacity for withdrawing into fantasy and escaping from brutal reality; because he knew how to abreact his intense feelings by pouring out details of his "case" in endless representations, metaphors, and flashes of self-knowledge; and because he was able to transform "horrible" situations into fairy tales and achieve a few glorious moments of relief during the act of creation. Once, however, the writing was done, he relapsed into an aching depression and feeling of deprivation. His most striking asset was his representational competence of the assimilative kind, so that he was both able to portray reality in some of its starkness and then change bad things into good things and sad endings into happy ones. The high degree of competence he demonstrated was related to the taking in of a disturbing chunk of reality, reshaping it imaginatively in accordance with wish fulfillments, and then, creatively, retelling the idiosyncratic fantasy as a universal story or fairy tale. In the process (to use Andersen's most famous metaphor), the "ugly duckling" of reality was changed into a "beautiful swan," and the act of transformation was one that had—and has—universal appeal. It was not a well-balanced cognitive exercise, and it was not a simple imitation of reality. It was an assimilative creation and not a construction.

Creative Competence: System Making

"One of the direct consequences of my mother's poor mental health," wrote Piaget (1952), "was that I started to forego playing for serious work very early in childhood; this I did as much to imitate my father (a scholar of painstaking and critical mind who taught me the value of systematic work) as to take refuse in a private and nonfictitious world. *I have always detested any departure from reality*, an attitude which I related to this important influential factor of my early life, namely my mother's poor mental state" (p. 237). From the age of 7 onward, he became successively preoccupied with mechanical inventions and with bird, fossil, and seashell collections; he even invented an automobile provided with a steam engine. By the age of 10, he was studying mollusks and classifying them, and at 15 he was already a recognized malacologist.

Between the ages of 15 and 20, he experienced a series of crises stemming from the disturbing family circumstances. He was torn between identifying with his father and developing a scientific frame of mind and identifying with his mother and following a religious bent. The inner representations were experienced as parts of the father and parts of the mother in constant and vehement conflict with each other; as a result, his own mental health broke down, and he was forced to spend a year recuperating in the Swiss mountains. Instead of completely relaxing, he wrote a novel depicting this intense inner struggle, the severe identity crisis, and the break from reality. His sheer logical competence was of such a high order that he used his writing to elaborate a comprehensive system, and as soon as he had done this, he recovered from his illness. The comprehensive system that Piaget elaborated was a truly creative synthesis and had to do, at all levels from cell to society, with the problem of relating parts to wholes: The various parts relate to one another and also relate to the whole, which in turn relates to itself. They are reciprocal relationships and reach a state of equilibrium.

These fundamental notions, conceptualized by an adolescent boy, determined Piaget's huge range of scientific activities for the next 60 years. He not only resolved the conflictual parts relating to his mother and father, but produced a life work. According to his own paridigm described earlier, he veered away from the purely assimilative mode, which led him dangerously into his mother's territory, but at the same time, he also kept off from the accommodative mode, which would have led him into his father's scholarly but largely imitative and identificative field. He sought, sometimes precariously, to maintain a balance between the inner and outer worlds so that his cognitive efforts could devote themselves to system making without hindrance. Whenever he finished one of his many books, like Virginia Woolf and like Hans Christian Andersen, he became a prey to overwhelming anxieties; his great compulsion was not to leave any vacancies in time that would render him vulnerable. This was his method for coping with the mental illness in his mother, and it led to a monumental productivity. His defenses, however, were not strong enough to deal with the anxieties that had accumulated since early life, and it was only through tremendous efforts of coping—coupled, once again, with an extraordinary representational competence—that he was able to continue his work. His autobiographical novel at adolescence described his predicament almost perfectly, and his efforts in this regard could be well described as self-chosen therapy (Anthony, 1974).

Retrospective Studies of Resilience in Children at High Risk for Schizophrenia

Although there have been many studies (Anthony, 1972) of children who later became schizophrenic, two stand out in particular because they both included "outstanding" outcomes (see Table 6-1). Kasanin and Veo (1932) looked into early school records and classified the children as "odd and peculiar," "mildly maladjusted," "average adjustment," "outstanding," and "shut-in" (i.e., schizoid). Of the children studied, 11.1% were judged to be "outstanding" and were clearly differentiated from those who made a normal adjustment. Bower, Shellhammer, Daily, and Bower (1960) used the same categories and almost the same methodology nearly 30 years later. Their findings were surprisingly congruent: There were also "outstanding" children in the 1960 sample, but in a smaller percentage (6.3%). If later prospective investigators had looked at these findings, the chances are that they would have included the class of "superphrenics" in their original designs.

Anna Freud (1969) has described the case of Jean Drew and the "unholy influence" on her development of parenting by a paranoid schizophrenic mother. The daughter was punished irrationally and unmercifully, relentlessly nagged, deprived of everyday pleasures, and constantly accused of every imaginable wickedness. With this "incomprehensible mixture of demandingness, love, hate and overwhelming injustice" (1969, p. 445), one might have expected Jean to turn out deeply maladjusted. Instead, in her adolescence, she became president of the student body, a leader on the campus, captain of the baseball team, and the best student in geometry. Anna Freud wonders how one can explain this type of resilience and the capacity to resume normal

Table 6-1. Clinical Groupings in Two Studies of Children Who Later Became Schizophrenic

Grouping	Percentage in Kasanin & Veo (1932)	Percentage in Bowers et al. (1960)
Type 1 ("odd, peculiar")	22.2	20.5
Type 2 ("mildly maladjusted")	29.6	43.2
Type 3 ("average adjustment")	9.3	20.5
Type 4 ("outstanding")	11.1	6.3
Type 5 ("shut-in")	27.8	9.0

development once the stressor has been removed, and she concludes that one can only assume that in addition to potentially "good genes," enough goodness was lavished on the child by her mother during her early years to compensate for the psychotic mismanagement. I have mentioned earlier that Bleuler (1984) linked Vreni's resilience to the fact that her living conditions with her mother and father had been normal for the first 2 years of her life. In Jean's case, the initial "symbiosis" did give her a good start in life, but then closed in on her development like the walls of a prison. As the symbiosis was threatened by the daughter's rebelliousness, the mother gradually became psychotic. She was too rigid to move with her child's development, having the capacity only to mother a dependent child within an anaclitic relationship.

In the case of Esther, an 11-year-old girl described by Winnicott (1965), the same question was posed: How was it possible for this child of a psychotic mother to publish a poem at the age of 11 conveying a "perfect picture of home life in a happy family setting" in which the family is "pulsating with potential living," and, as night falls and the dogs and owls take over, inside the home all is "quiet, safe and still?" The baby spent the first 5 months of her life with her mother, a highly intelligent woman whose "tramp-type" life had resulted in the illegitimate birth of Esther. During these 5 months, the infant was constantly with the mother, breast-fed by her, and idolized by her with what seems to have been a total maternal preoccupation. At the end of this time, the psychotic break ruptured this "perfect environment" that had been established. After a sleepless night, the psychotic mother threw her baby into a canal, making sure first that there were people around to rescue the infant. She was certified and hospitalized, and from then onward, Esther had an extremely hard time. She even had a psychotic foster father at one period. According to Winnicott; "A very ill mother like Esther's mother may have given her baby an exceptionally good start; this is not at all impossible. I think Esther's mother not only gave her a satisfactory breast-feeding experience, but also that ego support which babies need in the earliest stages, and which can be given only if the mother is identified with her baby. This baby was probably merged in with her mother to a high degree" (p. 71).

It would seem, therefore, that Bleuler, Anna Freud, and Winnicott all stress the importance of that early phase of the child's life for the development of good mental health and competence. Winnicott (1948) has emphasized the need for a "perfect" initial environment because, as he puts it, "The mental health of the human being is laid down in infancy by the mother who provides an environment in which complex but essential processes in the infant's self can become completed" (p. 160). What others have referred to as "ego" resilience has become an attribute of the "self" that underscores the personal aspect of nonvulnerability. When Freud speaks of the confidence and success of the mother's favorite, he too is talking in "self" rather than "ego" terms: It is the self that develops the sense of invulnerability.

But even before the neonatal and early infantile phase sets the child on his successful path, genetic robustness has already contributed an essential share. In his Icelandic studies, Karlsson (1968) described a group of "genetic carriers" with thought disorder who stemmed from schizophrenic stock several generations removed, but who currently showed unusual ability and high achievement in art, science and politics. He posed the question, similar to that of Lombroso in the preceding century, as to whether these creative individuals could be regarded as "nonpenetrant schizophrenics." Barron (1963) had suggested that the answer lay not in the genes, but in the degree of ego resilience and integration. The genetic factor, however, is difficult to discount. McNeil and Kaij (1984), in their research on adoptees with a schizophrenic biological parent, isolated a small number of cases in whom an impressive creative ability and achievement related to the mental health ratings of the biological and not of the adoptive parents.

A significant number of the cases in some samples of children at high genetic risk for schizophrenia were rendered more vulnerable as a result of prenatal and perinatal neurological deficit or damage, but even among these, Marcus (in press) has found infants who seemed to be, according to him, "impervious" to these organic insults and who developed successfully in the first year of life. He wondered whether they were the advanced cohort of "invulnerables" that other investigators were picking up later in their development.

It would appear as if one of the most consistent findings in both retrospective and prospective research has been the uncovering of this subsample of "outstanding" individuals, varying in size from 6% to 12% of the entire sample. It is a remarkable convergence of both investigative and single-case clinical studies that makes the postulate of a "superphrenic" category more supportable. As if to clinch the argument, Heston and Denney (1968) isolated a group of 21 children of schizophrenics who had been fostered immediately after birth and who were not only growing up "successfully" and becoming successful adults, but were much more spontaneous, colorful, imaginative, and creatively occupid than the controls. Unfortunately, this was another example of a serendipitous finding picked up later from the data, so that these intriguing outcome traits could not be subjected to systematic assessment.

So far, the focus has been on the children of schizophrenic parents; however, on an anecdotal level of inquiry, the offspring of manic-depressives have also shown a similar tendency in roughly similar percentages toward outstanding development. One of the prototypes presented earlier in this chapter, Hans Christian Andersen, had predominantly manic–depressive characteristics and a genealogy highly suggestive of manic–depressive disorder.

It is only in the St. Louis Risk Research Project (Worland, James, Anthony, McGinnis, & Cass, 1984) that the offspring of schizophrenics and mainc–depressives have been compared and contrasted, and it needs to be consulted as the only available source of data at the present time.

The St. Louis Project's Sample of "Invulnerables"

Although the children of psychotic parents often have "horrible" lives with many attendant sufferings (Bleuler, 1978), their reactions vary with the nature of the psychosis. The superadjusted children of schizophrenic parents, for example, tend to favor withdrawal and distancing as defenses and introversive preoccupations as coping mechanisms. The suppression of spontaneous affective responses may give the impression that these children are schizoid; however, as Bleuler (1978) has pointed out, once the clinician has established a trustful and friendly relationship with them over time, there is quite a degree of warmth behind the emotional mask. In contrast, the superadjusted offspring of manic–depressives display an abundance of energy that galvanizes their surroundings and produces mood changes in those they associate with and treat as audience. They are often charming, gregarious, excitable, and exciting to their friends, who learn to tolerate excesses of action and interaction.

The St. Louis Risk Research Project (Worland et al., 1984) made use of two experimental procedures that tested the level of interpersonal competence: the Affect Discrimination Test (ADT), involving the recognition and ascription of a subtle range of feelings, and the Family Relations Test (FRT), measuring the strength of cathexis to primary figures. As a group, the children of parents with affective disorders (bipolar or unipolar) started at a high level of discernment on the ADT and gradually became more highly attuned "emotional barometers," particularly those who had superior adjustment. The manic–depressive subgroup performed better as a whole on this test than the children of schizophrenic, physically ill, and normal parents. On the FRT, in the area of involvement with the sick parent, the children of manic–depressives maintained a similar developmental difference from the children of schizophrenic parents: As the manic–depressives' offspring grew out of early childhood into adolescence, they were able to dissociate themselves increasingly from the psychotic parents, while in contrast, the children of schizophrenic parents became more and more involved to the point of symbiosis. The distinctions between the two high-risk subgroups were remarkable and widened with developmental progression, but in the top 10% of a 6-point adjustment scale, with categories ranging from seriously maladjusted to well adjusted, the differences were both striking and subtle. On the ADT, the resilient individuals became exquisitely hypersensitive to the feelings of *others*, while the resilient children from the schizophrenic subsample moved in a characteristic introversive direction, becoming exquisitely hypersensitive to feelings stemming from *themselves*. On the FRT, the resilient children of those with affective disorders were almost clinically dispassionate and talked with sometimes a chilling degree of objectivity about the parental predicament. On the same test, the resilient children of schizophrenics appeared not so much uninvolved as defensively withdrawn from the psychotic situation and its ramifications within the family. On the basis of these findings, one would agree with Bleuler that the supposedly "schizoid" characterization overlies a welter of warm, concerned, and compassionate feelings from which the children are in constant retreat. The disposition to internalize represents an additional threat to the psyche, to be counteracted with alienation. The affective externalizers, on the other hand, can maintain their emotional distance effortlessly and can therefore function better in general.

The processes of emotional sensitivity and emotional involvement are overlapping and further entangled in complementary processes of empathy and identification, and, within the Piagetian framework, of assimilations and accommodations. From time to time, even the most competent and robust of high-risk children can become enmeshed in a welter of empathy and identification. To extricate themselves from these perils requires the exercise of all their consummately developed coping skills.

In the area of intellectual competence, wide discrepancies appeared within highly disorganized families with chaotic psychosis in a parent, so that test scores showed a wide scatter both within the individual respondents as well as within the group. Although the correlations with vulnerability scores were not significant between groups, there were instances within families when uneven testing was closely related to vulnerability scores: The high scorers tested well because they were able to focus lucidly on the tests presented to them, and low scorers generally tested considerably below their abilities. In several families, these superior and inferior test results on a standard battery (Franklin, Worland, Cass, Bass, & Anthony, 1978) corresponded to achievement and underachievement at school. The more vulnerable the children were, the more likely they were to exhibit high levels of classroom disturbance (inattentiveness, withdrawal, disruptiveness, impulsive-ness, etc.); the nonvulnerables, in contrast, showed high comprehen-sion, creative initiative, and relatedness to the teacher.

One of the families offered a clear illustration of how cognitive competences are scattered around lines of vulnerability, involvement, and identification within a family. In this particular family, the mother was a severely withdrawn schizophrenic who had undergone repeated psychotic attacks. In a problem-solving session, the family members as a group were confronted with the proverb "A rolling stone gathers no moss," and were invited to come to some conclusions about its meaning as a family.

The father, a well-adjusted and highly successful businessman and chief executive of a large business, opened with the following response: "If you want to get on in life, you cannot stand still; you cannot sit on your butt and do nothing; you've got to keep moving." His older son, who was currently presi-dent of his junior high school class and was rated as highly resilient and competent with good coping skills, gave the next response: "I am in complete agreement with Dad, because if I had not gone out actively and canvassed and taken advantage of the school assembly to speak, I would never have been elected president."

After some encouragement, the mother, currently in a state of remission, ventured a somewhat incoherent comment: "Nice to be quiet, to be still; to lie on soft moss." Her daughter, who was doing poorly in her sixth-grade class and receiving treatment for a learning disability, had this to say: "I lost all my friends when we moved, and although I know that Dad had to get on, I did not like moving; I did not know what to do in the new school; everything seemed so different." Finally, the younger son, who was also doing poorly in the fourth grade and waiting to receive treatment for his chronic anxiousness, gave his response: "I lost my fishing tackle when we left our home—I mean, our previous home—and I don't like it here; it would have been better to have stayed where we were; I knew where all my things were in the other home."

The vignette demonstrates how dichotomized families can become under conditions of psychosis. The levels of adaptation in this family ranged from superior to poor, as did the competences, the coping skills, and the degrees of achievement. It is clear that the older son was fully identified with his father, involved in his success, and earnestly at-tempting to walk in his footsteps. The two younger children were identified with the mother and involved not only with her but with her illness. The complete loss of drive on the part of the mother was closely paralleled by the striking loss of initiative in these two children.

The findings in the St. Louis Risk Research Project regarding the families agree with what Beisser, Glasser, and Grant (1967) had shown—namely that the range of adjustment in such families is quite wide, varying from normality to extreme psychopathology. In a study of the *folie à deux* phenomenon (Anthony, 1968), I pointed to the permeability of the psychological placental barrier that exists between the child and the psychotic parent and that governs the flow of morbid ideas between the two. The more vulnerable the child, the more undifferentiated he is, the greater his susceptibility will be to the parent's abnormal ideas. On the other hand, the more individuated and the more developmentally competent he is, the less receptive he will be to the psychotic influence. Mosher, Pollin, and Stabenau (1971), in their study of 11 pairs of identical twins in which one twin was schizophrenic, had found that in 10 pairs the vulnerable twin, who had become psychotic, identified with the "sicker" parent and tended to be more submissive.

Our group (Lander, Anthony, Cass, Franklin, & Bass, 1978) developed two separate vulnerability rating scales, one based on the psychiatric interview and the other on psychological ratings. In the psychiatric interview, the ratings were based on identification with the ill parent, credulity about his delusions, the influence of the parental illness on the child, the degree of submissiveness and suggestibility, and the extent of involvement with the ill parent as gauged by three small tests: the "three wishes," the "three houses," and "the three dreams." The first three items were scored from interview information derived from the well parent and the children. Submissiveness was measured by the child's willingness to perform certain unusual acts without prior explanation and his suggestibility by body sway and eye and fist closure. The "three wishes" tapped the child's inclusion of the ill parents in his wishes; the "three houses" expressed his desire to live far from or near to the ill parent; and the "three dreams" projected his involvement in the parent and his illness. Two groups of subjects were then drawn from the total number. One group consisted of those scoring at the higher end of the vulnerability scale and included the most highly vulnerable children ($n = 19$); the other consisted of those scoring at the lower end and included the very low-vulnerable, nonvulnerable, or invulnerable children ($n = 21$).

For the psychological evaluation of vulnerability, each subject was rated blindly by a team of three clinical psychologists on a quantitative "psychological rating scale." The scale was developed to access various areas of psychological functioning, using not only formal scores but also more complex data, such as content, sequence, and balance of responses from the test protocols. The 14 variables included diagnosis, severity of disturbance, logicality of thinking, reality testing, concreteness, efficiency of defenses, coping, pathology of content, object relations, anxiety, identity, impulse control, emotionality, and aggressivity. It was hypothesized that some of these variables would reflect more sharply the impact of the disorganized, primitive thinking of the psychotic parents on the vulnerable children, such as logicality of thinking, concreteness, and the severity of disturbance. The resilient children, it was thought, would show up well in the competence of their thinking, their reality testing, their efficient defenses and coping, their capacity to relate, their sense of identity, and their self-control (Franklin *et al.*, 1978). In Table 6-2, the low-vulnerable and high-vulnerable groups are compared descriptively. It is interesting to note that IQs did not differentiate the two groups significantly. There were equal numbers of children of manic–depressives and schizophrenics in both groups.

The cases were also scored on six psychiatric categories, each with a scale of 1–6, with the low scores indicating good adjustment and minimal pathology and the high scores various degrees of pathology. The categories included the risk of disturbance in childhood, the actual disturbance in childhood, the risk of disturbance in adulthood, the risk of psychosis in adulthood, the global rating of vulnerability, and the global rating of adjustment. The two groups differed markedly on all categories, with the high-vulnerable group showing more pathology on each measure than the low-vulnerable subjects (see Figure 6-2). The psychiatric variable "risk of psychosis in adulthood" demonstrated the marked difference between groups. None of the low-vulnerable children were seen to have prepsychotic symptomatology, while in contrast over 50% of the high-vulnerable group were rated as showing some prepsychotic symptoms. The number of well-adjusted children in the low-vulnerable groups was encouragingly high (62%). Only two of the high-vulnerable children were seen as showing no disturbance on psychiatric evaluation.

Table 6-2. High-Vulnerable and Low-Vulnerable Groups: Descriptive Data

	Low-vulnerable ($n = 21$)	High-vulnerable ($n = 19$)
$\bar{x}$ age in months	137.19	131.42
Fill-scale IQ	108.28	102.63
Number of male subjects	12	6
Number of female subjects	9	13
Number of subjects with mother psychotic	15	9
Number of subjects with father psychotic	6	10
Parental diagnosis: schizophrenia	14	12
Parental diagnosis: manic–depressive psychosis	7	7

Note. From "A measure of vulnerability to risk of parental psychosis" by Lander, H., Anthony, E. J., Cass, L., Franklin, L., & Bass, L. in E. J. Anthony, C. Koupernik, & C. Chiland (Eds.), *The Child in His Family: Vulnerable Children* (International Yearbook, Vol. 4), New York: Wiley. Reprinted by permission.

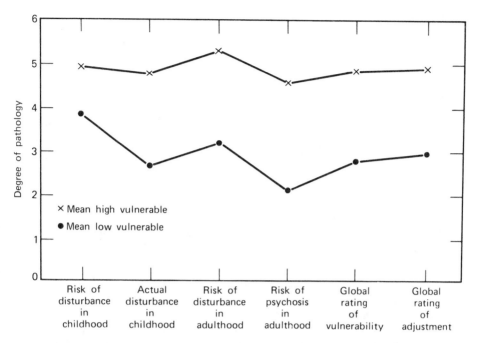

Figure 6-2. Psychiatric ratings of high and low vulnerability. (From "A measure of vulnerability to risk of parental psychosis," by H. Lander, E. J. Anthony, L. Cass, L. Franklin, and L. Bass, 1978, in E. J. Anthony, C. Koupernik, and C. Chiland [Eds.], *The Child in His Family: Vulnerable Children* [International Yearbook, Vol. 4], New York: Wiley: Reprinted by permission.)

In the psychological evaluation (see Figure 6-3), 37% of the high-vulnerable group were rated as showing "serious or incapacitating disturbance," whereas this was only true of 9% of the low-vulnerable subjects. Conversely, 43% of the low-vulnerables and only 31% of the high-vulnerables were rated as showing good adjustment. Of the high-vulnerable subjects, 20% showed "severe departures from stimulus accuracy, frequent tangential associations, percepts based on autistic thinking, and stimuli seen on the basis of patient's inner needs, conflicts and anxieties" (Franklin *et al.*, 1978, p. 330), while none of the low-vulnerables demonstrated this. However, significantly more of the low-vulnerable children were rated as having "creative and original responses but with high fidelity to the stimulus." All along the 14 variables, the low-vulnerable children were rated as showing no or only mild pathology, while the high-vulnerables were rated as showing serious or incapacitating pathology. When disturbances scored from all categories of the psychological ratings were summed, the high-vulnerable group scored significantly higher than the low-vulnerable group.

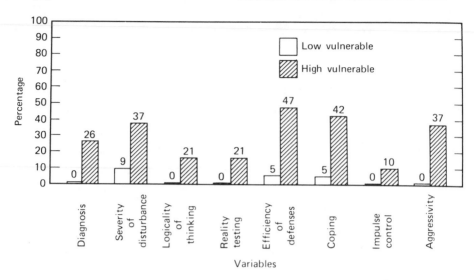

Figure 6-3. Psychological ratings: percentages of high- and low-vulnerable subjects. Rated as showing serious pathology. (From "A measure of vulnerability to risk of parental psychosis," by H. Lander, E. J. Anthony, L. Cass, L. Franklin, and L. Bass, 1978, in E. J. Anthony, C. Koupernik, and C. Chiland [Eds.], *The Child in His Family: Vulnerable Children* [International Yearbook, Vol. 4], New York: Wiley: Reprinted by permission.)

Several factors emerged in this project as being of value in protecting a child from the impact of parental psychosis. These included the child's ability to distance himself psychologically from the ill parent and to defend himself against the kind of submissive, receptive involvement with a psychotic parent that can lead to internalizing disturbed thought processes. Personality traits of confidence, nonsubmissiveness, and a kind of healthy skepticism seemed to be of considerable importance in the service of nonvulnerability.

The vignettes that follow provide examples of various types of competence that are evoked in the children of psychotic parents as a direct response to the psychotic influence.

Constructive Competence in the Accommodative Mode

M. was the male child of a paranoid schizophrenic father and a schizoid borderline mother. At the age of 6, he tested as hypervulnerable on both psychiatric and psychological evaluations, and the prediction was made that he would break down at some stage of his adolescence. He suffered from recurrent nightmares, micropsychotic episodes, and a severe learning disability, despite the fact that his IQ was in the above-average range. On clinical examination, he manifested loose associations, disorganized behavior, and vaguely paranoid ideation. Just prior to puberty, he developed juvenile diabetes and was admitted to the local children's hospital for setting up a remedial program. When he was seen again a few months later, there was a striking transformation in both his attitude and his behavior. He was now a self-sustaining diabetic. In the absence of any reliable supervision from his parents, he managed every aspect of the regimen: testing his urine daily; administering the insulin; planning the diet with a careful regard for calories, weights, and measures of food; maintaining the physician-prescribed course of exercise; and punctiliously attending the group meetings for young diabetics at the hospital. What was immediately apparent was that his vulnerability scores fell and his coping capacities increased. He presented very much as a self-assured, resilient child. He said that his aim was to be a model diabetic and that he was pleased at all the praise lavished on him at the hospital. He felt that his life depended upon himself and that it made him feel very grown-up. His new organizational drives were reflected in his school performance, and his teachers reported conspicuous across-the-board improvements. Toward the end of adolescence, he was shifted medically from the children's to the general hospital, and there was a setback. He was admitted for several diabetic crises, once in a coma, and his habits deteriorated. A young, enthusiastic resident physician took him in hand, showed a great interest in him, and gave him a book on diabetic heroes to read; as a result, he bounced back both physically and psychologically. In addition to finishing high school, he held several spare-time jobs and made enough money to become relatively independent of his parents. In his last checkup, he once again showed himself as a thriving and robust young man. In M.'s case, a good deal appeared to depend on the models to whom he attached himself and whom he imitated.

The G. family consisted of four children, all of whom had been grossly malparented by a violent manic–depressive father (who wrote poems during phases of remission) and a borderline mother with idiosyncratic but fundamentalistic religious beliefs and practices. All the children were rated as hypervulnerable, and all experienced a stormy childhood. The two older children pulled themselves together when they discovered themselves and their potentials through religion: in one instance, Scientology, and in the other, Jehovah's Witnesses. Both religions brought meaning, order, and dedication into their lives, so that their vulnerability scores fell dramatically as they became more confident and competent and developed a wide range of coping skills. The Scientologist not only did well within his religious circle, but also began to prosper as a businessman. The sister who had embraced the Jehovah's Witnesses not only brought up her own family extremely well, but took over the neglected, illegitimate child of her younger sister. She collected the Social Security of the parents and helped them to survive in what had been described originally as a "filthy hovel." She was very similar to Vreni as described by Bleuler (1984), and her compassion for her parents seemed to be endless. The Scientologist, who had moved to California, was also from time to time able to bring his parents to his comfortable residence there, but oddly enough, they both were uncomfortable in the setting and anxious to return to their "hovel." The two younger children had revolted bitterly against the religiosity of the parents and were both self-proclaimed atheists. They both went from bad to worse. They both made several suicidal attempts, and both were hospitalized frequently. On interview, both declared that they had no purpose in living and that they had no idea at all what to do with their lives. Even help from the two older children could not preserve them from further breakdowns.

The following is an excerpt from a self-report of a young girl recalling her childhood with her manic–depressive mother. Here she was describing the parent in a hypomanic phase:

> When she has little attacks, it's not so bad. She would be talking big, and we'd go into the stores and buy things and order all sorts of clothes and I'd feel like a princess. *She made me feel like a princess.* She'd say: "You don't have to think small." I'd sometimes go to school feeling grand and pretending I was some sort of princess and that all the children would know about it and stare at me and think I was great. Sometimes I began to feel so great that I got on everybody's nerves, and the kids soon started to tease me for putting on airs. I hate myself now when I think of it. But when mother was like that, she'd dress me up and do my hair. We'd sit for hours in front of the mirror, and she'd say that we were both beauties and that you couldn't find a pair like us in all the world. You know, I really believed it, and I began to think that I might become a film star or go on the stage. She always said: "You've got to think big because you are big." When she talked and talked and talked, I also talked and talked and talked and my friends at school thought that I talked too much, that I was too bossy, and that I wanted everything my way. If it weren't for the kids, I think I would have believed everything my mother told me. *She made me feel special, and they just made me feel ordinary.* (Anthony, 1975a, pp. 293–294; italics added)

It is clear that the narcissism and omnipotence of the mother were very gratifying to the developing child, and she found herself identifying with these exaggerated attributes in the mother. As she entered adult life and became successful as an announcer on the local TV station, she was conscious of being "above the crowd" but realized, with some insightfulness, that it stemmed from her mother's grandiosity. What she said was this: "One can be ordinary [that is, not crazy] and still feel that one can become something worthwhile." She had imagined herself becoming a famous painter, writer, or (even, less realistically) a saint, but she performed well at what she did, and a great deal of it was modeled on her mother.

Creative Imaginative Competence in the Assimilative Mode

Jim (described in Anthony, 1975a, pp. 306–309) was the only son of a manic-depressive father, a university professor. He could only be described as a phenomenon. Both parents reported on his "extraordinary babyhood," and some of the stories that sounded exaggerated turned out to be close to the facts. There were stories of his "insight" as an infant, his inventiveness as a toddler, and his industry and accomplishments after he got to school. He had always been a superconfident child with a strong belief that nothing was beyond his powers. His mother had sighed when she said that it was rough for a mere woman to live with two geniuses, her husband and her son, in the same household. She had married a genius, and they had produced a genius, and what more could a woman ask for in her life? The boy's energies during childhood matched these other attributes: "He seemed to be on the go everywhere all the time." Even now that he was older, there were parts of the wall, the ceiling, the stairway, and the furniture of the house that were almost worn down by his need to match his strength constantly against the world.

His mother remarked (with a certain amount of complacency) that what was so disturbing about her son was that he always had to show that he was the greatest. "Now, I do think that he is great, but not all that great, and certainly not as great as his father. He wants to be and to do everything. He has to be the strongest, the cleverest, and the brightest." It had begun during his infancy and childhood. As a baby, his thirst had been so insatiable that his mother alone had not been able to satisfy it, and that they had had to send out to the hospital for milk from other mothers to supplement her own. He had been toilet-trained overnight, his parents having pointed out the many and manifest advantages of urinating and defecating in the proper receptacle. As a toddler, he had awakened one night and had repainted the walls of the living room in a magnificent potpourri of color to the heights that he could reach, after his father had done the job during the day. Both parents had been flabbergasted and dismayed at first, but subsequently were excited and admiring; years later they recognized this as his earliest aspiration to outstrip his father.

Jim came in to his interview dressed eccentrically with all sorts of strange medallions hanging from his neck and waist. He clearly wanted admiration and blatantly "fished" for it. He remarked that he had read something in *Time* magazine about the interviewer and expressed pleasure that he was seeing somebody of some consequence:

> I might have ended up with some petty little shrink! He touched the large medallion on his chest and said that *as long as he had this around his neck, he could not be hurt.* (Not only did he have a legendary infancy and early childhood, but he created his own mythology as he went along.) The reference to his invulnerability reminded him of the time when he was very small and used to fancy that he could fly, and would occasionally take off from trees and buildings. *He never got hurt because something always seemed to be protecting him.* What was striking about Jim was not only that he had a sense of invulnerability, but that he garnered a huge amount of fantasy as he went along and that his internal stories about himself all had a prodigious quality about them. He said that he loved his daydreams because in them he could be "the cock of the walk" and do anything that he desired. "When I think what a dismal little place school is, I have to do something inside my head to make it bearable for me to live. All those stupid teachers just become puppets on my stage. (italics added)

Creative Systematizing Competence in the Assimilative and Accommodative Modes

George was the only son of a chronically schizophrenic father with severe thought disorder. His mother was a reasonable and reality-oriented woman who tried to provide a stable center for the household, although her husband's irrationality defeated most of her efforts. She turned frequently to her son for help in coping with the disorganization generated by her psychotic spouse, and she spoke with awe of his "wonderful ideas" that helped to keep some order in the household. There were three other children: an older girl who was extremely vulnerable and already showed evidence of thought disorder in early adolescence; and twin girls who were moderately vulnerable but clung to each other as transitional objects and to a large extent lived a private life of their own with a language peculiar to themselves. The son was an "invulnerable," and all his testing pointed to his adaptability, his robustness, and his wide range of coping that reflected the high level of his competence. His mother put it truly when she said, "Whenever we all feel messed up, he just has to come home and be with us and everything seems okay."

George had read up about his father's condition in various psychiatric textbooks, but found them more descriptive than explanatory. Eventually he produced a psychological theory of his own based on information theory. It had no emotional component to it. He postulated that something had gone wrong with his father's mind at the intake point and that its capacity to take in complex bits of information had gradually narrowed. As a result, there was a "crowding" at the entrance, with a consequent disorder in the items that were fed into the system. It became accidental as to which items followed which, with the result that at the point of emergence the action that ensued was generally unexpected and inappropriate. To deal with this, one had to recognize the limitation of the system and help it to deal with many fewer tasks, especially of the kind that required no internal disentanglement and were simple and concrete. Thus, for example, since his father awakened into a complex system of everyday demands, he very rapidly reduced his living arrangements to utter chaos. His son collected a series of cardboard boxes, colored them differently, and numbered them separately. Each box contained a task that needed to be completed before proceeding to the next box, and George felt that if his father followed the sequence, it would be possible for him to complete a day without disorganization. The father, George believed, was a "nice" psychotic who was ready to cooperate if he could be shown what to do.

The system worked well for 3 months; this, according to the son, supported his theory of schizophrenia. Toward the end of this time, however, the father lost interest and patience with the orderliness required, smashed up the boxes, and reverted to his usual life of disorder. What was striking in this case was that the son persisted in applying practice to theory, even though situations failed from time to time and even though the situation got so out of hand that the father needed to be hospitalized for a while. The son did extremely well at college and was admitted to a well-known institute of technology, where his further progress was described as "brilliant."

Competence in the Face of Terror

Elsewhere (Anthony, 1986), I have described microdisasters afflicting families when psychotic parents have run amok. These situations are associated with the "involving" type of psychosis, where the offspring themselves are deeply implicated in the delusional and hallucinatory notions of the deranged parent and are therefore liable to be violently attacked, abused, and seduced.

An act of paranoid terrorism took place in a black, lower-class family with eight children ranging from 5 to 16 years of age, with the second youngest being the only boy. Table 6-3 shows the evaluation of the children before the attack. Three of the children were in the high-risk category. One of them, Yvonne, was also deemed highly vulnerable to the psychotic process. Yvonne was also the poorest of the copers, while Telesie and Veronica were good copers and also moderately and highly competent respectively, Antoinette and her little sister Angela were clearly the family "stars," not only in having low risk scores but also in showing themselves to be the most resilient as well as the most competent of the children, coping extremely well in all the tasks presented to them. Among the predictions made, it was thought that the "invulnerables," Antoinette and Angela, would not be significantly disordered by any further psychotic developments and that they would continue to perform competently under all circumstances.

Some time after this basic assessment, while the mother was on night shift work, the father became acutely disordered and attacked the children murderously after first locking them up in the house. He said that he knew what they had done to him and what they were planning to do in the future. He could read their minds and there was nothing they could hide from him. He knew that

Table 6-3. Paranoid Terrorism (before the Attack)

Children (ages)	Risk[a]	Resilience–vulnerability[b]	Coping[b]	Competence[b]	Prediction
Telesie (16)	28	3	5	4	Neurotic ++
Veronica (14)	30	2	5	5	Neurotic +++
Edith (12)	24	2	4	3	Psychotic +
Hilary (10)	20	3	3	3	Psychotic +
Antoinette (9)	10	6	6	6	None 0
Yvonne (8)	36	1	1	2	Psychotic +++
Lenny (7)	18	4	4	3	Psychotic +
Angela (5)	14	5	5	5	None 0

[a]Risk scores: high (28–42), moderate (14–27), low (0–13).

[b]Resilience–vulnerability, coping, competence ratings: 1 (low) to 6 (high).

Note. From "Terrorizing attacks on children by psychotic parents" by E. J. Anthony, 1986, *Journal of the American Academy of Child Psychiatry, 25* (3), 326–335.

they and their mother were in league with "others" outside and were plotting to murder him. Throughout the night, he subjected them all to extreme abuse, demanding that they confess everything or else be killed. He lined them up by the window and hung some of them out by their hair, threatening to let them fall to their death. He chased them frantically around the room and shouted that he wanted to see them all dead. He turned Yvonne upside down, thumped her head against the floor, and threatened to throw her down the basement stairs. Somehow, the children managed to live through the night. At 6:30 A.M., the mother came home; the exhausted children threw themselves onto her, weeping helplessly and unable to speak. She phoned for the police as the clinging children clustered around, and they all watched as the ambulance came to take the father to the hospital.

In Table 6-4, the reactions of the children to "the night of terror" are tabulated in terms of a post-traumatic stress disorder (PTSD) and any emergent psychotic tendencies that might have been precipitated by the event. It looked as if two sets of vulnerabilities were involved: one related to the traumatic process, with antecedents in neurotic tendencies, and the other to the psychotic process, with antecedents in precursory psychotic propensities. Two of the children developed PTSD and one, Yvonne, showed a marked worsening of her prepsychosis. Antoinette and Angela both showed no evidence of PTSD and seemed completely free of any psychotic-like manifestations. Antoinette confirmed her superior level of global adjustment, with Angela just one notch below. What was striking was that the highly resilient children continued to thrive in 5- and 10-year follow-ups, and that the two vulnerable children who became more resilient as time went on also began to thrive, although not quite to the same extent. For a young black girl from a lower-class, disadvantaged family, Antoinette's "representational competence" was quite extraordinary.

Table 6-4. Paranoid Terrorism (after the Attack)

Children (ages)	PTSD[a]	Prepsychotic[a]	Global adjustment[b]
Telesie (16)	3	0	2
Veronica (14)	3	0	2
Edith (12)	1	1	3
Hilary (10)	1	1	3
Antoinette (9)	0	0	6
Yvonne (8)	0	3	1
Lenny (7)	0	1	3
Angela (5)	0	0	5

[a]PTSD, prepsychotic ratings: 0 (low) to 3 (high).

[b]Global adjustment rating: 1 (low) to 6 (high).

Note. From "Terrorizing attacks on children by psychotic parents" by E. J. Anthony, 1986, Journal of the American Academy of Child Psychiatry, 25 (3), 326–335.

Table 6-5. Type of Manic–Depressive Disorder in Parent and 10-Year Clinical Outcome in the Offspring

Outcome of offspring	Parental disorder		
	Bipolar	Unipolar	Total
Clinically disturbed			
Inpatient treatment	8	0	8
Outpatient treatment	10	1	11
Needing treatment	10	8	18
Total	28	9	37
Percentage	62.2	34.6	48.4
Not clinically disturbed	17	17	34

She provided the investigators with sensitive, comprehensive accounts of early family life, of family life following the psychosis, of the family's reactions to "the night of terror," and of family life during a period of long remission.

A 10-Year Follow-Up of Nonvulnerable Offspring of Manic–Depressive Parents

In a 10-year follow-up study, the difference between those who had been rated highly vulnerable and those who had been rated low in vulnerability was significant (see Tables 6-5 and 6-6). The type of manic–depressive disorder was of some importance: 37.8% of the bipolar parents and 65.4% of the unipolar parents had offspring who

Table 6-6. Spouses of Manic–Depressive Patients and 10-Year Clinical Outcome in the Offspring

Outcome of offspring	Diagnosis of nonproband parent		
	Not clinically disturbed (normal or "difficult")	Clinically disturbed (neurotic or psychopathic)	Total
Clinically disturbed			
Inpatient treatment	1	7	8
Outpatient treatment	1	10	11
Needing treatment	10	8	18
Total	12	25	37
Percentage	34.3	69.4	51.9
Not clinically disturbed	23	11	34

showed no sign of clinical disturbance and had not received any treatment. The influence of the nonpsychotic parent also was significant: The more normal the nonpsychotic parent was, the more likely the child was to be clinically undisturbed and without need to be treated. Unipolar manic–depressives more frequently tended to be married, to a significant degree, to spouses who were relatively normal. It would appear that resilience to the manic–depressive process, measured by the treatment criterion, held up well over a period of 10 years.

Conclusions

After 15 years of a prospective study, one is left, like Bleuler (1978), with the impression that "pain and suffering can have a steeling—a hardening—effect on some children, rendering them capable of mastering life with all its obstacles" (p. 409). Also, as Bleuler notes, it is important for future researchers to keep as careful a watch on the favorable development of these children at high genetic risk for psychosis as on that of the "sick minority."

So far, risk researchers can only speak of the first 30 to 35 years of life, with many years of possible breakdown lying still ahead. For this reason, it may be that the terms "resilience" or "stress resistance" are more appropriate than "invulnerability," especially if they are defined in terms of defense, coping, mastery, competence, and creativity. These terms can be and have been quantified, although the measures in use are still in a loose and rudimentary form. There is much need for newer and better methodologies.

It does seem, from the St. Louis sample, that the "invulnerables" do seem to pay a psychological price for their apparent immunity from psychiatric illness. First, the mechanisms that they utilize—distancing, isolation of affect, suppression, externalization, rationalization, and intellectualization—make it difficult for them to maintain good object relations with adequate levels of intimacy and generativity, particularly if the psychotic parent is of the opposite sex. As they have been longitudinally followed, many of them keep making relationships and breaking them when there is any hint of closeness. Second, they often search for relationships with problematical objects and dedicate themselves to the life task of helping them (many of them have joined the helping professions). Third, some of them have joined various religious and social groups, diffusing and diluting relationships although obtaining a good deal of ego support from the groups. Fourth, many relinquish objects for objectives and become involved in projects and life tasks that demand cooperation but not relationships. Finally, many of them seek treatment for reasons that they cannot specify, except that

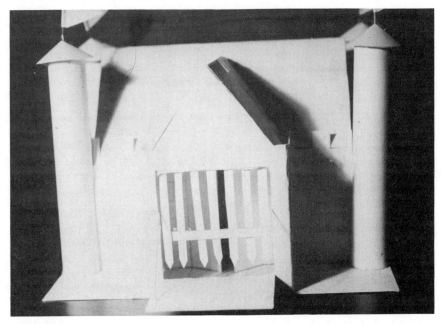

Figure 6-4. Ellen's "castle."

in the midst of all their successes and superachievements, they feel strangely unsatisfied.

In ending this presentation of "invulnerables," the creative aspects need to be emphasized.

Ellen was one of seven sisters subjected to the psychotic disturbances of a manic–depressive mother. Throughout her childhood and adolescence, she remained composed to the point of serenity amidst the wildest accusations, insinuations, and attacks of the mother, as well as the equally disagreeable reverberations from the psychopathic father, who had a strong sadistic streak in his personality. She thrived scholastically, emotionally, and interpersonally, to an extent that made her one of our favorite "invulnerables."

In one of the tasks in the research interview, she was asked to construct from materials provided an example of what it felt like to live with her sick mother at home. She came up with the "castle" shown in Figures 6-4 and 6-5. She described the castle as "the little space" that she had arranged for herself in the household and into which she could retreat when things were "rough" outside. She pointed to the most important part of the castle, the iron gate, which she could lift whenever she wanted to escape from the "enemies" on the outside and make it impossible for them to penetrate behind her defenses and disturb the even tenor of her development. When asked how it felt like to be

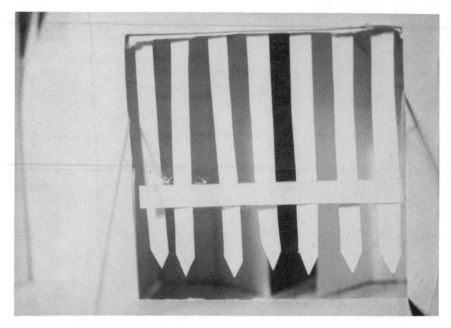

Figure 6-5. Closeup of the castle, showing the "iron gate."

inside the castle, she laughingly gave a lyrical response: "It was like being in a world in which everything worked and everyone worked together and where you had a job to do that was the job that you wanted to do and no one could stop you from doing it. I am the queen of this castle and I do not want anyone to enter who can spoil my life." The comment has certainly a narcissistic quality about it, but it does indicate how self-protective and self-preventative the egos of these resilient children can be.

ACKNOWLEDGMENT

This chapter is based on research funded by National Institute of Mental Health Grants No. MH-24819, No. MH-12043, and No. MH-50124.

REFERENCES

Andersen, H. C. (1847). *The true story of my life*. London: Longman, Brown, Green & Longman.
Anthony, E. J. (1968). The developmental precursors of adult schizophrenia. In D. Rosenthal & S. Kety (Eds.), *The transmission of schizophrenia*. New York: Pergamon Press.
Anthony, E. J. (1971). *Folie à deux*: A developmental failure in the process of separation-

individuation. In J. B. McDevitt & C. F. Settlage (Eds.), *Separation–individuation.* New York: International Universities Press.

Anthony, E. J. (1972). A clinical and experimental study of high-risk children and their schizophrenic parents. In A. R. Kaplan (Ed.), *Genetic factors in "schizophrenia."* Springfield, IL: Charles C Thomas.

Anthony, E. J. (1974). Self-therapy in adolescence. In S. C. Feinstein & P. L. Giovacchini (Eds.), *Adolescent psychiatry* (Vol. 3). New York: Basic Books.

Anthony, E. J. (1975a). Influence of a manic-depressive environment on the child. In E. J. Anthony & T. Benedek (Eds.), *Depression and human existence.* Boston: Little, Brown.

Anthony, E. J. (1975b). Naturalistic studies of disturbed families. In E. J. Anthony (Ed.), *Explorations in child psychiatry.* New York: Plenum Press.

Anthony, E. J. (1986). Terrorizing attacks on children by psychotic parents. *Journal of the American Academy of Child Psychiatry, 25*(3), 326–335.

Barron, F. (1963). The needs for order and for disorder as motives in creative activity. In C. W. Taylor & F. Barron (Eds.), *Scientific creativity.* New York: Wiley.

Beisser, A., Glasser, N., & Grant, M. (1967). Psychosocial adjustment in children of schizophrenic mothers. *Journal of Nervous and Mental Disease, 145*(6), 429–440.

Binswanger, L. (1959). Studies of the schizophrenia problem. *Proceedings of the Second International Congress of Psychiatry* (Vol. 2). Zurich: Orell Fussli.

Bleuler, M. (1978). *The schizophrenic disorders.* New Haven, CT: Yale University Press.

Bleuler, M. (1984). Different forms of childhood stress and patterns of adult psychiatric outcome. In N. F. Watt, E. J. Anthony, L. C. Wynne, & J. Rolf (Eds.), *Children at risk for schizophrenia: A longitudinal perspective.* Cambridge, England: Cambridge University Press.

Bower, E., Shellhammer, T., Daily, J., & Bower, M. (1960). High school students who later became schizophrenic. *Bulletin of the California Department of Education, 29*(8), 31–43.

Ey, H. (1959). The problem of defining and delimiting the group of schizophrenias. In *Proceedings of the Second International Congress of Psychiatry* (Vol. 2). Zurich: Orell Fussli. 2.

Ferenczi, S. (1913). Stages in the development of the sense of reality. In *First contributions to psychoanalysis.* London: Hogarth Press.

Franklin, L., Worland, J., Cass, L., Bass, L., & Anthony, E. J. (1978). Study of children at risk: Use of psychological test batteries. In E. J. Anthony, C. Koupernik, & C. Chiland (Eds.), *The child in his family: Vulnerable children* (International yearbook, Vol. 4). New York: Wiley.

Freud, A. (1969). *The writings of Anna Freud:* Vol. 5: Research at the Hampstead Child-Therapy Clinic and Other Papers (pp. 444–450). New York: International Universities Press.

Guilford, J. (1957). Creative ability in the arts. *Psychological Review, 64,* 110–118.

Hartmann, E. (1984). *The nightmare.* New York: Basic Books.

Heston, L., & Denney, D. (1968). Interactions between early life experience and biological factors in schizophrenia. In D. Rosenthal & S. Kety (Eds.), *The transmission of schizophrenia.* New York: Pergamon Press.

Jung, C. (1907). *On the psychology of dementia praecox.* New York: Nervous & Mental Disease Publishing Company.

Karlsson, J. (1968). Genealogical studies of schizophrenia. In D. Rosenthal & S. Kety (Eds.), *The transmission of schizophrenia.* New York: Pergamon Press.

Kasanin, J., & Veo, L. (1932). A study of the school adjustments of children who late in life become psychotic. *American Journal of Orthopsychiatry, 2,* 212–223.

Lander, H., Anthony, E. J., Cass, L., Franklin, L., & Bass, L. (1978). A measure of vulnerability to risk of parental psychosis. In E. J. Anthony, C. Koupernik, & C. Chiland (Eds.), *The child in his family: Vulnerable children* (International yearbook, Vol. 4). New York: Wiley.

Lidz, T., Fleck, S., & Cornelison, A. (1965). *Schizophrenia and the family.* New York: International Universities Press.

Lombroso, C. (1891). *The man of genius.* London: Walter Scott.

Marcus, J. (in press).

Minkowska, F. (1925). Essential difficulties of schizophrenics in their relationship with the givens of psychology and modern biology. *Evolutionary Psychiatry, 1,* 127–141.

Minkowski, E. (1927). *The schizophrenic.* Paris: Payot.

McNeil, T., & Kaij, L. (1984). Offspring of women with nonorganic psychoses. In N. F. Watt, E. J. Anthony, L. C. Wynne, & J. Rolf (Eds.), *Children at risk for schizophrenia: A longitudinal perspective.* Cambridge, England: Cambridge University Press.

Mosher, L., Pollin, W., & Stabenau, J. (1971). Families with identical twins discordant for schizophrenia. *British Journal of Psychiatry, 118,* 29–42.

Piaget, J. (1926). *The language and thought of the child.* London: Routledge & Kegan Paul.

Piaget, J. (1951). *Play, dreams and imitation of childhood.* (C. Gattegno & F. Hodgson, Trans.). London: Heinemann.

Piaget, J. (1952). Autobiography. In E. Boring, H. Langfeld, H. Werner, & R. Yerkes (Eds.), *A history of psychology in autobiography* (Vol. 4). Worcester, MA: Clark University Press.

Segal, J., & Yahraes, H. (1978). *A child's journey: Forces that shape the lives of our young.* New York: McGraw-Hill.

Winnicott, D. (1948). Paediatrics and psychiatry. In *Collected papers.* London: Tavistock, 1958.

Winnicott, D. (1965). The effect of psychotic parents on the emotional development of the child. In *The family and individual development.* London: Tavistock.

Worland, J., Janes, C., Anthony, E. J., McGinnis, M., & Cass, L. (1984). St. Louis Risk Research Project: Comprehensive progress report of experimental studies. In N. F. Watt, E. J. Anthony, L. C. Wynne, & J. Rolf (Eds.), *Children at risk for schizophrenia: A longitudinal perspective.* Cambridge, England: Cambridge University Press.

7

Predicting Mental Health in Children at Risk

JULIEN WORLAND
DAVID G. WEEKS
CYNTHIA L. JANES
Washington University School of Medicine

Children of parents with schizophrenia or affective disorder are as a group at high risk for the development of behavioral and emotional problems as they grow up. The proportional representation of such children eventually among the rosters of the disturbed may be as low as 25% (Bleuler, 1974) or as high as 50% (Heston, 1966), of whom a smaller number will fall victim at some point in their lives to a diagnosis of psychosis (10–14%). Thus has developed the interest in studying "children at risk"—to describe the development of pathology, or, put another way, the gradual fraying of the intertwined strands of personality, as the child at risk finally succumbs to the parental disease.

Although this familiar description is the rationale for numerous risk research projects both in the United States and overseas, it obscures more than it illuminates. Not only do only a small number of patients with psychosis actually have psychotic parents themselves (rendering fragile any generalizations we might hope to make on breakdown in risk samples), but most of the children at risk will lead relatively normal lives—free not only of psychosis itself, but free of pathology as well.

Clinical speculation abounds that a small number of such children not only will escape mental illness, but may even be endowed in life with an abundance of creative potential, academic proficiency, musical ability (Heston, 1966), or literary fecundity. Capturing these speculations for empirical test is the driving force behind the present volume.

Our interest here is more conservative. Since the test battery in the St. Louis Risk Research Project provides scant opportunity to tap unusual creativity or genuine "superphrenia," our more modest task has been to determine which children at risk are developing competently in adolescence and young adulthood, and whether any of the psychological assessments we made on these children when they were about 8 or 9 years of age could have predicted such competence.

Background Literature

Since risk research is as yet a young enterprise, it is not surprising that the majority of our information is cross-sectional, comparing children of mentally ill parents to variously composed groups of control children, rather than longitudinal. Here we combine recent cross-sectional studies from the risk research tradition with more classical studies on children of psychotic parents, as a method of providing background for the study we describe below.

A number of studies have demonstrated that, when compared with the offspring of normals, the offspring of schizophrenic parents demonstrate increased psychiatric and psychosocial symptoms, even when the offspring are adopted away in infancy (Heston, 1966); an increase in psychiatric diagnoses, including schizophrenia (Schulsinger, 1976); more academic problems (Higgins, 1966; Mednick & Schulsinger, 1968; Weintraub, Neale, & Liebert, 1975); and more behavior problems at home (Beisser, Glasser, & Grant, 1967; Cowie, 1961). Other reports have indicated that children of schizophrenic parents have lower intelligence than children in matched control groups (Mednick & Schulsinger, 1968) and that the intelligence test scores of children at risk for depression may be even lower (Cohler, Grunebaum, Weiss, Gamber, & Gallant, 1977). Visual–motor coordination skills may be an additional area of psychological functioning in which children of psychotic parents demonstrate diminished performance (Hanson, Gottesman, & Heston, 1976).

St. Louis Risk Research Project

Although a detailed description of the St. Louis Risk Research Project, from which we have drawn the data we describe below, is available elsewhere (Worland, Janes, Anthony, McGinnis, & Cass, 1984), a short description of our selection of families, our methods, and some cross-sectional findings on the offspring when they were children should acquaint the reader with our work, from which the study we present here has grown.

Sample Selection

We began our study in 1966 by recruiting psychotic inpatients, with hospital diagnoses of schizophrenia or manic–depressive illness, who had intact families with at least one child between 6 and 12 years of age, and who were willing to participate in a lengthy assessment of each family member. In this way, we recruited 34 probands with schizo-phrenia or manic–depressive illness. We also recruited 19 patients with a chronic physical illness, usually tuberculosis, plus 38 families with no parental history of emotional illness or prolonged hospitalization for a physical illness. The offspring of these parents provided our sample.

First Psychological Assessment

The first evaluation of offspring included what is considered in child guidance clinics as a "standard" battery of psychological tests. The battery included the Wechsler Intelligence Scale for Children (WISC; Wechsler, 1949), including all subtests except mazes. An additional cognitive measure was the Beery–Buktenica Developmental Form Se-quence (Beery, 1967), a pencil-and-paper test of visual–motor coordina-tion that requires children to copy 24 geometric designs of increasing difficulty. Personality measures included the 10-card Rorschach and the Thematic Apperception Test (TAT; Murray, 1943), cards 1, 2, 3BM, 6BM, 7BM, 7GF, 8BM, 10 and 16. Both of these personality measures are projective tests, on which children are asked to respond verbally both to ambiguous pictures with stories and to ambiguous designs with ideas of what they suggest to the children. We used the standard instructions for both of these personality measures.

There were numerous other assessments that we administered to offspring and their parents during this first barrage, but since we did not include them in the project reported here, we will pass over them. The reader is referred to our progress report (Worland *et al.*, 1984) for further information.

Data Available from First Assessment

From the cognitive assessment, we have available each child's verbal, performance, and full-scale IQ. From the Beery, we have for each child a developmental quotient (DQ) that was computed by dividing each child's "developmental age" according to Beery's norms by the child's chronological age, and multiplying the quotient by 100.

Data reduction from the projective tests was more difficult. From the Rorschach, we computed for each child a developmental level (DL) score according to Becker's (1956) adaptation of Friedman's (1952) system. This score is a qualitative measure of the maturity of a child's perceptions, and ranges from global, unarticulated, and inaccurate form level (at the least mature) to highly articulated, well-differentiated, and accurate form level (at the most mature). The DL score was the average of form level scores given for each Rorschach response. An additional Rorschach score was "Extended F+%," a simple measure of the accuracy that determined whether each response actually matched the ambiguous blot design, using tables provided by S. Beck, Beck, Levitt, and Molish (1961) and Hertz (1961). Further examination of the Rorschach tests also allowed us to identify a score for primitive Rorschach content, which was the total of such responses as food, fire, anatomy, blood, and so on.

Since we did not believe that these relatively simple scores would represent adequately all the available clinical material, each child's intelligence test, Rorschach, TAT, and Beery protocol were reviewed individually by a clinical psychologist, who made ratings representing 12 kinds of psychological functioning on a series of Likert-type scales. Selection of the 12 rated areas was made on the basis that each area had demonstrable importance in psychodynamic personality theory and could be rated from psychological test responses. The 12 areas were logicality of thinking; reality testing; concreteness; anxiety; object relationships; identity; conscience; emotionality; aggressivity; conflict and defenses; coping; and pathology of content.

The characteristics of test responses that raters used in making the ratings included both actual content and formal scores, codified into a formal manual (Cass, 1973). For each rated area, the psychologists established a score that represented a specific content or stylistic characteristic of a child's test protocol. For example, the description for a rating of "moderate pathology" in the area of reality testing was as follows: "Moderate departure from stimulus accuracy; Rorschach accuracy 10%–20% below norm for age; in TAT, one or two misperceptions in stimuli details; a few (two or three) instances of inaccurate elaboration on [intelligence test]" (Cass, 1973). A rating of "moderate pathology" would be made if more than half of these conditions were met.

The rating for pathology of content was a more clinical and informal judgment of the overall degree of disturbance seen in all the test protocols taken together, without requiring equal weight for all the variables.

The specification of methods for determining these ratings and the clinical maturity of the raters[1] were responsible for the unusually high degree of interrater reliability that we found on these measures. The average kappa (Cohen, 1960) based on 831 individual ratings was .61. When ratings were summed and compared among three pairs of raters, the Pearson correlations were quite respectable, r (63) = .94, .84, and .97 (Worland, Lander, & Hesselbrock, 1979).

1. We extend our thanks to Drs. Loretta Cass, Lois Franklin, Larry Bass, and Ruth Rosenthal for making these ratings.

When these separate ratings were subsequently factor-analyzed, we found that they were highly intercorrelated and could be represented by a single factor that we labeled "pathology."

From the TAT, research assistants[2] made ratings of the kind of coping (constructive, destructive, evasive, or no problem), interaction (positive, negative, both, or none), and affect (positive, negative, both, or none) shown in each TAT story. When factor-analyzed, we determined that these separate ratings could be reduced to a single factor, which we labeled "TAT aggression."

In summary, then, our assessment of the children netted us nine variables for study: verbal, performance, and full-scale IQ from the intellectual assessment; Beery DQ from the visual–motor assessment; DL, primitive content, and accuracy scores from the Rorschach; TAT aggression; and pathology, which was the psychologists' global rating of the whole test battery.

Effects of Parental Diagnosis on Children's Psychological Test Scores

We found that our children of psychotic parents did not have lower scores on intelligence tests than did children of nonpsychotic parents (Worland & Hesselbrock, 1980); however, our recent reanalysis of the intelligence test data, taken together with an intelligence re-evaluation in adolescence or young adulthood, provided evidence that, compared with children of psychotic fathers, children of psychotic mothers did have lower intelligence test scores (Worland, Weeks, Weiner, & Schechtman, 1982). Children of schizophrenic parents had higher scores on primitive Rorschach content. Furthermore, we determined that the pathology factor scores based on pathology ratings made by the psychologists at the first assessment reliably differentiated children at risk from children of nonpsychotic parents (Worland et al., 1979). The TAT aggression factor demonstrated a more complicated pattern. Children of schizophrenics had the lowest scores on this factor, children of manic–depressives had the highest scores, and children of normals fell in between. Finally, the Rorschach DL score showed more pathology in the young children of schizophrenic parents than in the children of normals (Worland, 1980), although this was no longer true when the children became adolescents (J. T. Beck & Worland, 1983). Incidentally, we found no differences in Beery scores between children in our different group—a fact that takes on added significance below.

---

2. We acknowledge the previous work of Linda Teal-Anthony and Patty Evans for making these assessments, and thank them for their work.

In summary, then, our cross-sectional evaluation of children determined that children of psychotic parents had more disturbance, as indexed by clinicians' ratings and projective test measures, but were not deficient in cognitive abilities—either in intellectual capability or in their visual–motor coordination. Clinically, they exhibited test behavior seen in children with immature emotional development, as well as problems in the control of their impulses. Children of schizophrenics dealt with the anxiety resulting from their difficulties in impulse control by emotional blunting or by overcontrol, resulting in a kind of psychological blandness or emptiness. The test results would suggest that children of parents with affective disorder would be more likely to act out this anxiety.

A major difficulty that could be pointed out in our studies and in the majority of the other studies cited is the issue of the reliability of the parental diagnoses, as noted by Hanson, Gottesman, and Meehl (1977). Since these studies were reported before the publication of the clear diagnostic criteria now available, it is reasonable to question whether these findings would be replicated if we assigned diagnoses from the third edition of the *Diagnostic and Statistical Manual of Mental Disorders* (DSM-III; American Psychiatric Association, 1980) to the psychotic parents and divided their children into groups on the basis of those diagnoses. A second issue is whether the same characteristic that differentiated children at high risk from those at lower risk would be able to predict later indices of mental health (McNeil & Kaij, 1979).

The Present Investigation

The purpose of the investigation we now present was to determine whether the same childhood measures of cognitive and emotional development that, as we explained above, could differentiate between children of psychotic parents and children of normals also could predict longitudinally a measure of mental health derived from a multimodal evaluation of the same offspring in young adulthood. We also wanted to determine whether they could predict later functioning at a level of certainty greater than could be predicted from demographic characteristics (race, social class) or parental diagnosis (using DSM-III criteria).

Method

SUBJECTS

There were 223 children involved in the analyses presented here, of whom 87 were the offspring either of parents with schizophrenic disorders ($n = 34$), of parents with affective disorders ($n = 27$), or of parents with schizoaffective disorders ($n = 26$), plus 136 children of nonpsychotic parents.

PARENTAL DIAGNOSIS

To determine the parental diagnoses using DSM-III criteria (American Psychiatric Association, 1980), one of us (J.W.) read the hospital index admission and discharge reports, which had been edited to delete the hospital diagnoses and therapy regimens. We had hospital records for 24 of 34 hospitalized parents that allowed for an unequivocal DSM-III diagnosis. For 5 other parents (who had 5 offspring), we did not have copies of the reports, so we examined all the diagnostic information available to us, including our project diagnosis and various hospital diagnoses without detailed records (from the hospitalization when the family had joined our project and from their other hospitalizations), and then classified them on the basis of this information. There were 5 additional parents (who had 13 offspring) whom we deleted from the analyses, either because we had inadequate information to work with, because the available diagnoses disagreed considerably from one another, or because they had definite nonpsychotic DSM-III diagnoses.

The result of this classification was the formation of three diagnostic groups and two nonpsychotic control groups. These are summarized in Table 7-1.

PREDICTOR VARIABLES

We wanted to know whether measures that had differentiated children of ill parents from children of parents who were not ill would also predict future pathology. That is, did children who later showed pathology look different as children from those who did not show pathology?

Our criterion for using a particular psychological test variable as a potential predictor was that the variable had yielded significant group differences when children at risk had been compared with children of nonpsychotic parents, either in our own work or in reports by other investigators.

The data from the initial psychological assessment that we used as predictor variables were the nine variables discussed above: intelligence (verbal, performance, and full-scale IQ) from the IQ tests; the accuracy, DL, and primitive Rorschach content factor scores, all from the Rorschach; the TAT aggression factor score; the Beery DQ; and finally the psychologists' ratings from a review of the entire battery (pathology).

In addition to these nine quantitative variables, we set up four coded variables to represent the diagnostic group each child's parent

Table 7-1. Parental Diagnoses, Number of Families, and Number of Offspring

Parental diagnosis	n	
	Families	Offspring
Children of parents with schizophrenic disorders (CSZ)		
1. Schizophrenic disorder, paranoid type	3	7
2. Schizophrenic disorder, residual type	4	11
3. Schizophreniform disorder	1	2
4. (Acute) paranoid disorder; paranoia	6	14
Total	14	34
Children of parents with affective disorders (CAFFD)		
5. Major depression with melancholia	2	5
6. Major depression, single episode	2	7
7. Bipolar disorder	5	10
8. Atypical depression	1	4
9. Cyclothymic disorder	1	1
Total	11	27
Children of parents with schizoaffective disorders (CSZAF)		
10. Major depression with psychotic features; schizoaffective disorder	6	17
11. Atypical depression	3	9
Total	9	26
Children of nonpsychotic parents		
12. Physical illness	18	43
13. Normal	38	93
Total	56	136

belonged to. These variables and the assigned values on them are given in Table 7-2. We set up these variables so that we could determine whether a parent's diagnosis predicted his or her child's later mental health. Additionally, we included three demographic variables—socioeconomic status (SES; Hollingshead, 1957), race, and age at the time of our follow-up evaluation—again, for the purpose of determining whether any of these would be related to a child's mental health.

Table 7-2. Coded Variables Representing Parental Diagnoses

Parent diagnosis	Coded variables			
	"Risk"	"CSZ"	"CAFFD"	"CSZAF"
Schizophrenia	1	1	0	0
Affective disorder	1	0	1	0
Schizoaffective disorder	1	0	0	1
Physical illness	−1	0	0	0
Control	−1	0	0	0

Note. Abbreviations in Table 7-1.

OUTCOME VARIABLES

Our problem in determining an outcome variable was to find a single score for each child in our sample that represented that child's overall mental health. With several hundred scores for each child to choose from, this was not an easy task. We present here a detailed explanation of and rationale for how we derived a score for each child, which we labeled "mental health." Some readers may wish to skip this section, in which case they should turn to "Design of Analyses," below. The intrepid are invited to read on.

We derived our outcome measure of mental health from our second assessment of the offspring conducted between 1975 and 1978, when the offspring averaged 16 years of age. This assessment included a wide variety of measures, including assessment of intelligence, psychopathology, social behaviors, and family relationships, garnered from self-report questionnaires and from individual ratings on each child provided by psychologists, parents, and teachers. The specific tests used and the way the data were combined are quite complicated and are described in detail here.

Repeated Tests
Several of the tests used during this second assessment of the offspring were repeated in substantially the same form as used during the first assessment, and do not require detailed explanation. The repeated tests included the Beery, the TAT, and the Rorschach. However, as an economy measure, the TAT and the Rorschach were shortened, with only five cards of each test being used during the second assessment.[3]

3. The TAT cards were 1, 2, 3BM, 7GF, and 8BM. The Rorschach cards used during the second assessment were I, II, IV, VII, and IX. We have determined that the DL score derived from the short Rorschach is highly correlated with the DL score derived in the traditional way ($r = .91$) (J. T. Beck & Worland, 1983).

Another small change from the first to the second assessment was the use of the Wechsler Intelligence Scale for Children—Revised (WISC-R; Wechsler, 1974) for those children less than 16 years of age during the assessment period. The older children received the Wechsler Adult Intelligence Scale (WAIS; Wechsler, 1955).

New Assessments

The focus of the assessment of children had broadened considerably from the first testing, as the research group developed an interest in gathering information about the actual behavioral functioning of our risk sample. For this reason, each child and each parent completed a General Information Questionnaire (GIQ; Janes, Gilpin, Lander, & Finn, 1975), an instrument designed to obtain specific information regarding the life patterns of offspring, with parallel forms for offspring and their parents. The GIQ is a pencil-and-paper test that is self-administered; it covers such areas as job and/or school functioning, family relationship, patterns of friendship, leisure-time activities, participation in peer group and community affairs, physical and mental health, and religious life. A majority of the questions are multiple-choice.

The Rochester Adaptive Behavior Inventory (RABI; Jones, 1977) is a structured interview administered to mothers about each child's academic, social, symptomatic, and family relationship behaviors. There are in excess of 120 questions on this protocol, with multiple-choice answers. The questions are slightly different in content from one child age to another. The style of interview is informal, with the interviewer asking questions as written but following up with multiple probes until the interviewer is satisfied that he or she understands the correct alternative and assigns an answer accordingly. Preliminary test–retest reliability was extremely high when raters listened to tape-recorded interviews and made independent ratings.

A measure of psychopathology included in the reassessment of offspring was the Minnesota Multiphasic Personality Inventory (MMPI; Hathaway & McKinney, 1942), which was completed by each child who was aged 16 years or older at the time of the follow-up assessment. The data that we included in the analyses reported below were the uncorrected T scores on the clinical scales, deleting any records from offspring who had invalid protocols (as determined by T scores greater than 70 on any of the validation scales).

Three forms completed by teachers on each child were used to collect information about behavior in school. These forms were the Devereux Elementary School Behavior Rating Scale (DESB; Spivack & Swift, 1967) for children who were in eighth grade or below at the time of this assessment, or the Hahnemann High School Behavior Rating

Scale (HHSB; Spivack & Swift, 1971) for children in high school. These two instruments include a wide variety of behavioral and academic items that a teacher is asked to respond to on clearly delineated, numerical scales. The individual items are combined into "factors," which are domains of behaviors that were of interest to the creators of the scales. In addition, each teacher was requested to fill out the Pupil Rating Form (PRF; Watt, Grubb, & Erlenmeyer-Kimling, 1982) for each child. The PRF is a pencil-and-paper task for teachers that asks them to select the best point along a bipolar scale that describes a particular child. For example, a behavior labeled "cooperation" is represented by a 5-point scale from "compliant" at one end to "negativistic" at the other end, and the teacher is asked to select the point between these two anchors that best describes the particular child.

One additional academic achievement assessment was the Wide Range Achievement Test (WRAT; Jastak, Bijou, & Jastak, 1963), which contains a series of spelling items, mathematics problems, and word recognition items. The test yields a standard score analogous to an IQ score according to the norms published for the test.

Categorization

In order to categorize the 235 outcome scores available into a comprehensive scheme, we divided scores into four areas of functioning and into four sources of information. We categorized the sources of information into self-reports, parents' reports, psychologists' tests, and teachers' reports. We categorized the area of functioning into intelligence, psychopathology, social behavior, and family relationships. When this scheme was completed, we could draw a 4 × 4 table with 16 pigeonholes into which we sorted the 235 test items. The reader is referred to Tables 7-3 and 7-4, which should help illustrate what is described below. As a matter of fact, readers will probably not understand this unless they study Tables 7-3 and 7-4 carefully.

The assignment of items to cells was straightforward, with the possible exception of differentiating between items that properly belonged in the social behavior category and those that belonged in the psychopathology category. In general, we made this distinction by classifying external behaviors into the social behavior cells while assigning to the psychopathology cells those items that apparently related more to internal states such as anxiety, mood problems, or disturbances in somatopsychological functioning (e.g., sleep disturbance).

Of the 16 available pigeonholes depicted in Table 7-3, 3 are empty because some sources could provide no information for them. The empty spaces were psychologists' reports of social behavior and family relationships, and teachers' reports of family relationships.

In order to create a single score for each subject in each of the 13

Table 7-3. Classification of Outcome Variables by Domain and Source, and Tests Contributing to Each Cell

Source	Intelligence	Psychopahtology	Social behavior	Family relations
Self	GIQ (Cell 1)	GIQ (Cell 2)	GIQ (Cell 3)	GIQ (Cell 4)
Parent	RABI (Cell 5)	RABI, GIQ (Cell 6)	RABI, GIQ (Cell 7)	RABI, GIQ (Cell 8)
Psychologist	WRAT, Beery, Wechsler (Cell 9)	Rorschach, TAT, MMPI (Cell 10)	(No data)	(No data)
Teacher	DESB, HHSB, PRF (Cell 13)	DESB, HHSB, PRF (Cell 14)	DESB, HHSB, PRF (Cell 15)	(No data)

Note. GIQ, General Information Questionnaire; RABI, Rochester Adaptive Behavior Inventory; WRAT, Wide Range Achievement Test; Beery, Beery–Buktenika Developmental Form Sequence; Wechsler, WAIS or WISC-R; TAT, Thematic Apperception Test; MMPI, Minnesota Multiphasic Personality Inventory; DESB, Devereux Elementary School Behavior Rating Scale; HHSB, Hahnemann High School Behavior Rating Scale; PRF, Pupil Rating Form.

Table 7-4. Examples of Variables in Each Cell (with Multiple-Choice Answers)

Variable	Source
Self-report	
Cell 1. *Intelligence* (2 items) "In general, how were [or are] your grades?" (A/B/C/D/F.)	GIQ
Cell 2. *Psychopathology* (47 items) "Have you ever had any of these symptoms . . . tiredness much of the time?" (This year/before/never.)	GIQ
Cell 3. *Social behavior* (32 items) "Have you ever been suspended or expelled [from school]?"	GIQ
Cell 4. *Family relationships* (19 items) "In the past year, have you and your parents argued (more than/the same as/less than) before?"	GIQ
Parent report	
Cell 5. *Intelligence* (6 items) "Does you child have trouble in reading? What is the problem?" (Yes, it is a major problem./Yes, he is a relatively slow reader./Not particularly./No, he reads well.)	RABI

Table 7-4. Continued

Variable		Source
	Parent-report	
Cell 6.	*Psychopathology* (20 items) "Have you ever heard your child say he/she was going to kill himself/herself?"	GIQ
	"Does your child have nightmares often?" (Yes, fre- quently, almost nightly; *or* a period during the pre- vious year of night terrors./Yes, perhaps a few times a week or more frequently over a short period of time./Occasionally./No.)	RABI
Cell 7.	*Social behavior* (26 items) "Does your child use drugs?" (Never/rarely/occasion- ally/frequently/often.)	GIQ
	"Does your child get into fights and quarrels more often than other kids at school?" (Yes, daily, a major problem./Yes, fairly often [weekly]./Occasionally, if pushed hard./Rarely, only if he cannot avoid it./Al- most never.)	RABI
Cell 8.	*Family relationships* (24 items) Same example as for Cell 4, phrased for parent.	GIQ
	"How often do you and your child get a chance to sit down and have a good talk together?" (Often, at least one a week./Occasionally, in the course of a month./ Seldom, a few times a year./Rarely, if ever.)	
	Clinical psychologist report	
Cell 9.	*Intelligence* (5 items) Reading, spelling, arithmetic standard scores Full-scale IQ Visual–motor integration	WRAT WAIS or WISC-R Beery
Cell 10.	*Psychopathology* (19 items) Extended F+% Constructive coping (number of stories in which con- structive solution to problem is given)[a] Mean of 10 uncorrected clinical scales	Rorschach TAT MMPI
	Teacher report	
Cell 13.	*Intelligence* (6 items) Comprehension Reasoning ability Achievement	DESB HHSB PRF
Cell 14.	*Psychopathology* (10 items) Inattentive–withdrawn General anxiety Mood	DESB HHSB PRF
Cell 15.	*Social behavior* (18 items) Classroom disturbance Verbal negativism Conduct	DESB HHSB PRF

Note. See Table 7-3 for explanation of abbreviations.

[a]See Worland *et al.* (1979) for explanation.

pigeonholes, we first transformed each available variable, if necessary, so that high scores would indicate competence or absence of symptoms. For example, some of the tests are designed so that high scores represent mental health or competence (e.g., intelligence) while others give high scores for mental illness (e.g., the MMPI). So we reversed some scores so that the high scores uniformly reflected mental health.

The next step was to transform each available variable in each cell into its z-score equivalent so that every score would have a mean of 0 and a standard deviation of 1. The purpose of this was to allow us to average scores from various tests. When tests are transformed into standard scores, they become comparable to one another, in much the same way as converting between metric and English systems of measurement allows comparisons to be made. Finally, we computed a cell score for each subject by averaging all of his or her available (transformed) scores in each of the 13 pigeonholes. We used all of the available data. If the particular offspring had less than complete data in one section, we computed an average score for that cell using all of the data available for that cell.

Where we had been heading with all this was to get one score for each child, and our last step was to compute the summary score, "mental health," for each offspring by averaging these 13 scores.

VALIDITY

A question that needs to be addressed about the mental health score we devised in the way just explained is whether it is a *valid* measure. There are several ways to answer this.

First, we can ask whether the measure has "construct validity." That is, does the way it has been derived validly relate to the concept that we are trying to measure? The concept of mental health has been defined by a number of researchers as a global feature that encompasses many subsidiary concepts, such as social competence (Rolf, 1972), or, to use Peterson and Kellam's (1977) term, "social adaptational status"; personal competence, which we have measured by such items as symptoms of illness; and academic competence, which we have indexed both in terms of actual grades and intellectual test performance. Consequently, we conclude that our measure of mental health reflects components of good personal and academic functioning.

Secondly, we can ask whether our measure has "concurrent validity." That is, does the mental health score relate to measures of similar constructs that supposedly measure the same thing? Ideally, this should be determined in a variety of different groups of individuals, which are not available to us at this point.

Within our own sample, though, we have available a measure of disturbance that can be checked for concordance with our mental health measure. This other measure is a Psychiatric Treatment Index that was assigned to each child. If children had received no mental health treatment, they were assigned on the Index a score of 0; if outpatient treatment only, a score of 1; and if inpatient, a score of 2. Theoretically, we could expect a significant negative correlation between the Psychiatric Treatment Index and the mental health measure (i.e., *high* scores on the Treatment Index should be associated with *low* scores on the mental health measure).

The correlation between these two measures ($r -.17$, $p < .001$) indicates that there is, indeed, an association in the expected direction between the two measures. The strength of the association, however, is weak, which can be explained by noting that factors other than a child's mental health might have entered into the decision to receive treatment (e.g., a family's tolerance for deviance, medical insurance coverage, or social stigma against treatment), and that many of the individuals who were identified as having poor mental health (i.e., low scores on the mental health measure) might not yet have received treatment. That is, the correlation between these two measures may increase as the children get older and have more opportunity to have received treatment.

In summary, we conclude that our mental health measure has construct validity and some limited evidence of concurrent validity.

DESIGN OF ANALYSES

Our goal was to determine whether any of the nine scores from the psychological tests that had been administered earlier in the lives of these children could reliably predict their later mental health scores, over and above any predictions we could make simply from parent diagnosis or family demographic characteristics alone. That is, could psychological testing predict who would be mentally healthy or unhealthy? We selected multiple regression as our method to answer these questions. What follows now is an explanation of the mechanics of multiple regression, which is not for everyone, but should make the results below more interpretable. If understanding statistics is not of concern to readers, they should skip to the "Results" section.

Before a regression procedure can begin, there must be a set of potentially predictive items, called "predictor variables" (in this case, our nine psychological variables from childhood, plus the parental diagnostic and family demographic variables), and a single outcome or "criterion variable" (in this case, mental health). The investigator prepares for the regression procedure by correlating (determining the degree of relationship between) each potential predictor variable and the criterion variable. (This degree of relationship is labeled "simple r" in the tables. Correlations, or "simple r's," vary between +1 [meaning perfect association], through 0 [meaning no association], to −1 [meaning perfect negative association].) In addition, the correlations or degrees of relationship that the predictors all have among themselves are also computed.

The regression procedure is begun by selecting the single predictor out of the list of potential predictors that is most highly associated (has the highest "simple r") with the criterion under study. It may be selected from the entire available group of predictors, or, if the researcher wishes, it may be selected from a limited set of predictors, in which case the procedure is called a "restricted stepwise regression procedure."

The procedure is called "stepwise" because it proceeds in sequential steps. When the first actual predictor is selected, it is removed from the list of potential predictors. This predictor explains (or accounts for) a portion of the variance in the criterion (in this case, in mental health), but not all of it. That is, the predictor partially (but not completely) explains why some individuals have high scores on the criterion (mental health) and others have low scores. The second step of the regression procedure selects a second predictor that explains (or accounts for) that portion of the variance remaining unexplained in the criterion (mental health) after the first step. When this second predictor is moved from the list of potential predictors to the list of actual predictors, the researcher has two predictors, a list of potential predictors (the original list minus the two selected), a measure of the variance in the criterion variable we have explained (called in the jargon its "squared multiple correlation," and listed in the tables as R^2), and a portion of variance still unexplained.

This procedure is repeated as more predictors are added one at a time to the list of actual predictors, with each predictor adding to the amount of variance in the criterion variable explained (i.e., with its squared multiple correlation gradually increasing). A point is reached finally when more predictors do not appreciably increase the squared multiple correlation; that is, more predictors will not account for more of the variance in the criterion. At this point the procedure is stopped.

When a regression procedure is complete, the final product is a "regression equation." The equation shows how the investigator can add together each selected predictor score (now linked with its own multiplier coefficient, called its "beta weight") to determine as closely as possible the criterion variable. Comparing the beta weight coefficients of the variable to one another provides a way of determining the relative importance of each predictor in computing the criterion. Predictors with large beta weights are more important in the prediction than are those with small beta weights.

The last detail is that the usefulness of final regression equation is determined by how large its R^2 is (i.e., how close to 1 it is), which is a measure of how much of the variance in the criterion can be explained (in this case, how perfectly high scores or low scores in mental health can be predicted). Also, the researcher can test the probability of whether the prediction equation chosen by this procedure is (or is not) based completely on a fluke of chance. This measure, called the "probability" of the equation, is abbreviated in the tables below as p. Generally, p's less than .05 (less than 5 chances in 100 of being a fluke) are considered statistically reliable (i.e., very unlikely to be based on chance).

For our prediction of mental health scores, we used a restricted stepwise regression procedure, wherein the parental diagnostic variables were selected first, family demographic variables were selected second, and psychological variables were selected third. We gave a higher priority to parental diagnosis and demographic variables because they indicated conditions in existence prior to the time we had administered the psychological tests. This assignment also provided a more conservative test of the hypothesis that the psychological variables would be predictive of later mental health, because it would show their ability to predict over and above the parents' illness or demographic variables alone.

It is well known by statisticians that multiple regression, particularly stepwise multiple regression, is somewhat unstable. Often results cannot be replicated because the procedure is sensitive to accidental characteristics specific to a single sample. To ameliorate this problem, we divided the total sample into two similar subsamples and computed separate regression analyses on each half. At each step, we retained only those predictors that were reliably predictive of mental health in both subsamples, using a very broad standard of significance in judging reliability ($p < .25$). That is, for these subsample regressions, we only required that there be less than 25% probability of a predictor's being selected by chance. Finally, we used the retained predictors in a regression analysis on the full samples, to obtain the most stable estimates of regression coefficients (beta weights) possible, using a more rigorous and traditional p level ($p < .05$, or less than a 5% probability of being selected by chance).

Results

We found in the first subsample, when the analysis was constrained to select only parental diagnostic variables, that having a schizophrenic parent or having a parent with schizoaffective illness was a significant predictor of mental health (Table 7-5). Children in these two groups both had *lower* mental health scores than other children. Among the

Table 7-5. Summary of Regression Analysis: Relationship of Predictor Variables to
Mental Health in Sample 1 and Sample 2

Variables considered[a] (and order)	Sample 1		Sample 2	
	r	Beta	r	Beta
Parental diagnostic variables				
CSZ	−.156	−.243	−.216	−.178
CAFFD				
CSZAF	−.091	−.195		
Risk				
Demographic variables				
SES[b]	−.291	−.006		
Age	−.010	+.127		
Race	−.070	+.132	−.212	−.139
Psychological variables				
Verbal IQ	+.363	+.245	+.348	+.180
Performance IQ				
Full-scale IQ				
Beery DQ	+.434	+.438	+.372	+.224
Extended F+%	−.086	−.151		
Pathology				
Primitive Rorschach content			+.075	+.138
TAT aggression				
Rorschach DL				

[a]Variables with no numerical entries were not related to later mental health.
[b]On SES, higher scores denote lower SES (Hollingshead, 1957).

demographic variables, the family's SES was a significant predictor: Lower-SES children had lower scores on the mental health factor. There was also a slight tendency for older offspring and black children to receive lower scores. In the second subsample, parental schizophrenia and race were significant predictors. Therefore, we retained only parental schizophrenia and race for our subsequent analyses.

In the next step, we wanted to know what psychological variables were important after parental diagnosis and race were accounted for. So, we "forced" parental schizophrenia and race into the analysis first and then allowed the psychological variables to enter. The result was that the Beery DQ and the Verbal IQ were significant in both samples, and were therefore retained. Children with high scores on these tests had higher mental health scores. In addition, accuracy from the Rorschach was a significant predictor in Sample 1 only and primitive Rorschach content was a significant predictor in Sample 2 only, and so both were dropped.

Thus, only four predictors were consistently related to mental health in both samples: parental schizophrenia, race, Beery DQ, and verbal IQ. Finally, we used these four as predictors of mental health for the combined sample, yielding a squared multiple correlation (R^2) of .237, F (3, 232) = 19.65, $p < .005$. That is, these four variables could together predict 23.7% of the variance in mental health, and the probability of selecting these variables by accident was less than 5 in 1,000. Actually, in the combined sample, race was unable to add to the predictive power of the other three variables, and so we concluded that race did not predict mental health. (See Table 7-6 for this summary.)

Discussion

Many issues need addressing before we can conclude that the findings of this investigation suggest that knowing a child's scores on psychometric instruments might really help predict who will later show good mental health (and who will not). The issues that we address here are, first, the limitations and strengths of our mental health score; second, the sample limitations, which affect the generalizations that we are able to make; and third, procedural and methodological limitations and strengths. We conclude with some general comments on the nature of prediction, especially the prediction of psychobehavioral functioning.

As derived, our mental health score presents some issues that the cautious reader should consider before making conclusions from our findings. For example, we used an *a priori* (as opposed to empirical) method for assigning particular test items to the 13 domains, which we then totaled and averaged to derive the summary mental health score for each child. Using such constructed factors involved several assumptions. We assumed that items that we pigeonholed into particular cells really did belong with one another. Furthermore, by using a process of averaging (both within individual pigeonholes, and finally among all the

Table 7-6. Summary Regression Procedure for Whole Sample, Simple Correlations, and Beta Weights of Predictors of Mental Health

Predictor	Simple r	Beta	Cumulative R^2
Beery DQ	+.414	+.311	.172
Verbal IQ	+.366	+.216	.209
CSZ	−.175	−.168	.237

pigeonholes together), we assumed that the items we average had equal importance. For example, it would make sense to average a child's verbal and nonverbal IQs to arrive at a summary intelligence quotient. However, it would not make sense to average a child's allowance and his parents' weekly income to arrive at an index of the family's SES. To do so would put a value too great on allowance and weaken the value of the parents' income as an index of the measure that would be derived.

Nevertheless, the process that we employed granted equal weight to the items within particular areas of interest (academic, behavioral, symptomatic, and familial) and, even more importantly, to the different respondents whose information we combined (self, parent, psychologist, teacher). Thus, for example, we decided that a child's own self-report should count the same as the parent's report in evaluating performance. For that matter, we also weighted equally a child's own report about his or her performance in school with the teacher's report. It could be argued that a teacher should be able to give more valid information about this particular area than a child would.

With these limitations, what are the alternatives? One commonly used alternative is to derive empirical factors rather than to design rational ones. The most common method for deriving empirical factors is factor analysis, in which the actual relationship among various variables is taken into account and factors are composed in such a way as to capture as much of the shared (common) variance among the variables as possible into separate (usually independent) factors that are presumed to underlie the actual scores obtained. If this had been done in the present situation, it is likely that we would have created a different measure of mental health than we did.

Are there any benefits to employing rational factors? The greatest benefit in the use of rational factors is that rational factors are in no way bound by accidental (rather than real) relationships among the actual variables that happen to have been sampled. When a group of variables is assessed in a certain sample, some relationships among variables will be real, and other variables, which appear to be highly associated, will only be accidentally correlated. Employing an empirical (factor-analytic) approach capitalizes on these accidental relationships between variables, and thus factor-analytic results tend to be highly unstable. That is, they do not replicate well when different samples are employed. On the other hand, the rational factors used here did not capitalize on such chance factors within a particular sample.

Additionally, the issue of whether it was correct to average all 13 cells in our matrix to derive the mental health score, which assumed that they were all equally important, may be a moot point. As a matter of fact, the cell scores were highly correlated with one another; consequently, if they had been weighted (e.g., by giving more importance to teacher reports than self-reports), the resulting mental health score would have been very similar to the one we actually derived.

We conclude, then, that our mental health score is a strong measure of competence and one that is not dependent on accidental sampling characteristics in the particular group of children that we happen to be following.

This leads us to other characteristics of our sample that the cautious reader will want to consider. It would not be appropriate to generalize the results of this study to all children of psychotic parents, and especially not to children of psychotic parents who might come in contact with mental health workers (e.g., in a child guidance clinic). First, we selected only intact families at the time the study began, so generalizations to nonintact families are questionable. Presumably, other factors in nonintact families could have much more importance in predicting later disturbance than the particular psychometric properties we isolated here. Also, the families that we studied and that were available for follow-up all had some willingness to participate in an extremely rigorous investigation over many years' time; this is certainly not a characteristic of many families that arrive at the door of the neighborhood child guidance clinic. In addition, the children that we evaluated early in their lives were, by and large, showing no overt signs of disturbance, although a few were. Children in a child guidance clinic sample, on the other hand, will almost universally be showing signs of disturbance. Consequently, caution must be employed before assuming that these particular signs of psychometric functioning are good markers of later development in other samples.

The statistical procedure that we employed, and the way that we employed it, however, lead us to have some faith in the conclusions to which our process led us, subject to the limitations mentioned. Dividing the sample into two comparable subsamples and applying the multiple-regression procedure separately in each had the same effect as developing a hypothesis on the basis of the first multiple regression and confirming the hypothesis by means of the second multiple regression. Finding that the Beery DQ, verbal IQ, and parental schizophrenia in each sample correlated with later mental health provided strong evidence that these measures of functioning and parental illness are indeed associated with how well children function in their adolescent and young adult lives. Of course, as has been pointed out by McNeil and Kaij (1979), predicting future functioning at this particular point in the lives of children at risk is suggestive but certainly not conclusive evidence of what may occur in the future. For example, while we might hope that the offspring who were exhibiting high mental health at this particular time will maintain their pre-eminence, it would be irrational to conclude that none of these offspring will later be psychotic themselves. The data prove nothing about how well the particular children who had high scores on the mental health measure will themselves function as they progress through adulthood. Only further investigation of this sample will answer that question.

What of the predictors we isolated? To a clinician performing psychological evaluations of children, cognitive measures of functioning (intelligence and visual–motor coordination) by themselves usually do not sway the clinician to make assumptions either about mental health or about mental illness. It is much more likely that the clinician will make those assumptions from and be swayed by projective test measures. Cognitive measures (at least in terms of the summary scores used in this investigation) are considered as facilitators for a particular child to overcome problems seen in the projective tests. For example, a child with blatantly pathological projective test performance who has low intelligence would be considered by many clinicians to be more at risk than a child with pathological projective measures but fair to good intelligence. The latter child would be assumed to have a higher range of coping mechanisms, more likelihood of achieving competently in his or her major life occupation (school), and more ability to benefit from psychotherapeutic experiences and thus to work out the problems that the projective tests might imply. However, even in making these assumptions, most clinicians would not give very much importance to the measure of visual–motor coordination. It was a surprise, therefore, that the Beery DQ, a measure of visual–motor coordination, explained alone so much of the variance in later mental health functioning, at least as indexed in this investigation.

The meaning of high (or low) scores on the Beery has several possible interpretations. At a most descriptive level, good functioning merely means that a child has mastered the complex tasks of visual perception, visual analysis, small muscle coordination, and self-scrutiny of his or her own performance, and manages to coordinate all of these skills into one smooth-flowing procedure. Things that interfere with good Beery performance and cause poor visual–motor coordination include inadequate visual perception, poor motor control, impulsivity, carelessness, and an incautious approach to the task. Since erasures are not allowed on this test, a child either does well on the first try or fails an item.

It has been found that adult schizophrenics do poorly on tests of visual–motor coordination. Whether this is due to a neurological interference in their performance or can be linked more specifically to a particular aspect of personality functioning seems unclear. Taking the hypothesis that visual perception is the culprit in the lower performance of adult schizophrenics on visual–motor coordination tasks, we have some corroborating information from the Rorschach performance of adult schizophrenics. On this test, which requires visual perception (like the Beery) but does not require motor control (unlike the Beery), adult schizophrenics usually perform in a way that is considered to be less perceptually mature than normal adults, even when differences in social class or intelligence are taken into consideration (Lerner, 1968).

This might lead the reader to be tempted to conclude that the reason we found a good prediction of later mental health from a child's earlier visual–motor test performance may be that the Beery tapped one emerging aspect of the psychometric test performance of later psychotics. Thus, this reasoning would continue, we isolated a group of future psychotics who had low scores on the Beery, and as future schizophrenics, they exhibited poorer mental health in adolescence. There are two fallacies lurking in this argument.

First, we have no evidence that our poorly functioning adolescents will later be schizophrenic (or that the better-functioning ones are immune). Second, our most rational and parsimonious interpretation of differences in mental health must be environmental rather than genetic. That is, it is far more likely that differences in mental health are the result of disturbances in family environmental factors than that they are the result of emerging psychosis. Again, not until we successfully follow these same individuals into their adult lives will we know whether we have been identifying genetic markers (which is probably unlikely) or have been finding psychometric signs of poor family functioning or some other nongenetic contributor to disturbance.

While our reasoning may seem extremely cautious, let us point out a possible pathway. If parents are concerned about the development of their offspring (either in families with a psychotic parent or otherwise), and thereby interact with their children in a way that teaches impulse control, pride in workmanship, and maintenance of attention on a particular task, it is likely that we are going to observe better visual–motor coordination from the children in these families than in other families. Furthermore, if the same families are interested in reading and read to the children or otherwise stimulate the children's verbal skills, we are likely to see higher verbal scores for these children on the intelligence test. These same families are likely to produce competent, self-confident, and well-functioning adolescents. Consequently, the whole relationship that we have identified between childhood indicators and later functioning could easily, and as a matter of fact most likely, be explained by family environmental variables, with no need to assume any individual genetic predisposition toward competence (or mental illness, for that matter). That SES alone did not predict later mental health scores implies that family relationship variables (which admittedly were hypothesized here but not directly observed) are more important than class membership. This is certainly a hopeful but testable theory (Caldwell & Bradley, no date).

One final comment is in order. Of all individual attributes, the most stable is intelligence. Although there is certainly considerable variability in measures of intellectual performance that an individual may display at different points in life, this disparity is nothing in comparison to the disparity that a person may show in behavioral functioning, emotional tone, mood, or any other attribute of psychological functioning. In this context, it consequently becomes more understandable why cognitive measures, rather than projective test measures, proved to be the most predictive of later mental health. That is, the particular component of mental health that is easiest to predict is the cognitive component. Furthermore, it is understandable that earlier cognitive ability will predict later cognitive ability. For this reason, it may be most reasonable to assume that the relationship that we have identified is a relationship between earlier cognitive competence (indexed by the Beery DQ and verbal IQ) and later cognitive competence (indexed by mental health). As the reader will recall, we were successful in explaining only 23.7% of the variance in our mental health measure, and we submit that the other 76% of the variance (less an amount attributable to error) probably contains the less cognitive and more affective components of good mental health functioning.

ACKNOWLEDGMENTS

This research was supported by National Institute of Mental Health Research Grants No. MH-12043 and No. MH-24819. The assistance of the staff of the Harry Edison Child Development Research Center is greatly appreciated, especially the help of Janice Hensiek in preparing this manuscript.

REFERENCES

American Psychiatric Association. (1980). *Diagnostic and statistical manual of mental disorders* (3rd ed.). Washington, DC: Author.

Beck, J. T., & Worland, J. (1983). Rorschach developmental level and its relationship to subsequent psychiatric treatment. *Journal of Personality Assessment, 47*, 238–242.

Beck, S., Beck, A., Levitt, E., & Molish, H. (1961). *Rorschach's test: I. Basic processes.* New York: Grune & Stratton.

Becker, W. (1956). Genetic approach to the interpretation and evaluation of the process-reactive distinction in schizophrenia. *Journal of Abnormal and Social Psychology, 53*, 229–236.

Beery, K. E. (1967). *Developmental Test of Visual–Motor Integration: Administration and scoring manual.* Chicago: Follett.

Beisser, A., Glasser, N., & Grant, M. (1967). Psychosocial adjustment in children of schizophrenic mothers. *Journal of Nervous and Mental Disease, 145*, 429–440.

Bleuler, M. (1974). The offspring of schizophrenics. *Schizophrenia Bulletin, 8*, 93–107.

Caldwell, B. M., & Bradley, R. H. (no date). *Home observations for the measurement of the environment.* (Available from the Center for Child Development and Education, 33rd and University Avenue, Little Rock, AR 72204)

Cass, L. (1973). *Manual for ratings from psychological evaluation.* Unpublished manual.

Cohen, J. A. (1960). A coefficient of agreement for nominal scales. *Educational and Psychological Measurement, 20*, 37–46.

Cohler, B., Grunebaum, H., Weiss, J., Gamber, E., & Gallant, D. (1977). Disturbance of attention among schizophrenic, depressed and well mothers and their young children. *Journal of Child Psychology and Psychiatry, 18*, 115–135.

Cowie, V. (1961). The incidence of neurosis in the children of psychotics. *Acta Psychiatrica Scandinavica, 37*, 37–87.

Friedman, H. (1952). Perceptual regression in schizophrenics: An hypothesis suggested by use of Rorschach's test. *Journal of Genetic Psychology, 81*, 63–98.

Hanson, D. R., Gottesman, I. I., & Heston, L. (1976). Some possible childhood indicators of adult schizophrenia inferred from children of schizophrenics. *British Journal of Psychiatry, 129*, 142–154.

Hanson, D. R., Gottesman, I. I., & Meehl, P. E. (1977). Genetic theories and the validation of psychiatric diagnoses: Implications for the study of children of schizophrenics. *Journal of Abnormal Psychology, 86*, 575–588.

Hathaway, S. R., & McKinney, J. C. (1942). *The Minnesota Multiphasic Personality Inventory.* Minneapolis: University of Minnesota Press.

Hertz, M. (1961). *Frequency tables for scoring Rorschach responses* (4th ed.). Beverly Hills, CA: Western Psychological Services.

Heston, L. L. (1966). Psychiatric disorders in foster home reared children of schizophrenic mothers. *British Journal of Psychiatry, 112*, 819–825.

Higgins, J. (1966). Effects of child rearing by schizophrenic mothers. *Journal of Psychiatric Research, 4*, 153–167.

Hollingshead, A. B. (1957). *The two-factor index of social position.* Unpublished manuscript, Yale University.

Janes, C. L., Gilpin, D., Lander, H., & Finn, S. (1975). *The General Information Questionnaire.* Unpublished manuscript.

Jastak, J. F., Bijou, S. W., & Jastak, S. R. (1963). *The Wide Range Achievement Test.* Wilmington, DE: Guidance Associates.

Jones, F. H. (1977). The Rochester Adaptive Behavior Inventory: A parallel series of instruments for assessing social competence during early and middle childhood and adolescence. In J. S. Strauss, H. M. Babigian, & M. Roff (Eds.), *The origins and course of psychopathology.* New York: Plenum Press.

Lerner, P. M. (1968). Correlation of social competence and level of cognitive perceptual functioning in male schizophrenics. *Journal of Nervous and Mental Disease, 146*, 412–416.

McNeil, T. F., & Kaij, L. (1979). Etiological relevance of comparisons of high-risk and low-risk groups. *Acta Psychiatrica Scandinavica, 59*, 545–560.

Mednick, S. A., Schulsinger, F. (1968). Some premorbid characteristics related to breakdown in children with schizophrenic mothers. In D. Rosenthal & S. Kety (Eds.), *The transmission of schizophrenia.* Oxford: Pergamon Press.

Murray, H. (1943). *Thematic Apperception Test manual.* Los Angeles: Western Psychological Services.

Petersen, A. C., & Kellam, S. G. (1977). Measurement of the psychological well-being of adolescents: The psychometric properties and assessment procedures of the How I Feel. *Journal of Youth and Adolescence, 6*, 229–248.

Rolf, J. E. (1972). The social and academic competence of children vulnerable to schizophrenia and other behavior pathologies. *Journal of Abnormal Psychology, 80*, 225–243.

Schulsinger, H. (1976). A ten-year follow-up of children of schizophrenic mothers. *Acta Psychiatrica Scandinavica, 53*, 371–386.

Spivack, G., & Swift, M. (1967). *Devereux Elementary School Behavior Rating Scale.* Devon, PA: Devereux Foundation.

Spivack, G., & Swift, M. (1971). *Hahnemann High School Behavior Rating Scale.* Philadelphia: Hahnemann Medical College.

Watt, N. F., Grubb, T. W., & Erlenmeyer-Kimling, L. (1982). Social, emotional, and intellectual behavior at school among children at high risk for schizophrenia. *Journal of Consulting and Clinical Psychology, 50*, 171–181.

Wechsler, D. (1949). *The Wechsler Intelligence Scale for Children.* New York: Psychological Corp.

Wechsler, D. (1955). *The Wechsler Adult Intelligence Scale.* New York: Psychological Corp.

Wechsler, D. (1974). *Manual for the Wechsler Intelligence Scale for Children—Revised.* New York: Psychological Corp.

Weintraub, S., Neale, J., & Liebert, D. (1975). Teacher ratings of children vulnerable to psychopathology. *American Journal of Orthopsychiatry, 45*, 838–844.

Worland, J. (1980). Rorschach developmental level in children of patients with schizophrenia and affective illness. *Journal of Personality Assessment, 43*, 591–594.

Worland, J., & Hesselbrock, V. (1980). Intelligence of children and their parents with schizophrenia and affective illness. *Journal of Child Psychology and Psychiatry, 21*, 191–201.

Worland, J., Janes, C. L., Anthony, E. J., McGinnis, M., & Cass, L. (1984). St. Louis Risk Research Project: Comprehensive report of experimental studies. In N. F. Watt, E. J. Anthony, L. C. Wynne, & J. Rolf (Eds.), *Children at risk for schizophrenia: A longitudinal perspective.* Cambridge, England: Cambridge University Press.

Worland, J., Lander, H., & Hesselbrock, V. (1979). Psychological evaluation of clinical disturbance in children at risk for psychopathology. *Journal of Abnormal Psychology, 88*(1), 13–26.

Worland, J., Weeks, D., Weiner, S., & Schechtman, J. (1982). Longitudinal, prospective evaluation of intelligence of children at risk. *Schizophrenia Bulletin, 8*, 135–141.

8

Competent Children at Risk: A Study of Well-Functioning Offspring of Disturbed Parents

LAWRENCE FISHER
RONALD F. KOKES
University of California at San Francisco

ROBERT E. COLE
PATRICIA M. PERKINS
LYMAN C. WYNNE
University of Rochester

The study of the etiology of psychopathology and the study of the determinants of competence and health have developed in parallel but divergent courses. Although there is little question that the primary emphasis of most clinical research in the behavioral sciences has been on the study of the course and development of psychological disorder, interest in successful adults (Terman & Oden, 1947), in the roots of creativity (Maddi, Propst, & Feldinger, 1965), and in the factors that lead to successful outcome with respect to a variety of human problems and dilemmas is well documented (Escalona, 1965; Murphy & Moriarty, 1976).

The current shift in emphasis away from disease to health, from maladaptation to competence, is probably the result of a confluence of factors that have influenced the health sciences in the last two to three decades. First, medicine in general has shifted from an emphasis on infection epidemics and chronic disease and has entered what Evans (1982) has labeled a third phase, a period characterized by a focus on social and environmental pathology and a concern for health promotion and disease prevention. Second, greater focus on large-scale social and educational intervention programs has emphasized assisting individuals through normal developmental periods or crises. Such efforts have become commonplace, as evidenced by child rearing programs for new parents, sex education for adolescents, and retirement programs for aging Americans.

A third factor in the shift in emphasis from disease to health is the development of a variety of programs for populations at risk for particular forms of disability (e.g., Intagliata, 1978; Visher & Visher, 1979). The risk research paradigm has focused on identifying samples of individuals who are at high risk for disability but who, at the point of contact, are symptom-free. These individuals are then followed over time so that the precursors of disability can be identified, the development and course of the disability can be monitored, and outcome data can be related to a host of premorbid and morbid variables. The paradigm avoids the problem of retrospective analysis and provides a rich source of developmental data on both normal and pathological development (Garmezy with Streitman, 1974).

Interest in the risk paradigm as a strategy for studying pathology has had two interesting side effects. Rather than maintaining the focus on pathology and the etiology of disease alone, several risk researchers have now begun to focus on methods of preventing the disorder under study and are devoting considerable resources to areas of secondary prevention. For example, Watt, Shay, Grubb, and Riddle (1982) have intervened with emotionally vulnerable children in the school setting, using variables that were identified as contributory to negative outcome in previous studies. Likewise, Falloon, Boyd, McGill, Moss, and Guilderman (1982) have intervened using techniques of communications training in families of schizophrenics.

A second side effect of the risk paradigm—one of particular interest in the present context—is the growing awareness that, despite the presence of a number of risk indicators, a substantial percentage of individuals at risk for disorder manage to overcome their "handicaps" and to emerge with no diagnosable pathology. The presence of these groups was at one time viewed as a *negative* consequence of the risk research enterprise, because they reduced the percentage of subjects with diagnosable pathology, thus reducing the size of the sample on which potential etiological factors could be studied. Consequently, efforts were made to restrict the sample to those whose level of risk was inordinately high. Yet despite these efforts, these so-called "positive-outcome" subjects remained, in one sense confounding the etiological studies and in another sense drawing attention to the pervasive resiliency and fortitude of many individuals who are at risk.

In overview, it is apparent that the risk paradigm has provided a unique opportunity to study not only the development and course of pathology, but also those factors that influence health. Consequently, the conclusions that emerge from studies of individuals at risk for disorder have clear implications, not only in the area of vulnerability to disease, but also to that of coping, adaptation, and competence (broadly defined).

In this chapter, we present preliminary data from the University of Rochester Child and Family Study (URCAFS), a large-scale developmental study of approximately 145 families in which one adult member, usually the mother, was hospitalized for psychiatric disorder. In previous reports (Fisher, 1980; Fisher & Jones, 1980; Fisher & Kokes, 1980; Fisher, Kokes, Harder, & Jones, 1980; Harder, Kokes, Fisher, & Strauss, 1980; Kokes, Harder, Fisher, & Strauss, 1980), we have identified aspects of adult, family, and child functioning that have covaried with incompetence in the offspring. In the present report, we reverse the process of investigation and study the competent functioning of these high-risk offspring, in an effort to identify factors that can be associated with "positive outcome."

University of Rochester Child and Family Study

URCAFS is a programmatic research project comprised of groups of investigators with expertise in various aspects of child, adult, and family health and pathology, under the direction of Lyman C. Wynne. Patient records were gathered from various inpatient settings around Rochester, New York. These were matched with county birth records so as to identify those patients with male offspring who would be 4, 7, or 10 years of age at the time of the study. Male offspring were selected as index subjects because sample size precluded sex of child as a major study variable. Because school competence was selected as a major dependent–independent variable, only data on the 7- and 10-year-old samples are reported here.

The case record of each hospitalized adult was scanned to ensure that the disorder was functional with no evidence of chronic brain syndrome, that the family was living together, and that the family fell within socioeconomic class I to IV. The interval between last hospitalization and the study evaluation was an average of 3.9 years. DSM-III (*Diagnostic and Statistical Manual of Mental Disorders*, third edition) diagnoses were based upon clinical interviews, the World Health Organization (1973) Psychiatric History Scales, and the Case Record Rating Form (Strauss & Harder, 1980) for assessing social functioning and symptomatology. For the sake of consistency, only families in which the mother was the patient were included in the present analysis. The breakdown of patient families by age of child and diagnosis of mother is presented in Table 8-1.

Following identification and recruitment, each family spent approximately 40 hours over several weeks with the various research teams. The measures that were used included studies of psychophysiology; studies of family interaction; child and adult intellectual and projective evaluations; ratings of parental psychopathology, child functioning, and marital discord; measures of school competence and parent–child interaction; and a host of more specific measures of cognitive and emotional functioning. The project provided a comprehensive as-

Table 8-1. Diagnosis of Mother by Age of Index Child

Diagnosis	Age of child		Total
	7	10	
Schizophrenia	5	1	6
Schizoaffective disorder	3	4	7
Major depression	3	3	6
Bipolar psychotic disorder	5	12	17
Severe personality disorder	4	2	6
Moderate personality disorder	5	5	10
Depressive disorder with melancholia	1	5	6
Depressive disorder without melancholia	9	7	16
Bipolar nonpsychotic disorder	3	0	3
Totals	38	39	77

sessment of a range of behaviors that the literature had previously indicated to be potential contributors to outcome in these children at risk (Fisher & Jones, 1978), as well as measures to assess age-appropriate competencies for all family members. A limited number of these variables have been selected for study within the present context.

The overall goals of the project are multiple. Children of parents hospitalized for psychiatric disorder are at higher statistical risk for receiving a similar diagnosis at some time in their lives than are children at large. Such children are at even higher risk for emotional disability or behavioral disorder in general. These probabilities, however, refer to the emergence of problems throughout the life span or at critical developmental periods, so that the vast majority of children function reasonably well at any point in time. Consequently, the first goal of the research was to assess "intermediate outcomes" in these children, using a competence–incompetence as opposed to a health–sickness model. A second goal was to associate a variety of family and adult measures with current offspring competence and incompetence. These children and their families are being followed longitudinally to assess additional outcomes at crucial developmental stages. In this way, concurrent and predictive associations can be ascertained.

The Study of "Invulnerability" in At-Risk Samples

Anthony (1974) has articulated four strategies for the study of invulnerability. In the first approach, "invulnerability" is implied as the antithesis of "vulnerability." This strategy is similar to defining "health" as the absence of disease, or to defining "invulnerability" as a listing of positive outcomes. This follows the concept that if no symptoms are present, the individual must be healthy. A second approach to the definition of "invulnerability" relates not to innate predispositions, traits, or characterological tendencies, but to an acquired flexibility in reaction to circumstance. This characteristic is viewed as enabling an individual to adapt readily to fluctuating environmental demands, thus increasing the flexibility and range of response to stressful life circumstances. A third approach involves definitions that focus on identifying an active mastery of the environment by labeling adaptive and successful defensive styles. For example, Murphy and Moriarty (1976) have undertaken extensive studies of the development of patterns of coping and the ways in which children learn to deal with difficulties in their environment.

A fourth approach to the definition of "invulnerability" is really an extension of the third and has to do with the development of competence (White, 1959). Garmezy (1974) has emphasized this aspect in studying children who are offspring of schizophrenic parents. The rationale here is that children display competence in many areas of endeavor, and studies of the development of competent behavior become sources for understanding mastery and success.

In the present study, "invulnerability" has been defined as the display of competent behavior in spite of deleterious circumstances (i.e., being an offspring of a seriously disturbed parent). Consequently, any child who displays competent behavior at this stage of development could be viewed as "invulnerable," or, alternatively, as competent while at risk. This strategy of analysis calls for starting with a group of children defined as vulnerable, dividing them into competent and incompetent subgroups, and looking at selected family and adult variables that distinguish group membership.

The primary dependent variable in the study of intermediate outcomes in URCAFS is school competence. Children spend a substantial percentage of their waking hours in the school setting, where their behavior can be observed directly without family influence and where comparisons with same-age classmates can be undertaken (see Fisher, 1980, for a discussion of school competence and risk). In addition, early school performance has been associated with psychiatric outcome in later years (Cowen, Pederson, & Babigian, 1973). URCAFS has employed several measures of school functioning, including ratings of grades, achievement test scores, anecdotal teacher records, and teacher and peer judgments.

The Rochester Teacher Rating Scale is a 35-item teacher scale on which students are rated on cognitive competence, social compliance, social competence, and motivation. Such ratings are then standardized on same-sex classmates. Similiarly, the Rochester Peer Rating Scale is a 25-item sociometric procedure in which children are selected for roles classified as brightness/compliance, intrusiveness, friendliness, and dullness. The development and standardization of these scales have been presented in Fisher (1980).

For the purposes of the present study, we were interested in dividing the risk sample (total $n = 77$) into competent and incompetent subgroups. To achieve this end, the summary Rochester Teacher Rating Scale and Rochester Peer Rating Scale scores were combined into a Grand Teacher-Peer Score (GTP), which reflected child functioning at school on a global level. Children scoring 0.5 standard deviations or more above the mean were labeled "competent" or high functioning ($n = 29$), and those scoring 0.5 standard deviations or more below the mean were labeled "incompetent" or low functioning ($n = 26$).

To assess the stability of the two-group dichotomy, the same 77 children were also divided on the basis of their score on a second dependent variable: a global index of the Rochester Adaptive Behavior Inventory (RABI), a parent rating form based on developmental criteria developed by Jones (1977) and analyzed statistically by Prentky, Fisher, and Cipro (1982). In its present form, the scale consists of 71 items on which the parent, usually the mother, rates the child. Items related to school behavior or academic functioning were omitted in the present study. Three statistically derived dimensions based on 12 rational factors were developed: social interaction, fearfulness–somatization, and motivation–obsessiveness. These were combined into a single global index of competence and standardized by age on the total risk sample. The same criteria of 0.5 standard deviations or more above or below the mean were used as the dividing points to establish the high- and low-functioning subgroups. These ratings served as an independent assessment of child competence outside the school setting.

The groups defined by the school and by the parental rating criteria then were compared on two adult and three family variables in order to identify factors that were associated with positive, competent functioning amidst generally adverse circumstances.

Results

Adult Variables

The DSM-III diagnoses of the hospitalized parents were reviewed for the high- and low-functioning groups, using both the GTP and the RABI scores as criteria. Analyses were undertaken for 7- and 10-year-old index children both separately and together. Chi-square analyses using the GTP scores yielded nonsignificant findings, in part due to the low n's of the various diagnostic groups. However, offspring of parents with a DSM-III diagnosis of bipolar disorder fell more frequently in the high-functioning than in the low-functioning group ($\chi^2 = 4.57$, $p < .05$). Moreover, offspring of all affectively disturbed psychotic parents (schizoaffective, bipolars, and unipolars combined) tended to fall more frequently into the high-functioning than into the low-functioning group ($\chi^2 = 3.20$, $p < .10$), although this finding did not reach statistical significance. Somewhat surprisingly, there was a similar though nonsignificant trend for offspring of psychotic parents to display more competent school behavior than offspring of nonpsychotic parents ($\chi^2 = 3.79$, $p < .10$).

Similar findings emerged when global parental ratings (RABI) were used to divide the high- and low-functioning groups. Offspring of parents with bipolar disorder were found more frequently in the high-than low-competence group ($\chi^2 = 4.45$, $p < .05$); offspring of affectively disturbed parents combined were more frequently in the high than the low groups ($\chi^2 = 4.47$, $p < .05$); and, similarly, offspring of psychotics were more frequently in the high than the low groups as well ($\chi^2 = 4.67$, $p < .05$). These data appeared to be consistent, regardless of which of the two independent variables were used. Although diagnosis per se was not related to competence, specific clusters of diagnoses, particularly those having to do with affective disturbance, were related to competence in offspring.

The second adult variable under consideration was chronicity of parental disorder. Rutter (1978) has spoken of the impact of parental disorder on the child when the pathology is chronic and is present over long periods of the child's development. Indeed, our own experience (Harder et al., 1980) has underlined the fact that single or infrequent psychotic episodes in the parent appear to have little or no measurable influence on offspring functioning as compared to repeated and/or chronic parental disability. With this in mind, one of us (P. M. P.) scaled all hospitalized adults on a 6-point rating of chronicity, as presented in Table 8-2. For purposes of the present analysis, ratings of 5 or 6 on the chronicity scale were considered chronic and all others were considered episodic. It should be emphasized that this rating characterized symptomatology over time. Those with the most hospitalizations were not necessarily the most chronic as scaled by this measure.

We performed t tests between the high- and low-competence groups, based on chronicity level of parent; these were significant for the GTP ($t = 3.20$, $p < .002$) and for the RABI ($t = 2.47$, $p < .002$) data. It would appear, therefore, that children at risk perform relatively well with respect to these two criteria when their parents' disorder is brief or intermittent rather than prolonged or chronic.

Table 8-2. Perkins's Chronicity Rating Scale

1—Single episode with full recovery or onset within 2 years of study and asymptomatic prior to episode.

2—Single episode with mild intermittent symptoms thereafter, or, if onset within 2 years, mild intermittent symptoms prior.

3—More than one episode; essentially asymptomatic between episodes.

4—More than one episode with mild intermittent symptoms between episodes.

5—Chronic, mild symptoms, with or without acute episodes, for a period of at least 2 years prior to interview.

6—Chronic, moderate to severe symptoms with or without.acute exacerbations, for at least 2 years prior to interview.

Note. Mild, moderate, or severe ratings were based on the Global Assessment Scale (GAS; Endicott, Spitzer, Fleiss, & Cohen, 1976). Mild = expectable GAS in 60-70 range; moderate to severe = expectable GAS less than 60.

Family Variables

Family theories of psychopathology (e.g., those of Bateson, Lidz, and Wynne) have emphasized faulty and confusing communication, marital discord, and familial uses of guilt (Leff & Vaughn, 1985) as crucial influences on the development of offspring. Family factors, however, can also have ameliorative and protective influences in settings where particular members display circumscribed or limited pathology. For example, Rutter (1978) has discussed the role of the nondisturbed parent in providing a source of support and consistency in this regard.

To study the interaction among families with relatively young children, Alfred and Clara Baldwin, together with one of us (R. E. C.), developed a standardized but unstructured family task. The mother, father, and index child were observed in a free play setting and the parents were encouraged to interact with their child as they would at home if they had an uninterrupted half hour. The laboratory was a quiet, comfortable room containing a variety of toys appropriate to the age of the child. The interaction was narrated by a trained observer and recorded on audiotape. The resulting descriptions were then coded by computer into categories and types of social and nonsocial interaction. For example, the program provides accurate counts of child to parent and parent to child initiations of activity as well as qualitative ratings of the content and tone of these initiations and activities. A fuller description of this task along with scoring and reliability data are presented in Baldwin, Baldwin and Cole (1982).

For purposes of the present study, each family dyad was coded on an index of the activity, balance, and warmth of the interaction. This index reflected at least moderate rates of interaction initiated relatively equally by each dyad member with both members communicating at least moderate warmth in their interchanges. The rating reflected the overall tone of the interchange and, by extrapolation, the relationship. Three balance scores were selected: mother to child (M-C), father to child (F-C), and parents to child (P-C) (this latter being the arithmetic sum of M-C and F-C).

An analysis of the GTP data yielded generally significant findings in the predicted direction. High-GTP children had more balanced M-C relationships than low-GTP children, although this finding only approached significance ($t = 1.90$, $p < .06$). However, significance was reached in comparisons between high- and low-GTP groups on F-C ($t = 2.36$, $p < .02$) and P-C ($t = 2.91$, $p < .006$) measures. In general, there were more balanced/warm family relationships in the high-GTP group than in the low-GTP group.

The analyses using the RABI data were not as definitive. Although all three group means in the M-C, F-C, and P-C comparisons were in the predicted direction, none reached or approached statistical significance.

The findings that competence was related to M-C, F-C, and P-C, at least when using the GTP data, led us to question what effect an active/warm father had on his offspring's competence when the mother was rated negatively in her ability to maintain a qualitatively and quantitatively adequate relationship with the child. That is, we wished to determine whether or not positively interacting fathers could "compensate" for negatively interacting mothers. To test this "compensatory hypothesis," we divided the sample into four groups on the basis of M-C and F-C scores: (1) positive mothers and negative fathers; (2) positive mothers and positive fathers; (3) negative mothers and negative fathers; and (4) negative mothers and positive fathers. A one-way analysis of variance yielded significant findings using the GTP data ($F = 4.54$, $p < .006$) but not the RABI data, although the order of the means was the same in both analyses. The crucial test, however, was whether the GTP and/or the RABI scores differed between the negative-mother/positive-father and the negative-mother/negative-father groups. Our prediction was that, given families with negative mothers, those with positive fathers would have more competent offspring than those with negative fathers. The resulting t test yielded means in the predicted direction for both the GTP and the RABI data; however, only the GTP comparison reached significance ($t = 3.15$, $p < .003$).

Additional Analyses

Several sources of data, as well as our own, have indicated that chronicity of parental impairment and age of child at the first acute episode of parental disorder are crucial influences on offspring development. It follows, therefore, that one way to identify a particularly high-risk sample would be to search for a subgroup of children whose mothers not only were chronically disturbed, but, in addition, suffered acutely very early in the children's lives. This process would identify a cohort of children who had been exposed to the influence of maternal psychopathology starting early in their lives and continuing relatively constantly thereafter.

A decision was made to divide the sample into early-onset and late-onset groups, based on the age of the child at the mother's first hospitalization. A natural break in the distribution of child age at mother's first admission occurred at 0–1 years of age, and, consequently, this was established as the dividing line. A total of 13 mother patient families were identified in which the first admission had occurred prior to the child's first birthday. A late-onset group of 13 families also was identified by selecting mothers with the most recent first admissions. No differences in parental diagnosis between these two groups were noted.

Utilizing the high versus low GTP and RABI dichotomies described above, we were able to classify the families according to (1) early-onset/chronic mothers versus late-onset/nonchronic mothers, and (2) high versus low child scores on the GTP and the RABI. The resulting 2 × 2 breakdowns are presented in Table 8-3. The chi-squared analysis using the GTP data was significant ($\chi^2 = 3.85$, $p < .05$), and the arrangement of the subjects within the cells was congruent with our initial speculations. Only four early-onset subjects were in the high-GTP group whereas nine were in the low-GTP group. The same pattern was found in the late-onset group (i.e., better-functioning children in the late-than in the early-onset group).

The contingency table based on the RABI data, however, was inconclusive and did not replicate the GTP data discussed above. In fact, there was very little difference among all four cells.

Notwithstanding the lack of agreement on data based on these two independent variables, we decided to look more closely at the four children of early-onset/chronic mothers who had high GTP scores—children categorized as competent despite very adverse circumstances as defined by these criteria ("invulnerable"). Because the sample size was too low for statistical analysis, a descriptive summary was undertaken, and data from several sources were reviewed in an effort to characterize these children. The results were quite surprising and unexpected. Two of the "invulnerable" children identified by the GTP data were similarly identified by the RABI data, so our discussion here focuses on these two as representative of the subgroup.

Although both of these children appeared to perform competently, according to global measures of school competence and global behav-

Table 8-3. Early or Late Onset versus High or Low Scores on Child Competence Criteria

Onset	High scores	Low scores
School competence criterion (GTP)		
Early	4	9
Late	9	4
Parental report criterion (RABI)		
Early	6	7
Late	7	6

ioral ratings based on parent report, considerable variability existed on subtest scores. For example, the first child was rated as quite friendly by both teachers and peers, but teachers and peers also agreed that his academic skills were weak, even though his IQ was well above average. Indeed, his arithmetic grades and verbal achievement test scores were well below average. In addition, his mother rated him as fearful with a tendency toward somatization. Teacher anecdotal comments were basically nondescript, but a tendency toward underachievement was noted at previous grade levels.

The second child displayed a similar pattern of variable performances not reflected by the global scores. This second child excelled in academic areas, with high ratings by both teachers and peers and average to above-average grades and achievement test scores. However, teachers, peers, and parents rated him variably low on social skills and friendliness. On a follow-up 3 years after this assessment, it was learned that he had been referred for psychotherapy. A review of the data on the remaining two children in the "invulnerable" GTP group revealed a similar pattern of strengths and deficits not reflected by the global index. In this light, variable performance existed among all four of these children who emerged following a statistically significant analysis of the data.

Discussion

We wish to begin this section by first discussing strategic issues and problems of definition with respect to studying "invulnerability." Second, we shall summarize the findings presented above in light of these considerations.

Issues of Strategy and Definition

By and large, the vast majority of research studies in the area of invulnerability have employed a research strategy similar to our own. Perhaps the largest and most comprehensive investigation to date in this area is that by Werner and Smith (1982). These researchers studied 690 multiracial children who grew up in poverty and who were exposed to a series of stressful life events on the Hawaiian island of Kauai. Their approach was to follow these competent and incompetent children, who were identified by their severe environmental circumstances over the years, in order to determine which aspects of their early experiences appeared to buffer or protect them through their formative years. The large sample size permitted a variety of analyses (e.g., sex differences, social class, etc.), as well as cross-sectional comparisons at varying developmental levels.

This strategy can raise particular difficulties, however. First, the use of multiple criteria to discriminate high from low competence groups may lead to puzzling inconsistencies. For example, although there tended to be general agreement in the present data when both the GTP and RABI criteria were utilized, some differences did occur. The GTP data yielded significant differences on the family variables, whereas the RABI data did not. Although we could easily generate potentially testable explanations for these differences, the fact remains that when multiple criteria are used to define competent and incompetent functioning so that environmental or parental factors can be identified, inconsistencies and discrepancies develop. The children identified as competent or incompetent using one criterion may be different from those identified when another criterion is used. There is little doubt that single indices of competence are insufficient to reflect the complexity of adequate adjustment; yet it becomes clear that the use of multiple criteria produce discrepant results when used singly or reduce sample size considerably if used in combination.

A second problem that emerges when this strategy is employed relates to the selection of appropriate control groups. The use of control groups has been notably lacking in invulnerability research, most likely because (1) most studies have been generally clinical in nature and (2) questions regarding variables to control for have not been clearly articulated in the literature. In the present research, comparisons were made between so-called "competent" and "incompetent" children at risk, but an argument could have been developed to justify the use of other control groups of children. Potential controls could have included children (1) exposed to different kinds of risk, (2) exposed at different ages, and (3) exposed under different environmental circumstances. For example, Werner and Smith (1982) found that the competent children in their sample tended to have (1) younger parents, (2) fewer siblings, (3) many caretakers, (4) a cohesive sibling group, and (5) fewer illnesses, among others. Are such indicators equally applicable when "risk" is defined as being an offspring of a psychiatrically disturbed parent or when it is defined on the basis of a chronic disability? In addition, are these indicators as influential throughout the formative years, or only at certain points in time? Finally, how do these indicators relate to different familial, social, and cultural contexts? Although there is a large amount of current clinical and empirical data on all three of these questions, future research in invulnerability and on the growth of adaptive, coping, and mastery behaviors in general will need to focus more concertedly on an integration of knowledge across settings through the use of appropriate comparison groups.

A third problem emerges with respect to the timing of child assessment. Anthony (1974) has emphasized the need to observe children at risk as they pass through crucial developmental stages, rather than viewing them only at one point in time. Unfortunately, a competent child at risk observed at point A will most likely display less competent behavior when assessed at point B, simply due to the effects of regression to the mean. In this way, statistical and probability issues come into play in attempts to understand competence over time, as one might expect in most forms of longitudinal research.

Fourth, difficulties emerge from research in which an extreme group is identified in the hopes of labeling variables that will be generalizable to the sample as a whole or to other samples or populations as well. Such was the case in describing our groups of particularly vulnerable or high-risk offspring. Although not directly tested in our research, issues of generalizability of outcome data are paramount in utilizing special groups with quite circumscribed characteristics.

A fifth problem refers to the use of single global indices that purportedly typify overall functioning. It is readily apparent that variability in development is more the rule than the exception, and that development occurs differentially for different skills and behaviors. Yet there appears to be a pervasive myth that "superkids" or children labeled as "invulnerable" excel in all areas: socially, cognitively, emotionally, and so on. As is the case with most myths, this one may be based more on wish than substance. However, to acknowledge that a child at risk has areas of strength and weakness may, by definition, remove him/her from the category of "invulnerable" to begin with. Where one draws the line depends on a precise definition of terms and a realization that no living object is truely "invulnerable."

In the present study, the data generated utilizing the very high-risk subgroups also point out that our myths about invulnerability are not bounded by time or setting. There appears to be the belief that "once invulnerable, always invulnerable," without accounting for Anthony's (1974) valuable comment that individuals who appear invulnerable at early stages of development may develop negative outcomes at later stages or periods of increased risk. Also, invulnerability, as most frequently defined, is expected to generalize to all settings without reference to the fact that the display of competent behavior is at least in part dependent upon the setting of its display. Consequently, it should not be surprising, for example, that children may display competent behavior in school but not at home, irrespective of the issues of comparability of raters or methods of assessment.

In overview, the use of the term "invulnerable" may be unrealistic and potentially misleading. The term brings with it a series of myths and expectations that may reflect a hypothesized but nonexistent state of excellence and invincibility more applicable to myth than to reality.

What we seek at a more fundamental level are individual characteristics and environmental circumstances that are related to an individual's ability to overcome the influences of stressful or negative life circumstances, be they natural occurrences of short duration or biological–social stresses of considerable duration. Consequently, we are engaged in a search for explanatory variables, ones that will help us understand why some individuals succumb to these events in a negative fashion and why others are able to adapt and to continue to grow. To label this process as a search for "invulnerable" individuals clouds the issue and biases our perspective. Given this discussion of strategic issues and problems of definition, let us now proceed with a discussion of findings based upon the data reported above.

Competent Children at Risk

An overview of the data reported above leads to the following conclusions within the constraints of our sample and design. First, the higher-functioning children tended to come from families where the previously hospitalized mothers had some form of affective pathology. Second, these children tended to have mothers whose disorder was not chronic and the onset of the disorder occurred generally later in the children's developmental career. Third, such children tended to reside in families that, in spite of the disorder, were still able to manage an active/warm series of interrelationships among members. Last, competence was generally maintained in settings where the mothers were not active/warm if the fathers were able to "compensate" effectively in an interactive manner.

These data tend to confirm the findings of other studies of children at risk. Kauffman, Grunebaum, Cohler, and Gamer (1979) reported that competent children at risk tended to come from families where (1) the children had an opportunity to interact with extrafamilial adults and (2) the mothers functioned at an adequate level of social interaction. Their findings also indicated that in some cases offspring of schizophrenic women performed more competently than offspring of depressed women. These authors speculated that offspring of schizophrenic mothers may have been able to interact with their mothers in a warm, positive fashion despite the mothers' cognitive distortions, whereas offspring of depressed mothers were unable to receive such warm, positive interactions because of the mothers' emotional withdrawal and unavailability. These data may be at some variance with our own, in that we found that offspring of affectively disordered mothers performed more competently than did offspring of schizophrenic mothers. It is not clear from our data or theirs, however, what impact the following variables may have had on these outcomes: mania versus depression in the respective samples; the relative severity of depressive episodes; and the frequency of depressive episodes. Our group of "affectively disordered" patients included schizoaffectives, manics, and depressives, and the depressives varied in severity and chronicity. Consequently, this apparent contrast in findings may have been due to the interaction of any number of the above variables. Efforts are now being focused on refining these data to isolate relevant interacting variables.

Kauffman *et al.*'s data also indicated that the mother's level of social functioning may be more important in influencing child outcome than her diagnosis per se. Our data support this view if one accounts for the dimensions of chronicity and affective involvement across diagnosis, as mentioned above. It may be the case that the use of diagnosis alone as a primary discriminator is too global and diffuse a variable to reflect the more subtle nuances of parent–child interaction. Perhaps a dimensional approach to adult assessment, as suggested by Strauss, Bartko, and Carpenter (1973), may be more sensitive to the kinds of issues raised in this context.

Several studies have pointed to the role of the nondisturbed parent in compensating for the disturbed parent's deficits in parenting (Rutter, 1978). Anthony (1974) stressed the need for "support, encouragement and candor from an adequately functioning parent" (p. 542), and Kellam, Ensminger, and Turner (1977) found that even the simple presence of a nondisturbed parent had a positive influence on outcome. In addition, Werner and Smith (1982) found that the presence of many caretakers tended to influence positive outcome as well.

It is unclear, however, what mechanisms mediate the nondisturbed parent's influence on the child. Three independent sources of comment, however, may shed some light on this subject, albeit speculative. First, at a conference on risk research held in Puerto Rico in 1980, Manfred Bleuler presented a striking clinical vignette. In describing Vreni, a remarkably "sane" offspring of a severely disturbed, chronic schizophrenic mother, Bleuler (1980) commented on her need for mastery over an otherwise intolerable situation. This was a young woman who clearly was not a "superkid," but who managed to cope well, to care for her ill mother and her siblings, and later to marry and have children of her own. What comes across in Bleuler's description, however, is the competent offspring's ability to see the disorder or the circumstances as outside of herself, to seek out ways of understanding her parent's problems, and to conceptualize them within a manageable, reality-focused framework.

Second, Anthony (1974) commented in a similar fashion in reviewing the attributes of the well-functioning offspring of disturbed parents in his sample. He stated that these offspring "had a stubborn resistance to the process of being engulfed by the illness; a curiosity in studying the etiology, diagnosis, symptoms and treatment of the illness . . . ; [and] a capacity to develop an objective, realistic, somewhat distant and yet distinctly compassionate approach to the parental illness, neither retreating from it nor being intimidated by it" (p. 540).

Finally, Space and Cromwell (1978) have described what they call the "unique personal construct structure" of the healthy offspring of a schizophrenic parent. In their view, such an individual does not accept the conceptual structure of the psychotic parent, but instead formulates a conceptual structure based on an internal locus of control.

All three of these sources of data uniformly point to the capacity of the child to objectify the disturbed parent and to view her as outside the self. This view also characterizes the child's continuing desire to master an understanding of the parent's pathology—in essence, to deal with the aberrant behavior or circumstances through learning and other more objective and reality-based approaches. In this light, perhaps the role of the nondisturbed parent is to foster this objective stance, in which mastery of the situation in a developmentally appropriate fashion is encouraged and reinforced through a warm and active interchange.

This research has focused on identifying variables that are associated with positive outcomes in children at risk. Problems of variability of child functioning, the use of multiple criteria for defining "competence," and the selection of appropriate controls also have been mentioned. These data indicate (as one would expect) that long-term continuous exposure to severe circumstances leads to the lowest probability of positive outcome, but, at the same time, that positive, supportive figures can compensate for these negative influences in some as yet unclear fashion. Our future work will center on identifying other factors in family, personal, intellectual, and social life that also may affect positive outcome in these children at risk.

REFERENCES

Anthony, E. J. (1974). The syndrome of the psychologically invulnerable child. In E. J. Anthony & C. Koupernik (Eds.), *The child in his family: Children at psychiatric risk* (International yearbook, Vol. 3). New York: Wiley.

Babigian, H., Gardner, E., Miles, H., & Ramano, J. (1965). Diagnostic consistency and change in a follow-up study of 1215 patients. *American Journal of Psychiatry, 121,* 895–901.

Baldwin, A. L., Baldwin, C. P., & Cole, R. E. (1982). Family free-play interaction: Setting and methods. In A. L. Baldwin, R. E. Cole, & C. P. Baldwin (Eds.), Parental pathology, family interaction and the competence of the child in school. *Monographs of the Society for Research in Child Development, 47*(5, Serial No. 197).

Bleuler, M. (1984). Different forms of childhood stress and patterns of adult psychiatric illness. In N. F. Watt, E. J. Anthony, L. C. Wynne, & J. E. Rolf (Eds.), *Children at risk for schizophrenia.* Cambridge: Cambridge University Press.

Cowen, E., Pederson, A., & Babigian, H. (1973). Long term follow-up of early detected vulnerable children. *Journal of Clinical and Consulting Psychology, 41,* 438–446.

Endicott, J., Spitzer, R. L., Fleiss, J. L., & Cohen, J. (1976). The global assessment scale. *Archives of General Psychiatry, 33,* 766–771.

Escalona, S. K. (1968). *The roots of individuality.* Chicago: Aldine.

Evans, J. R. (1982). Measurement and management in medicine and health services. In M. Lipkin, Jr., & W. A. Lybrand (Eds.), *Population based medicine.* New York: Praeger.

Falloon, I. R., Boyd, J. L., McGill, C. W., Razini, J., Moss, H. B., & Guilderman, A. M. (1982). Family management in prevention of exacerbations of schizophrenia. *The New England Journal of Medicine, 306,* 1437–1440.

Fisher, L., & Jones, F. (1978). Planning for the next generation of risk studies. *Schizophrenia Bulletin, 4,* 223–235.

Fisher, L. (1980). Child competence and psychiatric risk: I. Model and method. *Journal of Nervous and Mental Disease, 168,* 323–331.

Fisher, L., & Jones, J. E. (1980). Child competence and psychiatric risk: II. Areas of relationship between child and family functioning. *Journal of Nervous and Mental Disease, 168,* 332–337.

Fisher, L., & Kokes, R. F. (1980). Child competence and psychiatric risk: III. Comparisons based on diagnosis of hospitalized parent. *Journal of Nervous and Mental Disease, 168,* 338–342.

Fisher, L., Kokes, R. F., Harder, D. W., & Jones, J. E. (1980). Child competence and psychiatric risk: VI. Summary and integration of findings. *Journal of Nervous and Mental Disease, 168,* 353–355.

Garmezy, N. (1974). Competence and adaptation in adult schizophrenic patients and children at risk. In S. Dean (Ed.), *Prize lectures in schizophrenia: The first ten Dean Awards.* New York: MSS Publications.

Garmezy, N., with Streitman, S. (1974). Children at risk: The search for the antecedents of schizophrenia. Part I. Conceptual models and research methods. *Schizophrenia Bulletin, 8,* 14–90.

Harder, D. W., Kokes, R. F., Fisher, L., & Strauss, J. S. (1980). Child competence and psychiatric risk: IV. Relationships of parent psychopathology severity to child functioning. *Journal of Nervous and Mental Disease, 168,* 343–347.

Intagliata, J. (1978). Increasing the interpersonal problem-solving skills of an alcoholic population. *Journal of Consulting and Clinical Psychology, 46*, 489–498.

Jones, F. (1977). The Rochester Adaptive Behavior Inventory: A parallel series of instruments for assessing social competence during early and middle childhood and adolescence. In J. S. Strauss, H. M. Babigian, & M. Roff (Eds.), *The origins and course of psychopathology.* New York: Plenum Press.

Kauffman, C., Grunebaum, H., Cohler, B., & Gamer, E. (1979). Superkids: Competent children of psychotic mothers. *American Journal of Psychiatry, 136*, 1398–1402.

Kellam, S. G., Ensminger, M. A., & Turner, J. (1977). Family structure and the mental health of children. *Archives of General Psychiatry, 34*, 1012–1022.

Kokes, R. F., Harder, D. W., Fisher, L., & Strauss, J. S. (1980). Child competence and psychiatric risk: V. Sex of patient parent and dimension of psychopathology. *Journal of Nervous and Mental Disease, 168*, 348–352.

Leff, J., & Vaughn, C. (1985). *Expressed emotion in families.* New York: Guilford Press.

Maddi, S., Propst, B. S., & Feldinger, I. (1965). Three expressions of need for variety. *Journal of Personality, 33*, 82–98.

Murphy, L. B., & Moriarty, A. E. (1976). *Vulnerability, coping and growth.* New Haven, CT: Yale University Press.

Prentky, R., Fisher, L., & Cipro, C. (1982). *Competence at home and school in children at risk: Instrumentation and comparisons.* Unpublished manuscript.

Rutter, M. (1978). Early sources of security and competence. In J. S. Bruner & A. Garten (Eds.), *Human growth and development.* Oxford: Clarendon Press.

Space, L., & Cromwell, R. L. (1978). Personal constructs among schizophrenic patients. In S. Schwartz (Ed.), *Language and cognition in schizophrenia.* Hillsdale, NJ: Erlbaum.

Strauss, J. S., Bartko, J. J., & Carpenter, W. T. (1973). The use of clustering techniques for the classification of psychiatric patients. *British Journal of Psychiatry, 122*, 531–540.

Strauss, J. S., & Harder, D. W. (1981). The Case Record Rating Scale: A method for rating symptom and social functioning data from case records. *Psychiatry Research, 4*(3), 333–345.

Terman, L. M., & Oden, M. H. (1947). *The gifted child grows up.* Stanford, CA: Stanford University Press.

Visher, E., & Visher, J. (1979). *Stepfamilies: A guide to working with stepfamilies and stepchildren.* New York: Brunner/Mazel.

Watt, N. F., Shay, J. J., Grubb, T. W., & Riddle, M. (1982). Early identification and intervention with emotionally vulnerable children through the public schools. In M. J. Goldstein (Ed.), *Preventive intervention in schizophrenia.* Washington, DC: U.S. Department of Health and Human Services.

Werner, E., & Smith, R. (1982). *Vulnerable but invincible: A longitudinal study of resilient children and youth.* New York: McGraw-Hill.

White, R. (1959). Motivation reconsidered: The concept of competence. *Psychological Review, 66*, 297–333.

World Health Organization. (1973). *The International Pilot Study of Schizophrenia* (Vol. 1). Geneva: Author.

9

Maternal Factors Related to Vulnerability and Resiliency in Young Children at Risk

JUDITH S. MUSICK
Ounce of Prevention Fund

FRANCES M. STOTT
Erikson Institute

KATHERINE KLEHR SPENCER
Northwestern University

JUDITH GOLDMAN
Erikson Institute

BERTRAM J. COHLER
University of Chicago

Introduction

While there has been extensive study of the development of children of psychiatrically impaired mothers, the findings from these studies lead to somewhat ambiguous conclusions. Much of this research has assumed a continuity between infancy, early childhood, and later adjustment that is not warranted on the basis of studies of cognitive and socioemotional development across the first 2 years of life (Kagan, 1980). This research has also neglected the self-righting tendencies of young children (Sameroff & Chandler, 1975), and has generally failed to consider the range of outcomes that preserve or destroy such self-righting tendencies.

The majority of studies conducted to date on the children of seriously disturbed parents have been based primarily on research strategies that seek to identify potential psychiatric patients prior to the onset of illness; they have not been as concerned with the study of parenting itself and of the impact of variations in parenting upon the developing child. This "high-risk" tradition (Mednick & McNeil, 1968) is concerned with identifying persons likely to succumb to the major mental disorders on the basis of increased genetic loading for psychopathology, with the dual goals of isolating the etiology of these disorders and of providing prevention before the manifestation of psychiatric symptoms.

The term "risk" denotes a statistical concept, indicating that a child of a parent with a major psychiatric disorder (e.g., manic–depressive illness or schizophrenia) has a greater probability of subsequently developing mental disorder than the child of a well parent. For example, 10–15% of the offspring of schizophrenic parents become schizophrenic, while 35–50% have some form of emotional disturbance. The problem with this notion is precisely that it is statistical rather than psychological in nature, and more recent investigators have preferred to use the concept of "vulnerability" (Anthony, 1974; Garmezy, 1974). The notion of vulnerability implies that the children of mentally ill parents may be negatively influenced by a *variety* of factors, including genetic predispositions, prenatal and perinatal complications, and ongoing interaction with a disturbed parent. These factors may lead to lowered capacity for coping with adverse life events, as well as to increased potential for cognitive and social–emotional dysfunction. The concept of vulnerability makes no assumptions about the "causes" of this impairment in coping ability (Zubin & Spring, 1977), but only asserts that such impairment exists.

While earlier investigations of risk and vulnerability tended to focus somewhat narrowly on attentional and cognitive capacities, more recent studies have extended the notion of competence to include developmentally appropriate measures of childhood adjustment (Rolf, 1972). Most of these studies have targeted school-age and early adolescent children (Baldwin, Cole, & Baldwin, 1982; Fisher, Harder, Kokes, & Strauss, 1980; Watt, Grubb, & Erlenmeyer-Kimling, 1982; Weintraub, Prinz, & Neale, 1978), using the classroom setting as the primary arena. Fisher (1980) and Rolf (1972, 1976) found few differences between high-risk and control children on *teacher* ratings, but differences were found on ratings of *peers*, who viewed the high-risk children as more intrusive, selected them less frequently for positive roles, and selected them more frequently for externalizing negative roles. Watt *et al.* (1982) found that the 12- to 15-year-old children of schizophrenic parents were rated by teachers as showing greater interpersonal disharmony, less scholastic motivation, more emotional instability, and lower intelligence than a comparison group. Weintraub and colleagues (Neale & Weintraub, 1975; Weintraub, Neale, & Leibert, 1975; Weintraub *et al.*, 1978) compared children (second through ninth grades) of schizophrenic and depressed parents with a well comparison group. They reported that the combined risk sample scored more poorly on a variety of teacher-rated behavioral dimensions and on peer evaluations (Weintraub *et al.*, 1978). This group of investigators has noted that children with an affectively ill parent and those with a schizophrenic parent show lower academic and social competence than children of well parents. The considerable overlap between the two risk groups on almost every dimension assessed (Weintraub, Winters, & Neale, 1982) suggests that the general stress and upheaval associated with living with a mentally ill parent may be of greater significance in determining future maladjustment than the specific form of the parental psychiatric illness. Indeed, reliability of diagnostic categories has traditionally been hard to ascertain, and many studies indicate that overall parental disorder as reflected by chronicity and severity may be more important than the specific diagnostic classification in predisposing a child to future disorder.

As noted earlier, the majority of studies of children at risk have sought to identify potential psychiatric disorder prior to the onset of illness. This focus on adult disturbance has resulted in more intensive study of the high-risk age period of early adolescence through adulthood, in order to shorten the time between assessment and pathological outcome (Watt, Anthony, Wynne, & Rolf, 1984). Few investigations have targeted the earliest years of life (Marcus, Auerbach, Wilkinson, & Burack, 1981; Musick & Cohler, 1983; Sameroff, Barocas, & Seifer, 1984; Sameroff, Seifer, & Zax, 1982; Silverton, Finello, & Mednick, 1983), and few of these have explored the impact of variations in child-rearing patterns upon the course of the young child's development.

This chapter describes such a study, and reflects an approach to assessment that views the capacity to maintain development as the premier task of childhood. While the concept of vulnerability has determined the particular children to be studied in this investigation, notions of competence and vulnerability in infancy and early childhood have been expanded beyond those of attention and cognition to encompass other developmentally appropriate measures of adjustment, such as interactive behavior and motivation for learning. Variations in these markers of child competence have been evaluated within the context of the early social and caregiving environment provided by the mother. For, while we acknowledge that risk and vulnerability are certainly functions of multiple biological and environmental factors in a changing organism, we also recognize that the mother represents a most salient factor in the infant's and young child's developing competence and sense of self.

The Thresholds Mothers' Project

Description of the Project

As a result of what was known about the vulnerability of the children of severely disturbed mothers, and about the critical role of the mother–child relationship in affecting both the child's development and the mother's own conception of herself as a woman and a mother, a novel research and clinical intervention program was undertaken in the fall of 1976. This program, the Thresholds Mothers' Project, was designed to treat and study mentally ill mothers and their children under 5 years of age. There were five basic and interlocking components of this project:

1. A multifaceted treatment package, with aspects designed specifically for the *mother's* own psychiatric rehabilitation; a special therapeutic nursery program for the *child*; ongoing evaluation and clinical efforts with the *mother–child relationship itself*; and, finally, involvement and treatment of the *larger family system*. (See Table 9-1.)

2. The comparison of this program with a home-based aftercare/ intervention program. This program was structured to include weekly home visits by a psychiatric nurse or clinical social worker, who offered therapeutic treatment based on the individual needs of the mother and family.

3. An in-depth comparative study of mentally ill and well mothers and their young children. (See Tables 9-2 and 9-3.)

4. The development, utilization, and analysis of treatment methods and knowledge that could be shared with others seeking ways to treat these challenging families.

5. A study of children's response to the therapeutic nursery experience, as related to issues of vulnerability, competence, and resiliency

---

Table 9-1. Treatment Components of the Thresholds Mothers' Project

1. Vocational rehabilitation, including job placement should a mother choose this option.

2. Social rehabilitation in a group setting, including some evening and weekend programs and therapeutic camping in the summer.

3. Academic preparation for the high school general equivalency diploma or college-level courses.

4. Prevention of rehospitalization through a medication maintenance program for those mothers on medication.

5. Mothers' therapy group.

6. Child development course.

7. "Mothers' time in the nursery."

8. Staff-assisted lunchtime with children, plus one "moms' lunch out" per week when the children are fed in the nursery.

9. A 4-day-per-week therapeutic nursery program for the children.

10. Videotape intervention program utilized in counseling sessions with the mother concerning issues of child care and relationship with her child.

11. Individual and/or family treatment for mothers and spouses or grandparents where feasible.

12. Individual child treatment, where required.

Table 9-2. Measures Used in Evaluation of Mothers and Children at Admission and Discharge

Mothers (mentally ill and well)

Structured Scaled Interview to Assess Maladjustment

Maternal Attitude Scale

Life event stress

Interpersonal Apperception Technique

Shipley Institute of Living IQ Screening Measure

Witkin Embedded Figure Test

Three 5-minute videotapes of mother–child interaction. (Rated with the Mothers' Project Rating Scales [Clark, Musick, Stott, & Klehr, 1980]. Well-established interrater reliability. Currently in use in a variety of settings across the country.)

Children (of mentally ill and well mothers)

Bayley Scales of Infant Development (under 1 year)

Infant and Child Behavior Scales; Mothers' Project Coping Child Scale (over 1 year)

Harvard Preschool Scale of Social Competence (over 1 year)

Assessment Outline of Early Child Development (Revised)

Bayley Scales; Stanford–Binet; Wechsler Preschool and Primary Scale of Development; Wechsler Intelligence Scale for Children—Revised

Landmark testing

Hunt–Uzgiris Object Permanence (1-year-olds)

Preschool Embedded Figures Test (3-year-olds)

Rorschach (5-year-olds)

in early childhood. The results of this study are the special focus of this chapter.

Between the fall of 1976 and the project's termination in the fall of 1981, this National Institute of Mental Health (NIMH) research and demonstration project treated and studied 65 mentally ill women and their children: 39 mothers in the Thresholds program and 26 in the home care program. Numbers of schizophrenic women and women with affective disorders were approximately equal. Additionally, we treated some severely character-disordered and borderline women, as well as a number of women having postpartum psychoses with no previous history of mental illness. These mothers constituted a heterogeneous group in terms of their ages, socioeconomic factors, ethnicity, and severity of illness. In addition to the 65 mentally ill mothers in the two treatment groups, a control group of "well mothers" (women who had never experienced a psychiatric hospitalization) were recruited from the community. Of the pool of approximately 300 women who

Table 9-3. Additional Clinical Data on Mothers and Children in the Thresholds Mothers' Project

These forms have been utilized in recording additional clinical data and progress during and after participation in the project.[a]

Intake Form

Monthly Progress Notes

New Member Rehabilitation Plan

Thresholds Evaluation

Thresholds Rehospitalization Report

Group Evaluation

Monthly Work Evaluation

Mother–Child Interaction Video Data

Treatment Plan for the Mother–Child Dyad/Staffing Report

Mother–Child Separation Report

Mothers' Project Video Intervention—Form I & Form II

Mothers in the Nursery Evaluation

Nursery Observations (including Nursery Assessment Forms, Early Childhood Notes Assessment Form, and Anthony Child Psychiatric Report)

Pediatric Nurse Report

Mothers' Interview

Risk and Protective Factors (Prenatal and Perinatal)

Demographic Checklist

Closing Form

Follow-Up Status Report

[a]In addition to the forms listed here, notebooks were kept to record mothers' participation and progress in the mothers' therapy group and the child development group.

agreed to participate as a control group, 36 were successfully matched with the experimental group of mentally ill mothers on six demographic variables: age and sex of youngest child, age of mother, race, socioeconomic status, (SES; mother's education and father's occupation), and marital status.

Findings from the 5-Year Study

No significant differences were found between the two treatment groups on any of the child measures. Nevertheless, both treatment groups did show improvement over time on developmental quotient (DQ) and IQ measures, social competence, and adaptive skills. For example, the Thresholds group moved from a mean IQ score of 98.7 to 107.6, and the home care group moved from a mean IQ score of 79.7 to

94.1, an increase of 9 and 15 points, respectively. It is important to note that this improvement represented for the home care children a movement from the borderline retarded to the normal range of intellectual functioning, and speaks to the efficacy of even minimal intervention with this apparently understimulated group of children. Additionally, positive changes over time in attentional skills, overall social adjustment, and adjustment to work and parenting roles were found for both treatment groups of mothers. Although no significant group differences were found on any measure, it appears that both treatment programs had an important impact on their participants.

In terms of the comparison of the children of both groups of mentally ill women to the children of their well counterparts, a number of differences were found at the initial testing period. The children of mentally ill mothers were characterized by lowered intellectual capacities and delayed normative development. Their coping style during testing sessions was less adaptive; for example, they demonstrated more anxiety, greater emotional lability, more attentional difficulties, and less cooperation with the examiner. In terms of outward appearance (cleanliness and dress), children of mentally ill mothers appeared to be less well cared for than children of well mothers. This was one index of the quality of care available to the child in his home. The children of well mothers were more socially competent; that is, they sought the attention of adults more often, responded more to social initiatives, displayed more positive affect, and sent clearer signals. The children of mentally ill mothers were somewhat angrier, more apathetic, less enthusiastic, and more anxious than the children of well mothers. All these differences remained after the effects due to SES were removed. These differences may have reflected an impoverished social environment within the homes of the children of mentally ill mothers, which somehow hindered normal development and was implicated in the "developmental arrest" found in many of the children.

In looking at both groups of mentally ill women in comparison to their well counterparts, we found significant differences on almost all variables at the initial testing period. Well mothers showed better overall social adjustment than mentally ill mothers, as well as higher levels of adjustment to specific work, leisure, marital, parental, and extended-family roles. Well mothers had also experienced fewer stressful life events. Although mentally ill and well mothers had roughly equivalent verbal scores, mentally ill mothers had much lower scores on abstract thinking and IQ equivalence. Mentally ill mothers also displayed greater attentional problems than their well counterparts and tended to perceive child rearing as requiring control and separation rather than mother–child reciprocity. While SES was definitely found to be related to intellectual and social performance, it did not account for what may be essential differences between the two groups. The number and consistent direction of the differences found supports other research identifying intellectual and social deficits associated with mental illness. These deficits were noted among higher-SES as well as lower-SES mentally ill women and may reflect an inability of the mentally ill to draw upon the benefits of education and SES. It appears, therefore, that the social deficit associated with psychiatric disorder may outweigh to some degree the advantages normally provided by education and higher SES.

The results of the Thresholds study thus showed initially lower intellectual capacities, social competence, and normative development in the children of mentally ill mothers as compared with their well counterparts. These differences were found on standardized measures of child competence; our clinical data, gathered over 5 years of work with these families, complemented these research findings. Many of these children fell into the general categories of learning disabilities with language dysfunction, borderline mental retardation, emotional disturbance, and early or precursor signs of behavior disorders of the acting-out type. Although the range and severity of problematic aspects of development was wide, four major areas of concern did clearly emerge. The first area was the interpersonal domain. The children often had unresolved attachment and separation issues; expectations that adults would be distant, denying, or punishing; immature ways of dealing with impulses and feelings; and, concomitantly, poor self-concepts. The second area was that of verbal–conceptual functioning. Language was often delayed, restricted, or used ineffectively or inappropriately for communication. In addition, the children often showed immaturity of those thought processes that go beyond concrete immediate experience; poor discrimination; lack of information; and lack of symbolic or "as-if" experience to encourage abstract thought. A third area was that of attentional skills. The children often lacked the ability to focus or sustain attention to relevant stimuli in the environment, both animate and inanimate. The final area of concern was that of mood and effect. The children lacked spontaneity or *joie de vivre*, seemed depressed, and lacked the urge to explore (Stott, Musick, Clark, & Cohler, 1983).

At discharge, approximately half these children did demonstrate significant gains across a variety of measures. The other half either remained the same or showed losses over time. Since programs of this kind are costly, and since many of the children who did not improve would be unable to function adequately within the normal school environment, it was felt to be important to investigate those factors that may have contributed to treatment outcome.

The Risk and Recovery Study

Rationale

Although the research design of the 5-year NIMH-funded study had included the analysis of developmental data, as well as comparisons of treatment outcome between our experimental (Thresholds) and comparison (home care) groups, there was neither the time nor the funding available to undertake the in-depth analyses that could help us to understand why some children responded so well to treatment, while others did not. Additionally, since the primary focus of the original NIMH-funded study was on the rehabilitation of mentally ill *mothers*, many data were collected toward this end; there was originally an emphasis on maternal assessments, with child and dyadic assessments as secondary. However, as the project evolved, staff attention was increasingly drawn toward the *children*, and toward the *mother–child relationships* as these relate both to the ontogenesis of childhood psychopathology and to the children's responses to the therapeutic nursery experience.

A second study, Risk and Recovery in the Children of Mentally Ill Mothers (Musick, Cohler, & Dincin, 1982), was initiated under a grant from the Illinois Department of Mental Health and Developmental Disabilities. This study called for analysis of child outcome as related to key factors within the children themselves as these interacted with maternal factors, and with the mother–child relationships over time. It sought to clarify the relationship between risk for psychopathology and recovery from developmental delay or deviation—that is, "resiliency." Research measures used in evaluation of mothers and children were integrated with selected additional ratings of systematic data collected during the treatment process, in order to develop composite profiles of these children and to give a clearer understanding of factors surrounding vulnerability, resiliency, and response to intervention efforts in this population.

The Thresholds Mothers' Project was the largest long-term clinical research study specifically focused on mothers of infants and young children. As such, it became a laboratory for the study not only of treatment and intervention, but also of developmental issues such as competence and vulnerability in this "at-risk" population. Moreover, it was unusual in the heterogeneity of its population in terms of ethnicity, SES, ages of mothers and children, and diagnostic categories. Because families were not drawn from one SES group, as has generally been the case in other studies of mental illness, we were better able to study the influences of the psychiatric disturbance apart from the effects of the other factors surrounding and within the mother–child relationship. Prior clinical findings from Anthony's (1969, 1971, 1975) series of detailed observational reports of schizophrenic and depressed mothers and their children indicated a number of subtle ways in which the caretaking environment provided by a mentally ill mother may have an impact on the adjustment of her offspring. Problems include failure in realizing self–other distinctions, in overcoming magical thinking, and in dealing with pervasive feelings of becoming "defective" like the mentally ill parent. Among a number of children, minibreakdowns appeared already to have taken place, representing, at least in part, identification with the parents' own illness. Anthony's reports present an excellent description of a subgroup of more troubled children who may be particularly at risk for psychopathology. What they do not reveal are the pictures of the considerable number of children, even those of multiply hospitalized parents, who do not show such problems in adjustment. This issue we also chose to address.

Description of the Study

The sample for the Risk and Recovery Study consisted of the 25 mother–child dyads in the Thresholds Mothers' Project who had been posttested by July 1, 1981. We chose to use only participants from the more intensive agency-based program, because far more clinical data on this group were available. Measures (listed in Table 9-2) were integrated with selected additional ratings (listed in Table 9-3) to develop composite profiles of these children.

Initially, we examined the change scores from pretesting to post-testing on the following *child* measures:

1. DQ-IQ: Bayley Scales of Infant Development, Stanford–Binet, Wechsler Preschool and Primary Scale of Development.
2. Mothers' Project Coping Child Scale (based on Gallant and Gamer's [1977] Infant and Child Behavior Scales).
3. Harvard Preschool Scale of Social Competence.

Using these change scores as outcome measures to assess which children improved or declined (and the degree to which they did so), we found that the majority of our sample fell into two basic groups: (1) children who showed significant improvement (no less than one standard deviation) in DQ-IQ and at least one other domain (n = 14), and (2) children who showed significant decreases (no less than one standard deviation) in DQ-IQ and at least one other domain (n = 11).

The next step was to refine certain of our more clinical assessments in order to better evaluate mothers' and children's use of the multifaceted treatment program. For example, data from the various therapeutic nursery assessments were restructured into the following general domains, each of which was scored as "normal," "delayed/ deviant," or "precocious":

- *Cognition*
  Attention
  Language
  Motivational factors (e.g., eagerness to explore, learn; goal-directedness; persistence). Evidence of thought disorder (present/ absent only), differentiation (e.g., reality testing).
- *Social behavior*
  Peers
  Parents
  Other adults
- *Emotional lability*
  Mood swings, impulsivity (*no* lability would be as deviant as too much)
- *Development over time*
  (in the sense of maintenance vs. loss)
- *Overall clinical rating*
  Rigid versus flexible behavior; diffuse versus complex behavior; organized behavior (in response to what sorts of stimuli?)

Findings and Comments

Using a case-by-case method to examine the match between standardized and clinical *child* measures, we found no simple relationship. For instance, a child might have gone up in IQ and social competence, but still (clinically) might display problems in the affective area. This was found with a number of children who had improved cognitively and even socially.

For the purposes of this study, the concepts of competence, resiliency, and relative invulnerability were defined in terms of a child's ability to use the therapeutic nursery experience to catch up with development. Indeed, over half of our sample did improve significantly on standardized measures from the time they entered the program until they left. While we acknowledge that each child had a unique array of cognitive and social–emotional abilities, the children who showed marked increases in competence did seem to form a group (albeit heterogeneous) that was currently functioning at closer to their "potential."

However, when we asked why only *certain* children had improved, we at first found no easily discernible patterns. Well-functioning, competent children at posttesting were found across all SES and ethnic groups, in homes with single or married, schizophrenic or affectively disordered mothers. Their mothers had participated in the program for anywhere from 9 to 30 months and seemed, as a group, to have about the same degree of severity or chronicity of illness. The mothers of these more resilient children were not more highly educated than some of the mothers of the children doing far less well, several of whom had at least bachelor's degrees. How were we to interpret these results? Were there truly no patterns to give meaning to our findings, no linkages between child and maternal factors?

Finally, we turned to the clinical information we had gathered while treating the *mothers*, and integrated it with standardized assessments of maternal psychosocial functioning and mother–child interactions. The profiles derived from the use of this material on the mothers allowed us to make sense of what was initially a puzzling picture. Without in-depth clinical knowledge of these mothers as well as their children, we would have been unable to understand the meaning of our child outcome findings.

Could it be that particular patterns of maternal caretaking behavior were related to particular areas of vulnerability and resiliency in the children? Certainly the notion of one-to-one correspondence between a dimension of child competence and a particular pattern of maternal behavior denotes a degree of causality and specificity of influence that is clearly unwarranted. Beyond this, such a view disregards the bidirectionality of the influence of the dyad, and fails to recognize what the child brings to the transactions between himself and his caretaking environment. On the other hand, our extensive knowledge of the character of the mother–child relationships and the flavor of the children's everyday life led us to a constellation of maternal factors that seemed to be related to the children's capacity to seek and use growth-fostering influences beyond their mothers' orbit. This constellation of maternal factors is best described by the term "enablement": The children who improved were those whose mothers enabled them to turn to significant others within the therapeutic nursery environment, and to "use" positively what was offered to enhance their own development.

In our investigation, the primary factor in a child's ability to make use of the intervention program was the *enabling quality of his relationship with his mother*. In general, those children who did better had mothers characterized by the following traits:

1. They used the treatment program well and showed improvement in at least some aspects of psychosocial functioning.

2. They were less involved and, interestingly, more "likeable"; they had friends, thought of others apart from themselves, and generally were interested in other people.

3. They displayed more positive affect and emotional availability (even though they may have been depressed) toward their children; they were able at some times to enjoy their children and become actively involved with them in an activity requiring joint attention and engagement.

4. They may have viewed their children as burdens, but did not see them as victimizing agents to be blamed for their mental illness and other troubles. They were able at least some of the time to relate to their children as separate beings, and to differentiate the children's needs from their own. They could therefore recognize that their children needed help in order to develop to their fullest capacity. Amazingly, these women were keenly aware that many of their children's problems were to some degree the results of understimulation, repeated separations, and exposure to a somewhat unpredictable environment. Nevertheless, they could join with the project staff in encouraging their children to get *their* needs met, even if it sometimes hurt that others had to provide what they themselves had been unable to give. Their active willingness to share their children with the teacher therapist (without competing with the children for her attention, as the other mothers did) gave the children permission to seek and use help from other caring adults. Although they may have been quite openly jealous of the teacher's capabilities, position, and relationship to their children, they could nonetheless join with her to improve their own parenting skills, and could look to her for approval when they succeeded.

Simply speaking, these mothers had been able, to some degree, to form an appropriate attachment to their children that allowed them to let them go in a positive, encouraging, and growth-fostering way. At the risk of oversimplification, it seems accurate to say that these mothers were less "selfish," and consequently better able to care for others. They did not "use" people, their children included, solely to meet their own needs. Nowhere within our study sample was this capacity for moving beyond oneself better exemplified than in the contrasts observed between two mothers who at first appeared quite similar.

Two Mothers and their Daughters

The two women selected to illustrate maternal issues surrounding child competence and vulnerability had many characteristics in common, but also differed in a number of subtle and critically important ways. Both women were white, middle-class, married, and in their mid-20s. They both had experienced successful and satisfactory career paths and had good premorbid histories. Each one, soon after the birth of her first child, had suffered a severe postpartum psychosis marked by delusional thinking, profound depression, and homicidal ideation directed toward the baby. Both families had initially resisted psychiatric hospitalization for the new mothers. Their psychiatrists had then referred them to the Thresholds Mothers' Project as an alternative to hospitalization. In both cases, however, the mothers did require hospitalization shortly after entering the program. They returned to the Mothers' Project after a 2-month hospitalization in one case, and a 3-month stay in the other.

Carol and Nancy

Carol was the second child of immigrant parents whose conflicting values had strongly influenced the manner in which they raised their children. For example, while it was extremely important to Carol's father that the family maintain the traditions of the "old country," Carol's mother subtly conveyed the message that it was of greater importance to become assimilated into the American culture. Carol's reaction to these mixed parental messages had led to the development of a conflictual relationship with her mother, characterized by rebellious acting out. This included dating inappropriate men, and ongoing struggles over issues related to autonomy and control. While there was a less overtly conflictual relationship with her father, there were indeed differences with this parent as well. Mr. B.'s suspected involvement in a number of acts of voyeurism in the neighborhood had embarrassed the family and exacerbated the normal problems of assimilating to an alien culture. Later, after a tentatively negotiated adolescent identity struggle, Carol married a man from a similar ethnic background. Although her husband was a somewhat rigid and controlled man who tended to become helpless during any crisis, he was capable of genuine caring and concern for his family.

Despite the family members' problems, they immediately drew together when Carol became ill. Although distrustful of American institutions, they would bring Carol and 4-month-old Nancy to the Mothers' Project, and were able to deal with their apprehension by staying for the morning and observing in the nursery each time they came to the agency. When it became apparent that Carol could no longer avoid psychiatric hospitalization, the family reluctantly agreed to continue to bring Nancy to the Mothers' Project nursery three times a week, respecting Carol's expressed wishes.

Toward the end of her 3-month hospitalization, Carol was able to leave the hospital for several hours at a time. During this period, she made frequent trips to the agency to visit with Nancy. It was very important to Carol to have Nancy brought to the nursery, not only for the sake of continuity of care but also to reduce her own feelings of inferiority in relation to her family, all of whom she perceived as being "better" caregivers than she. While very tenuous with Nancy at first, Carol was always concerned about her well-being and about the effect of the separation on their relationship. She gradually assumed more and more responsibility for her daughter's care and was greatly encouraged by Nancy's increasing responsiveness. Mother and daughter remained with the Mothers' Project for 1 year following Carol's discharge from the hospital.

Initial testing at 4 months had indicated that Nancy was motorically delayed, although she did have good visual abilities. A passive baby, she would respond to social interactions, but did not initiate these exchanges or actively reach out to interact with the world of objects. This passivity contributed to some degree to her below-average DQ.

After being in the program for a year, Nancy's development showed considerable improvement in both cognitive and social domains, despite the fact that she continued to manifest extreme separation anxiety. Her coping ability during the developmental assessment changed considerably from the first hour, when she was severely inhibited and literally inseparable from her mother, to the end of the session, when she began to be more independent and to explore freely. Nursery observations at this time also indicated separation issues to be of greatest concern. Although characterized as a shy and anxious child, Nancy was able to relate to her teachers and had good attentional abilities, and (when not anxious) a productive learning style. During follow-up testing at 28 months, Nancy continued to show separation problems. Her score of 114 on the Stanford–Binet was considered to be an underestimate of her intellectual abilities and was attributed to her separation anxiety and test inhibition.

Both Nancy and Carol benefited markedly from treatment during their participation in the Mothers' Project. As noted earlier, Nancy was able to make use of the therapeutic nursery, and Carol was able to permit this to occur. While somewhat hesitant to form relationships, Nancy was able to use them, once she did so, as a supportive foundation from which to learn and grow. Mother and child together responded quite well to the child development specialist, who worked with them to facilitate the development of their relationship—first by enabling Carol to "get to know" Nancy, and then by allowing Carol to slowly take over caretaking and stimulation functions. Carol was a thoughtful member of the child development group, as well as the more therapeutically oriented mothers' therapy group. She was able to identify with issues raised by other mothers and to model herself after the leaders. Carol continued her individual therapy with the psychiatrist who originally saw her in the hospital and kept in contact with former project staff, calling with appropriate questions about Nancy's developmental needs. These periodic calls were indicative of Carol's capacity to form attachments and to make use of outside resources, not only for herself but for her child as well.

Cindy and Martha

Cindy was the younger of two daughters in a family where both parents had experienced depressions, although neither had required psychiatric hospitalization. Her father was described as having the pattern of cyclical mood swings characteristic of a bipolar disorder, while her mother had suffered a postpartum depression that remitted only after she had returned to work, leaving Cindy in someone else's care. The emotional climate in which Cindy developed was simultaneously cold and intrusive. The resulting deprivation was a theme that was to run through the narrative of all of Cindy's subsequent relationships.

Cindy's husband, Paul, was a rigidly defended man whose history bore a striking resemblance to her own. Mental illness existed within the family, but was denied because of the family's strong investment in maintaining the image of their newly acquired upper-middle-class status. As we came to know Paul better, we began to see his struggles with his own unmet dependency needs, and his defenses against them became understandable as a false show of competence and autonomy. Cindy and Paul had a fragile marriage that was highly dependent upon keeping up appearances. This brittle marital system shattered with the birth of their daughter, Martha, because Cindy's depleted emotional resources could be stretched no further. Paul became enraged at Cindy's inability to care adequately for their child, largely because he viewed her illness as a betrayal of their mutual facade. At this time, Paul took over Cindy's mother's deprecating role by belittling her and physically abusing her on occasion. He and his family denied the existence of any significant emotional disturbance and insisted that Cindy could "cure herself" through will power. It was only when Cindy's suicidal ideation became homicidal and began to incorporate Martha that Paul could be persuaded to permit her to be hospitalized. Cindy's parents offered as little support as her husband. Indeed, when Cindy's illness could no longer be denied, *her* mother had said, "Paul, if I had known, I wouldn't have let you marry her."

In contrast to Carol and her family, Cindy's family did not allow, nor did Cindy desire, Martha to come to the therapeutic nursery during her mother's hospitalization. Cindy did, however, return to the program with Martha soon after her discharge. Invested in maintaining her image as a healthy, functioning person, Cindy had difficulty identifying with a program that was designed to serve psychiatrically ill people. Consequently, she would come to the agency only on those days when she could receive individual attention from the project social worker. This self-absorption acted to prevent her child from benefiting from the consistency and regularity that is such a critical aspect of the therapeutic nursery experience.

Martha's 7-month Bayley score at entrance to the program showed the wide variability of performance so characteristic of early developmental disorder: Her Psychomotor Development Index (PDI) was 117, while her Mental Development Index (MDI) was 150. At posttesting 1 year later, her MDI had fallen two standard deviations, remaining at that level at follow-up testing 2 years later. Clinical data from the nursery indicated that while Martha was in some ways a very bright and friendly child, she had very poor attentional skills and was unable to remain with a task beyond the briefest period of time. This worrisome aspect of her development was again noted in her test-taking behavior at her follow-up examination, when she was almost 2½ years old. At that time it was difficult to elicit or maintain her attention, and so she was unable to complete the Stanford–Binet. This, to some degree, accounted for the underestimate of her IQ (120), given her superior verbal skills.

Comparison of Carol and Cindy

Regardless of the etiology of their disturbance, both mothers had exhibited psychotic behavior following the birth of their daughters, and both had been separated from their infants because of a psychiatric hospitalization. Finally, both could be said to have low self-esteem, long-standing life adjustment problems related to poorly resolved issues from their own childhoods, and troubled relationships with their spouses and families of origin.

Beneath these similarities lay critical differences in the characters of these two women, as well as in the basic nature of their relationships to their children. Our projective testing had shown both women to be anxious in regard to intimate relationships, distant and denying of their feelings toward others, and significantly concerned about issues of separation. Nevertheless, Carol was able to see others as dependable and trustworthy, and even to experience strong, positive maternal and nurturing feelings, although she did have some difficulty expressing them. In contrast, Cindy was more rigidly defended, brittle, and immature, relying more on defense mechanisms such as "splitting" and magical thinking to cope with the threats of her overwhelming anxiety.

Highly ambivalent about her role as a mother, Cindy experienced few maternal or nurturing feelings.

Assessment of mother–child interaction using the Mothers' Project Rating Scales (Clark, Musick, Stott, & Klehr, 1980) highlighted possible linkages between internal conflict around mothering and actual mothering behaviors. Two examples of this are particularly striking, and serve to illustrate interesting differences between these two women in their roles as caretakers and nurturers. Cindy was rated as more intrusive than Carol during three videotaped sequences involving feeding, a structured task, and free play with her infant daughter. The variable of "intrusiveness" was designed to assess a mother's interference with and domination of her child, and includes overstructuring, overcontrolling, and active interfering to such a degree that the child's initiative is often thwarted. In this case, it seemed to capture the flavor of Cindy's insensitivity and unresponsiveness to her child as an individual with needs that might be different from her own. Related to this were the differences between the two mothers on "mirroring," the variable that measures the behavioral indicators of maternal emotional availability. This can be observed in a mother's reflection of her child's affect and behavior through imitating, echoing (with smaller infants), gazing, smiling, and confirming the child's behavior with approval, encouragement, and praise. Carol was rated as engaging in more "mirroring" behaviors than was Cindy. This was not an unexpected finding, in view of Cindy's general unavailability to her child, but it does give a confirming sense or the relationship between the psychological capacity for parenting and observed parenting behavior. It has been observed (McCowan, 1977) that the prognosis for recovery from postpartum disturbance is, to a great degree, dependent on the environmental and interpersonal supports available to the mother. Here again we can see an important difference between the two women. While both could certainly be said to have had troubled relationships with their own mothers, Carol's problems appeared to center primarily around the not-so-unusual mother–daughter issues of control and autonomy. On the other hand, Cindy's issues with her mother involved serious conflict over dependency, as well as powerful (but denied) hostility toward the nonsupportive and deprecating mother. Although the pathological aspect of each woman's relationship with her husband served to replicate the pathology within her family of origin, Carol's was clearly of a far less toxic nature. It seemed to be "closer to the surface," and restricted to only a few domains of daily existence, whereas Cindy's was both deeper and more pervasive.

As indicated earlier, Carol and Cindy differed markedly in terms of their use of treatment, both for themselves and for their children. Carol actively strove to use her individual treatment as well as the groups and classes to develop some insight and to be able to relate to

Nancy as separate from herself. For example, she was able to speak of how angry she felt at Nancy for her passivity and shyness with strangers, and she came to realize the projective nature of this feeling by recognizing her anger at herself for having these same qualities. Carol's understanding of this process indiciated an awareness of herself and her child as two individuals, connected yet separate.

In contrast, Cindy was never able to move beyond a narcissistically rooted perception of Martha as an extension of herself. Initially, during the most acute phase of her illness, she had believed that her child had caused her to become sick, and was now somehow trying to deprive her of all that she valued. After her release from the hospital, Cindy began to treat Martha as though the child's needs were identical to her own. This naturally resulted in gross misinterpretations of normal behavior and the attribution of her own needs and motives to her infant daughter. A striking example of this was Cindy's frequent interpretation of Martha's behavior (crying, exploratory behavior, etc.) as indicating that "she needs time away from me," when clearly it was her wish to be away from her child that she was expressing.

Cindy remained highly ambivalent about her participation in the program; her limited use of the groups centered primarily on her self-chosen role as "model mother" and advice giver to others. Martha's latest developmental accomplishment was often used to illustrate her mother's skill at parenting, and by (unspoken) implication her own superior mental health. She was unable to sustain a therapeutic relationship either with her psychiatrist or with staff members of the Mothers' Project, and repeatedly annoyed the other mothers by her attitude of superiority.

Because Carol was able to differentiate her own needs from those of her daughter, she understood that Nancy needed to be in the nursery on a regular basis. Lacking this capacity, Cindy brought Martha to the nursery only when *she* had a session with the project social worker, thus depriving her child of the therapeutic benefits of the continuity and regularity of the nursery experience. As a result of these mother-based differences in attendance, the two children were to have very different experiences in the program. Nancy began to use the nursery to form attachments to the teachers, which in turn allowed her to "catch up" in a number of aspects of cognitive and social–emotional development. It became apparent that her developmental delay was due more to the early separation than to a pathological parent–child relationship. Nancy is doing well today, several years after her participation in the program, although she is still a very shy child with noticeable difficulties in regard to separation. While it is far too early to know what life will be like for her, we know that she has parents (and grandparents) who are able to respond appropriately to her needs.

Martha, who was not brought to the nursery on a regular basis, showed declines in both cognitive and social–emotional performance at posttesting. While a portion of this could possibly be accounted for by artificial inflation of her initial test scores, it seems more likely that her increasingly severe attentional problems were at the root of these dysfunctions. It is not possible to know the degree to which her poor attentional skills are a function of genetic factors, the separation from her mother, or adverse environmental effects. What does seem clear, however, is that, like her mother, Martha will have increasing problems related to being the child of parents who are unable to differentiate their needs from her own.

In summary, it appears that although both infants were exposed to severe maternal depression and early separation, Nancy's experience of caretaking was actually quite different from Martha's. These differing experiences can most clearly be observed in the presence or absence of several critical (and related) factors that represent "compensatory aspects of caretaking" (Sameroff, Seifer, & Zax 1982) in these children's lives. These factors are fathers, grandparents, regularity of nursery attendance, and *maternal sensitivity*. Nancy had a loving and attentive father and grandparents, who were interested in both Carol's and Nancy's well-being. This caring manifested itself in the special efforts they took to make certain that Nancy could fully benefit from the therapeutic nursery experience. This was done in agreement and accordance with the expressed wishes of her mother. In contrast, Martha's father and grandparents treated her selfishly, as they had always treated Cindy, seeing no need for the baby to receive the comfort and growth-enhancing stimulation of the nursery. Since Cindy was also not sensitive to Martha's needs in this regard, there was little impetus toward regular nursery attendance either during or after Cindy's hospitalization.

Werner's view of the role of grandparents as "resistance resources" seems particularly apt here. Grandparents, she says, "can provide continuity and support in an otherwise unstable situation and can buffer the effects of family strife and the dissolution of marital ties" (Werner & Smith, 1982, p. 160); we might add that they can buffer the effects of maternal psychopathology.

Conclusion

The finding of these studies, like those of Head Start, bring into question the wisdom of relying too heavily on the use of standardized tests in intervention research; by doing so, the researcher not only loses the richness and complexity of a child's response to intervention, but, more seriously, may be left with what are basically invalid and misleading findings. In relation to the results discussed in this chapter, had we relied solely on standardized assessments, we would have missed what Vygotsky (1978) has called the child's "zone of proximal development," or the distance between a child's actual developmental level as determined by independent problem solving, and the level of his/her *potential* development as determined through problem solving under guidance. The zone of proximal development will differ for each child, and we think it will do so partially because of the mother's previous and ongoing role in what Bruner and his colleagues have referred to as the "scaffolding" process (Wood, Bruner, & Ross, 1976). This consists essentially of the adult's "controlling" those elements of the task that are initially beyond the learner's capacity, thus allowing the child to concentrate upon and complete only those elements that are within his range of competence. It is this process that enables the child to solve a problem or achieve a goal that would be beyond his unassisted efforts. Notions such as the zone of proximal development and scaffolding are helpful to our understanding of the ways in which maternal behavior may be implicated in child outcomes, either by facilitating self-righting tendencies or by blocking adaptive routes for children already at risk or somewhat vulnerable (Musick, Stott, Spencer, Goldman, & Cohler, 1984).

The interactional history of the more resilient children seems to have given them the expectation that adults could be turned to for guidance, nurturance, knowledge, and even particular cognitive, social, and affective needs that could not always be met by their mothers. These children had a more facilitating relationship with their mothers, which manifested itself in two observable ways: (1) their active reaching out to others, and (2) their mothers' support and permission to do just that. Our observations tend to confirm those of Werner and Smith (1982) and Anthony (1983) that one of the key environmental factors in developmental resiliency among children at risk is a good mother-child relationship during the first year of life.

Although our resilient children certainly experienced separation and family discord during their earliest months and years, they were nonetheless partners in a relationship characterized, at least some of the time, by maternal responsiveness, availability, and warmth, regardless of the psychiatric illness. Indeed, the factors involved in a mother's ability to foster this kind of relationship are tied far more to her character than to the presence or absence of mental illness per se. Rather, the capacity for motherliness is dependent on enough psychological distance from the child to enable the mother to move in the direction of making the right choice for the sake of that child (Benedek, 1970). It seems clear that certain aspects of Cindy's character mitigated against her being able to respond positively and empathetically to her child's needs, and to make the right choices for her sake. We do not refer here to the minor failures of empathy that are a natural part of the process of parenting, and that are essential to helping a child achieve the development of inner regulation. As Kohut (1977) notes, the basis of the child's self-pathology is the parent's own lack of empathy, not just occasionally, but pervasively in the parent–child relationship. The parent fails not by simply providing too much to too little stimulation, but by providing tasks that are not appropriate to the child's developmental needs. Maternal defects of this nature in our sample manifested themselves on a number of levels—from a mother's specific inability to read a child's cues, to her more general lack of awareness of the child's needs for positive experience in order to reduce the effects of the early separation and family discord related to her illness. Positive experiences such as those offered in the therapeutic nursery environment can go a long way toward ameliorating the effects of early trauma, whether this trauma is biological (Sameroff & Chandler, 1975) or psychological in nature. The mother who enables her child to make use of growth-enhancing alternative caretaking environments has given that child the unselfish and loving gift of a second chance.

Finally, we need to recognize that good therapeutic settings allow children to "bounce back" because they remove some of the barriers to realization of developmental potential (Stott et al., 1984). Naturally, they will do their best for children whose potential has merely been *suppressed* rather than truly thwarted. Here the difference between delay and deviation, and the environmental (as opposed to organic) factors that may be implicated, are especially pertinent. It seems likely that the majority of our more resilient children were primarily affected by multiple separations, rather by the ongoing effect of being enmeshed in a psychopathological system. This serves to bring our attention once more to the complexity involved in the studying of development in children at risk and to remind us that psychopathology does not necessarily manifest itself in the mother–child relationship in a continuous and negative manner.

ACKNOWLEDGMENTS

The research reported in this chapter was made possible by grant No. IRO1MH28143 from the National Institute of Mental Health and R & D Grant No. 8252-01 from the Illinois Department of Mental Health and Developmental Disabilities.

REFERENCES

Anthony, E. J. (1969). A clinical evaluation of children with psychotic parents. *American Journal of Psychiatry, 126,* 177–184.

Anthony, E. J. (1971). *Folie à deux*: A developmental failure in the process of separation-individuation. In J. McDevitt & C. F. Settlage (Eds.), *Separation–Individuation: Essays in honor of Margaret S. Mahler* (pp. 253–273). New York: International Universities Press.

Anthony, E. J. (1974). The syndrome of the psychologically invulnerable child. In E. Anthony & C. Koupernik (Eds.), *The child in his family: Children at psychiatric risk* (International yearbook, Vol. 3). New York: Wiley.

Anthony, E. J. (1975). The influence of a manic–depressive environment on the developing child. In E. J. Anthony & T. Benedek (Eds.), *Depression and human existence.* Boston: Little, Brown.

Anthony, E. J. (1983). Infancy in a crazy environment. In J. D. Call, E. Galenson, & R. Tyson (Eds.), *Frontiers of infant psychiatry.* New York: Basic Books.

Baldwin, A. I., Cole, R. E., & Baldwin, C. P. (Eds.). (1982). Parental pathology, family interaction, and the competence of the child in school. *Monographs of the Society for Research in Child Development, 47,* (5, Serial No. 197).

Benedek, T. (1970). Motherhood and nurturing. In E. J. Anthony & T. Benedek (Eds.), *Parenthood: Its psychology and psychopathology.* Boston: Little, Brown.

Clark, R., Musick, J., Stott, F., & Klehr, K. (1980). *The Mothers' Project Rating Scales of Mother–Child Interaction.* Unpublished manuscript.

Fisher, L. (1980). (Ed.) Child competence and psychiatric risk: I. Model and method. *Journal of Nervous and Mental Disease, 6,* 323–331.

Fisher, L., Harder, D., Kokes, R., & Strauss, J. (1980). Child competence and psychiatric risk: III. Comparisons based on diagnosis of hospitalized parents. *Journal of Nervous and Mental Disease, 168,* 338–342.

Gallant, D., & Gamer, E. (1977). *Infant and child behavior scales: Ratings from developmental examinations.* Unpublished manuscript, Massachusetts Mental Health Center, Boston, MA.

Garmezy, N. (1974). Children at risk: The search for antecedents of schizophrenia: Part I. Conceptual models and research methods. *Schizophrenia Bulletin, 8,* 14–90.

Kagan, J. (1980). Perspectives on continuity. In O.C. Brim, Jr., & J. Kagan (Eds.), *Constancy and change in human development.* Cambridge, MA: Harvard University Press.

Kohut, H. (1977). *The restoration of the self.* New York: International Universities Press.

Marcus, J., Auerbach, J., Wilkinson, L., & Burack, C. (1981). Infants at risk for schizophrenia: The Jerusalem Infant Development Study. *Archives of General Psychiatry, 38,* 703–713.

McCowan, M. N. (1977). Post partum disturbance: A review of the literature in terms of stress response. *Journal of Nurse-Midwifery, 22*(2), 27–34.

Mednick, S., & McNeil, T. (1968). Current methodology in research on the etiology of schizophrenia. *Psychological Bulletin, 70,* 681–693.

Musick, J., & Cohler, B. (Eds.). (1983). Parental psychopathology and infant development [Special issue]. *Infant Mental Health Journal, 4*(3).

Musick, J., Cohler, B., & Dincin, J. (1982). *Risk and recovery in the children of mentally ill mothers* (R & D Grant No. 8252-01). Chicago: Illinois Department of Mental Health and Developmental Disabilities.

Musick, J., Stott, F., Spencer, K., Goldman, J., & Cohler, B. (1984). The capacity for enabling in mentally ill mothers. *Zero to Three, 4*(4), 1–6.

Neale, J., & Weintraub, S. (1975). Children vulnerable to psychopathology: The Stony Brook High-Risk Project. *Journal of Abnormal Child Psychology, 3,* 95–113.

Rolf, J. (1972). The social and academic competence of children vulnerable to schizophrenia and other behavior pathologies. *Journal of Abnormal Psychology, 80,* 225–243.

Rolf, J. (1976). Peer status and the directionality of symptomatic behavior: Prime social competency predictors of outcome for vulnerable children. *American Journal of Orthopsychiatry, 46,* 74–88.

Sameroff, A. J., Barocas, R., & Seifer, R. (1984). The early development of children born to mentally ill women. In N. F. Watt, E. J. Anthony, L. C. Wynne, & J. E. Rolf (Eds.), *Children at risk for schizophrenia*. Cambridge: Cambridge University Press.

Sameroff, A. J., & Chandler, M. J. (1975). Reproductive risk and the continuum of caretaking causality. In F. D. Horowitz (Ed.), *Review of child development research* (Vol. 4). Chicago: University of Chicago Press.

Sameroff, A. J., Seifer, R., & Zax, M. (1982). Early development of children at risk for emotional disorder. *Monographs of the Society for Research in Child Development, 47* (7, Serial No. 199).

Silverton, L., Finello, K., & Mednick, S. (1983). Early factors predictive of schizophrenia. *Infant Mental Health Journal, 4*(3), 202–216.

Stott, F. M., Musick, J. S., Clark, R., & Cohler, B. J. (1983). Developmental patterns in the infants and young children of mentally ill mothers. *Infant Mental Health Journal, 4*(3), 217–235.

Stott, F., Musick, F., Cohler, B., Spencer, K., Goldman, J., Clark, R., & Dincin, J. (1984). Intervention for the severely disturbed mother. In B. Cohler & J. Musick (Eds.), *New directions for mental health services: Intervention among psychiatrically impaired parents and their young children*. San Francisco: Jossey-Bass.

Vygotsky, L. S. (1978). *Mind in society*. Cambridge, MA: Harvard University Press.

Watt, N. F., Anthony, E. J., Wynne, L. C., & Rolf, J. E. (Eds.). (1984). *Children at risk for schizophrenia*. Cambridge: Cambridge University Press.

Watt, N. F., Grubb, T. W., & Erlenmeyer-Kimling, L. (1982). Social emotional, and intellectual behavior at school among children at high risk for schizophrenia. *Journal of Consulting and Clinical Psychology, 50*, 171–181.

Weintraub, S., Neale, J., & Leibert, D. (1975). Teacher ratings of children vulnerable to psychopathology. *American Journal of Orthopsychiatry, 45*, 838–845.

Weintraub, S., Prinz, R., & Neale, J. (1978). Peer evaluations of the competence of children vulnerable to psychopathology. *Journal of Abnormal Child Psychology, 6*, 461–473.

Weintraub, S., Winters, K. C., & Neale, J. M. (1982). *Competence and vulnerability in children with an affectively disordered parent*. Paper presented at the conference on Depression and Depressive Disorders: Developmental Perspectives, Temple University, Philadelphia.

Werner, E., & Smith, R. (1982). *Vulnerable but invincible: A longitudinal study of resilient children and youth*. New York: McGraw-Hill.

Wood, D., Bruner, J. S., & Ross, G. (1976). The role of tutoring in problem solving. *Journal of Child Psychology and Psychiatry, 17*.

Zubin, J., & Spring, B. (1977). Vulnerability—a new view of schizophrenia. *Journal of Abnormal Psychology, 86*, 103–126.

10

Invulnerability among Abused and Neglected Children

Ellen A. Farber
State University of New York, Buffalo

Byron Egeland
University of Minnesota

Since C. Kempe's (1962) seminal paper, which alerted health professionals to the extent of child abuse, numerous studies have investigated the effects of maltreatment on children. The results of these studies clearly indicate that child abuse has severe developmental consequences. This is true regardless of the particular area of development being studied.

The cognitive development of the abused child has been examined extensively. The findings across studies indicate that disproportionately large numbers of abused children fall below average on measures of intelligence (Morse, Sahler, & Friedman, 1970; Sandgrund, Gaines, & Green, 1974). The extent of retardation (IQ < 80) in the abused samples ranged from a low of 33% (Martin, 1972; Martin, Beezley, Conway, & Kempe, 1974) to a high of 57% (Elmer & Gregg, 1967). Averaging the scores of abused children can be deceptive, as the range of scores in each study is rather large. For example, Martin *et al.* (1974) reported the mean IQ in their sample of abused children to be 92; the standard deviation was 22; and the range was from 15 to 131. Few investigators have attempted to account for the large spread of scores, nor have they specifically examined the abused children who are functioning at the average or above-average level of intelligence.

Two studies did explore factors in the abused child's environment that account for the large variability in IQ scores. Martin *et al.* (1974) found that the stability of the family and the degree of parental "punitiveness" were highly related to the degree of retardation. Morse *et al.* (1970) examined a number of factors and found one related to outcome: Abused children who appeared to be developing normally had mothers who perceived the mother–child relationship positively. In many of the studies, it is impossible to separate the effects of abuse on the intellectual development of the child from the effects of the overall quality of

253

care and home environment experienced by the abused child. Children who have been abused are usually raised in an environment that hinders cognitive development, regardless of abuse.

The reported social and psychological consequences of abuse are also highly varied. Perhaps the most extensive observations are those by R. Kempe and Kempe (1978). They reported that some abused children were compliant and accepting of whatever happened to them, while others were aggressive, hyperactive, and lacking in trust and social skills. Other investigators have described abused children as having low self-esteem (Kinard, 1980; Martin & Beezley, 1977); as being withdrawn, passive, apathetic, and unresponsive to others (Martin & Beezley, 1977; Terr, 1970); and as lacking in the ability to comprehend social roles and believing that they had little power to alter their experiences (Barahal, Waterman, & Martin, 1981). George and Main (1979) found that abused preschool children were more aggressive and less socially interactive than their nonabused peers.

The conclusion based on the results from various investigations is that abused children display a wide range of social, emotional, and intellectual problems, and that these exceed the number of problems of nonabused children. There is no consistent or typical personality profile of abused children. It is not surprising that there is no predictable pattern of maladaptation, considering that the abusive situation and "abusive environment" are highly varied from one case to another. The consequences of abuse are mediated by caretaker characteristics, environmental circumstances, life stress, and support from family and friends, as well as by a child's own temperament and past developmental history. None of the outcome investigations have attempted to determine the factors that make the abused child more or less vulnerable to the effects of maltreatment.

In this chapter, we examine the development of a group of maltreated children from birth through preschool. The children are part of a prospective longitudinal study of families at risk for caretaking problems. From the detailed data regarding the development of the children, we identify those maltreated children who were functioning in a competent fashion at each assessment period. Using the comprehensive data regarding parental characteristics, infant temperament, parent–child interaction, life stress, support, and life circumstances, we attempt to determine those factors that seem to make a child less vulnerable to the effects of maltreatment. We begin by discussing the notion of the at-risk model of research as it applies to studies of child abuse. Next we provide some background information about the study, the Minnesota Mother–Child Interaction Project, and explain our theoretical and empirical approach to studying individual differences in adaptation. Then the results of previous investigations of group differences between abused and neglected and nonabused children in this sample are presented. With this understanding of the mean outcomes, it is possible to investigate within-group differences. In other words, do some children seem to be invulnerable to maternal abuse? Using both statistical analyses and case studies, we attempt to clarify how these children thrive.

Child Abuse Research and the At-Risk Model

Until recently, most of the studies in child abuse were retrospective. This approach involves gathering data on families with reported incidents of child abuse and then, in most instances, comparing them to a control group. The retrospective approach has been used by a number of investigators to identify the etiological factors involved in abuse. However, these studies have several limitations.

First, retrospective research, while it can identify characteristics of abusing families, cannot differentiate abusing families from similar families who do not abuse. For example, one consistent finding from these studies is that abused and neglected children are most likely to come from families experiencing large amounts of social and economic stress (Alvy, 1975; Garbarino, 1976). The conclusion from these studies is that poverty causes abuse. Certainly there is a relationship, but the majority of poor parents do not abuse their children. We need to identify the factors differentiating poor families that abuse their children from the similar families that provide adequate care.

A second limitation of retrospective research involves the issue of causality. Assessing differences between abused and nonabused children does not tell us whether the differences were causes or consequences of abuse. For example, several investigators (Gelles, 1973; Parker & Collmer, 1976) have suggested that abused children may be particularly difficult to care for. The important question here is this: Did the children's difficult temperaments cause them to be abused, or are their temperaments the result of previous abuse? Examining children only after abuse occurs makes it impossible to distinguish cause from consequence.

Risk research avoids the problems inherent in retrospective research. A prospective, at-risk approach follows children who are known, based on actuarial data, to have a higher probability of specific outcomes than a random sample of children. It is based on the assumption that a group can be identified in which a certain problem will occur with a frequency great enough to warrant extensive study of a large sample, most of whom will not share the particular pathology being studied. This basically healthy group referred to by Garmezy and others (Garmezy & Neuchterlein, 1972) as "invulnerable" serves as an appropriate comparison group, for it is only in contrast to good outcomes within the same sample that the major influences on the poor outcomes can be identified.

The at-risk approach allows both for statistical comparisons among groups and for detailed study of individual cases that examine the interaction of a number of factors. Garmezy and Devine (1975) note that the strength of the at-risk model "lies in the more accurate extension it permits of the developmental process as represented by the group, and, of equal importance, of individuals within the group." It not only provides measures of central tendency and dispersion at various ages; it also points out the atypical cases at any given age and permits one to trace the consequences of atypicality at one age upon later development (Garmezy & Devine, 1975). The failure to consider the cumulative effects of abuse is one shortcoming of many previous investigations. Abused children are usually examined at only one point in time.

A Prospective At-Risk Study of Abuse

The Minnesota Mother–Child Interaction Project is a prospective longitudinal study that has been following a group of mothers considered at risk for abuse and neglect. During their last trimester of pregnancy, 267 primiparous women receiving prenatal care at a public health clinic were enrolled in the study. The families were from low-socioeconomic-status backgrounds; the majority were on welfare. The base rate for abuse and neglect in the public health clinic population was approximately 2%, which was considerably higher than that for the state in general, thus defining the at-risk nature of the population (Egeland & Brunnquell, 1979). Risk factors, in addition to economic difficulty, included limited education, youth of the mothers, and generally chaotic and stressful living conditions. The mean age of the mothers was 20.5 (range = 12–34), and 40% of them had not graduated from high school. Moreover, 62% of the mothers were single; thus, it is not surprising that 86% of the pregnancies were unplanned.

Obtaining our sample prior to the actual births of the children allowed us to assess maternal personality characteristics and expectations about child rearing prior to the arrival of the children as well as in the years following. Shortly after the births, in the newborn nursery, we began assessments of the children's characteristics. We also periodically evaluated environmental circumstances. "Independent" assessments of maternal, child, and environmental characteristics, and observations of mother–child interactions over time, aided us in identifying etiological factors in abuse.

This approach is consistent with the transactional model (see Sameroff & Chandler, 1975; Seifer & Sameroff, Chapter 2, this volume). This model assumes plasticity of a child's environment and views the child as an active participant. The mother and child are continually influencing each other and creating, as well as being influenced by, their environment. It should be noted that the transactional model is in sharp contrast to the linear model used in many longitudinal studies. In the linear model, individuals with specific attributes (e.g., perinatal complications) are followed up to assess the outcomes (e.g., deviancy). The linear approach erroneously assumes direct cause and effect, thus ignoring intervening variables and intermediate outcomes. The transactional model is more relevant to studying the process of adaptation-maladaptation and the factors that shape its course.

A Developmental Model of Adaptation

To fully understand the consequences of abuse, researchers cannot be content with simple outcome variables such as aggression. Within a developmental framework, the crucial task is to formulate assessment procedures that are specifically appropriate to each age period. This involves determining the central issue for each developmental period and then constructing appropriate assessment procedures. Assessment within our prospective transactional study has been guided by organizational-developmental theory.

Organizational-developmental theory, a synthesis of several theories (evolutionary, ego-analytic, and cognitive-developmental), views development not as an incremental or linear process, but rather in terms of the organizations and reorganizations of behaviors. Behaviors are hierarchically organized into more complex patterns, at the core of which are the earlier modes of functioning. These reorganizations insure qualitative changes in the way the individual transacts with the environment. In infancy, physiological factors are very important in how the infant deals with the environment, but over time psychological factors take on increasing importance. The different systems—physiological, cognitive, affective, and so on—are interrelated, and advances or lags in one system will affect another (Sroufe, 1979b).

Of major importance in this theory is an emphasis on adaptation, an active process of the individual engaging the environment with respect to his needs and goals (Sroufe, 1979a). With respect to the quality of adaptation or the development of competence, the model suggests that the reorganizations take place in "response" to a series of salient issues that occur in an invariant sequence. Early experience is important in that it shapes the way the next issue is faced. The developmental model asserts that there are consistent individual differences in the ways that children organize their behavior to meet the environmental demands. Furthermore, behaviors may not be identical across situations, but behavior is coherent across situations and is organized with respect to the individual's goals (Sroufe, 1979a). This point addresses the vigorous controversy over intrapersonal consistency versus situational determinism. A basic premise of the theory is that we can predict future adaptation from knowledge of current adaptation; however, an intermeshing of the notions of continuity and stability has created a greater opposition to this view than may be necessary.

The use of identical measures (with or without age-appropriate content variations) has for the most part failed to show stability of personality traits and behaviors (e.g., Mischel, 1968). This type of assessment attempts to demonstrate complete continuity (e.g., Kagan, 1971)—stability in both the manifest behavior and its underlying psychological process or stability of discrete behaviors from Time 1 to Time 2. This type of continuity might be expected after puberty, when psychological organization nears completion. In the early years, when response systems are undergoing rapid change, heterotypic continuity (stability between two different response modalities as a function of a common underlying process or continuity of patterns of behavioral organization) would be a more reasonable expectation. Since environment and child are viewed as mutually influencing, it follows that behavior at Time 2 reflects not only quality of adaptation at Time 1, but also the intervening environmental inputs. Thus, we also expect predictable changes in quality of adaptation, based on changes in the environment.

Some of the developmental issues for the early years that we and others have studied are the formation of an effective attachment relationship toward the end of the first year of life and effective autonomous functioning by age 2. An expanded ability to organize and coordinate environmental resources to engage problems posed by the environment, and effective peer relations, are major issues during the preschool years. With the issues mentioned above, researchers have demonstrated continuity in adaptation from birth to 5 years (Arend, Gove, & Sroufe, 1979; Matas, Arend, & Sroufe, 1978; Waters, Wippman, & Sroufe, 1979). A discussion of some of the constructs and corresponding assessment procedures may help clarify the theory.

Assessment of Attachment at 12 and 18 Months

The development of an affective bond, an attachment between the infant and its mother, is the major developmental task in the first year of life. According to the ethological/evolutionary theory of attachment

(Bowlby, 1969), it is the natural course of events for an infant to become attached to a mother figure. This enduring affectional tie is a product of interaction over time, a function of the initial behaviors each brings to the relationship and the effects those behaviors have on each member.

Ainsworth and her associates have developed and validated a procedure, the "Strange Situation," for assessing individual differences in the organization of attachment behaviors (Ainsworth, Blehar, Waters, & Wall, 1978; Ainsworth & Wittig, 1969). The Strange Situation, which we used to assess attachment at 12 and 18 months, was designed to assess the balance of attachment and exploration behaviors in increasingly stressful circumstances. It consists of a series of episodes in which the infant's exploration of a novel environment in the presence of the mother, reaction to separation from the mother, and reunion with the mother are observed. In addition, the baby's reaction to a stranger with and without the mother present is observed. Primarily on the basis of behaviors seen upon reunion with their mothers after the separation, infants are assigned to classification groups reflecting both the patterning and the quality of observed attachment behaviors.

Infants are classified into three main groups. An infant is classified as secure in attachment (Group B) if the presence of the mother supports exploration of the room and the toys prior to separation and if the presence of the mother reduces distress and facilitates a return to exploration after separation. Even if not distressed by separation, securely attached infants actively greet and/or seek interaction with their mothers upon reunion. When the caregiver's presence does not support exploration or reduce distress following separation, an infant is said to be anxiously attached. There are two patterns of anxious attachment. Anxious/avoidant infants (Group A) explore with little affective interaction in preseparation episodes, treat their mothers and the stranger similarly, and avoid the mothers upon reunion. Anxious/resistant babies (Group C) demonstrate impoverished exploration and difficulty being comforted. Often they mix active comfort seeking with struggling, stiffness, and continued crying.

These individual differences in quality of attachment were found to be highly stable between 12 and 18 months of age for middle-class families. Frequencies and durations of particular behaviors were not stable (Waters, 1978). This finding is consistent with the view that attachment is a construct reflecting the organization of behavior rather than any particular behavior (Sroufe & Waters, 1977). In other words, specific behaviors, such as how much or how little contact an infant seeks or how much or how little it cries, will vary across time and are only meaningful within the overall patterns of behavior (Sroufe & Waters, 1977). In our study, involving a less stable, economically disadvantaged sample, patterns of attachment behavior observed in the Strange Situation were also significantly stable, although more changes occurred than did for middle-class samples (Egeland & Farber, 1984).

Assessment of Autonomous Functioning at 24 Months

In the second year of life, the well-functioning child is making great strides toward autonomous functioning (e.g., Erikson, 1963). Our procedure for assessing competence at age 2 involved a tool-using, problem-solving situation developed by Matas et al. (1978). In a problem-solving situation, movement toward autonomy is indicated by flexibility, resourcefulness, and ability to use adult assistance without being overly dependent on it. The competent toddler should also be affectively involved by showing pleasure in task solution and, in the face of frustration, remaining involved and examining alternative strategies before giving up all efforts at solving the problem.

In the procedure developed by Matas et al. (1978), the children, with their mothers present, are asked to work on four tasks. The first two are simple. The last two are increasingly difficult and somewhat beyond the capacity of a 2-year-old; only these are included in the scoring. Mothers are instructed to let the children work on the problem independently and then give any help needed. Like the Strange Situation, in which the infants are subjected to separation and stress, this procedure taxes the toddlers' capacities for maintaining organized behavior—for coordinating affect, cognition, and behavior—and for drawing on personal and environmental resources. Whether the children solve the problem or how quickly they solve it is unimportant. The tool-using situation was videotaped in our study, and each child was rated on a number of scales, including dependency, noncompliance, frustration, persistence, coping, enthusiasm, and positive and negative affect. From these ratings we were able to assess the child's competence along three dimensions: an emotional dimension (e.g., enthusiasm and the ability to face challenges when frustrated); motivation, reflected by the time spent on the task; and ability to use maternal assistance effectively, as indicated by the child's compliance or tantrums.

Assessment of Self-Awareness and Socialization at 42 Months

Competence during the preschool period revolves around issues of self-regulation, control of impulses, self-awareness, identity formation, and peer relations. The issue of control is particularly salient during this developmental phase. This issue is also important during earlier periods of development, but it is conceptualized in a much different form. In the toddler period, control revolves around parental demands for obedience and controlling impulses. During the preschool period, this external source of control gives way to self-control. By gaining self-control rather than experiencing external control, the child enhances his ability to function autonomously and effectively. The competent 3-year-old is neither too rigid in self-regulation of feelings nor at the mercy of impulses. His competence is reflected in a flexible, enthusiastic, and confident approach to problems.

An assessment procedure centering around a "Barrier Box" was devised in our study to measure a child's approach to a problem situation in a nonsocial context. The procedure involved allowing each child to play with a variety of attractive toys on the floor. After a short period of time, the toys were removed and placed in a latched Plexiglas box. For 10 minutes the child was allowed to try to open the box, play with uninteresting toys that remained on the floor, or wander around the room. At the end of the session, the child was allowed to play with the toys in the box. The session was videotaped, and the child was rated on scales of 1–3 or 1–7 on the following variables: self-esteem, ego control (how well the child was able to control impulses and modulate responses), apathy/withdrawal, flexibility, creativity, agency (the child's confidence and assertiveness in approaching the task), hyperactivity/distractibility, dependency on the project assistant for help and support, directness and intensity of help seeking, and positive and negative affect. In addition to these rating scales, the child's persistence was measured by computing the proportion of time spent on the task.

In addition to the Barrier Box task, the children were observed in a teaching situation at 42 months. The children were observed with their mothers in four learning tasks that were difficult enough to require that the mothers use some teaching strategies to enable the children to complete the tasks. The teaching session was videotaped, and the children were rated on their persistence, enthusiasm for the tasks, anger/negativity (directed at the mothers and/or the environment in general), compliance with mothers' directions, reliance on mothers for support, affection for mothers, and avoidance of mothers.

Assessment of Peer Relations and Socialization in Preschool

We also assessed competence in a preschool or day care setting for 90 of the children from our total sample. Of these children, 40 attended a special laboratory preschool at the University of Minnesota (Sroufe, 1983). The others attended a variety of school and day care centers throughout the Minneapolis metropolitan area. We were particularly interesting in the preschool children's social skills and relations with peers. We were interested in their prosocial behavior, compliance, independent functioning, and emotional responsivity. Using 7-point rating scales, observers assessed the children on the following variables: agency (how confidently and assertively the children dealt with the environment), ego control (how the children monitored impulses and modulated responses to the preschool environment), dependency on teachers for support and nurturance, social skills in the peer group, positive affect, negative emotional tone, and compliance with teachers' directions and suggestions. In addition, a preschool teacher or child care provider completed the Preschool Behavior Questionnaire (Behar & Stringfield, 1974), which consists of 31 items often associated with socioemotional problems in young children. The respondent was asked to check for each item: (1) "doesn't apply" (scored 0 points), (2) "applies sometimes" (1 point), or (3) "certainly applies" (2 points). A behavior problem checklist consisting of 31 items written by our staff was also completed by the teachers, using the same format as for the Preschool Behavior Questionnaire.

The assessment procedures just described, spanning the children's first 5 years of life, occurred in a variety of situations. Each child was observed with the mother, with peers, and alone. These procedures parallel the important developmental tasks as a child grows from infant to toddler to preschooler. Previous studies have demonstrated that securely attached infants are more likely to become competent, effective preschoolers than anxiously attached infants (Arend *et al.*, 1979; Waters *et al.*, 1979). The fact that the quality of adaptation was assessed in the preschool situation without the mother present is important. Although the quality of attachment is a product of mother–infant interaction, the continuity in adaptation between infancy and preschool cannot be attributed to maternal behavior in the assessment situations. Rather, any such continuity is attributable to the child's emerging personality. Thus,

> the infant who uses the caregiver as a base for moving out into the world, and as a haven when threatened or distressed, develops motor skills and a sense of himself as effective. In sharing his play with his caregiver at a distance, the infant evolves a new way of maintaining contact while operating independently. The infant is free to invest himself in challenging the environment because he is confident that he can maintain his tie with his caregiver while he is widening his world. . . . Children who have adapted well will look at challenging situations positively, and their expectations concerning people will also be positive. (Sroufe, 1978, p. 52)

It should be noted that the procedures described above are not assessments of specific skills (i.e., competencies). Competence—behavioral organization—has an affective core. For example, intelligence is not a critical variable in our model. Intelligence is a competency that may be an advantage in approaching the challenges of the environment, but it is not enough to ensure healthy functioning. Well-adapted children may be high or low on intelligence. In addition, we have found it more useful to develop profiles of behavioral organization, which describe patterns of adaptation, rather than analyzing rating scales individually. These profiles are obtained either from previously defined patterns, such as the attachment classifications, or through cluster analysis. With this review of the developmental model, it is now time to consider the developmental consequences of abuse and other forms of maltreatment.

Background for This Study: The Effects of Abuse

In previous investigations with this sample (Egeland & Sroufe, 1981; Egeland, Sroufe, & Erickson, 1984), four maltreatment groups were identified: "physically abusive," "hostile/verbally abusive," "psychologically unavailable," and "neglectful." A control group of mothers who clearly provided adequate care was also chosen from the at-risk sample. These groups were chosen based on information obtained and observed during visits to the mothers' homes, during laboratory assessments, and from public health records. In the initial investigation (Egeland & Sroufe, 1981), we examined development at 12, 18, and 24 months. We extended the follow-up to include the assessment of developmental adaptation at 42 months and preschool age (Egeland et al., 1984). The present investigation of "invulnerable" abused children involved examining the competent children in our abused sample from infancy through the preschool period.

Behaviors of mothers in the physically abusive group ranged from frequent and intense spanking while disciplining their children to unprovoked, angry outbursts resulting in serious injuries, such as cigarette burns. The mothers in the hostile/verbally abusive group chronically found fault with their children and criticized them in an overly harsh fashion. The difference between these mothers and the physically abusive mothers was in the chronic nature of their abuse; they continually berated their children.

The psychologically unavailable group consisted of detached, emotionally uninvolved mothers. They showed a lack of emotional responsiveness to their children and interacted only when necessary. They seldom would comfort or console the children when the children were distressed, nor would they respond to the children's attempts to elicit positive social interactions. These women appeared depressed and withdrawn.

Mothers in the neglectful group were irresponsible in managing the day-to-day activities of child rearing. They failed to provide the necessary physical and health care for their children and did not protect them from possible dangers in the home. Although these mothers often expressed interest in the well-being of their children, they did not have the skills or understanding to provide consistent adequate care (Egeland & Sroufe, 1981; Egeland *et al.*, 1984).

Although there was overlap among the groups, the purpose of trying to delineate four groups was to determine whether specific patterns of maltreatment resulted in specific developmental consequences. One reason for the range of outcomes in previous studies may have been differences in the patterns, frequencies, and severity of the behaviors labeled "abuse."

As noted above, a control group of mothers who provided adequate care was selected from the remaining sample. If there was some question whether a mother was mistreating a child, or if the mistreatment was borderline, the case was not included in the control group or any of the maltreatment groups. Of approximately 200 cases considered from the total at-risk sample on whom data were available across the first 2 years, 24 mothers were in the physically abusive group, 19 in the hostile/verbally abusive group, 19 in the psychologically unavailable group, 24 in the neglectful group, and 85 in the control group. Of the 19 hostile mothers, 15 were also in the physically abusive group. Of the 19 mothers in the psychologically unavailable group, 12 out of 19 were in the physically abusive group, and 13 of 24 mothers in the neglectful group also physically abused their children. In all, there were 44 mothers in the maltreatment group.

Effects of Physical Abuse

A larger proportion of the abused children than the control children were anxiously attached at both 12 and 18 months. This difference was statistically significant for the 18-month attachment classifications. In the tool-using, problem-solving situation at 24 months, physically abused children displayed more anger, frustration, noncompliance, and aggression, and less enthusiasm and positive affect, than did children in the control group. These two groups of children did not differ on measures of infant social behavior or on the Bayley Scales of Infant Development (BSID), administered at 9 and 24 months.

At 42 months in the Barrier Box task, physically abused children were hyperactive, distractible, and undercontrolled. They exhibited low self-esteem, low agency, and much negative affect. With their mothers in the teaching task, the abused children were negativistic and noncompliant and expressed little affection for them, compared to controls. They were more reliant on as well as more avoidant of their mothers and were less persistent and enthusiastic. In preschool, physically abused children had higher total scores than controls on the Preschool Behavior Questionnaire filled out by the teachers, indicating more adjustment problems. They were also rated by observers as having less adequate ego control, being less compliant, and expressing more negative emotions.

Effects of Hostility/Verbal Abuse

There were no observed differences between verbally abused and control children in the first year of life. By 18 months, though, a majority of the infants in the verbally abused group were anxiously attached. At 24 months, these children expressed more anger and frustration and were more noncompliant than children in the control group. Children subjected to both verbal and physical abuse had a significantly lower BSID developmental quotient than control children. There were only two significant differences—ego undercontrol and negative affect— between verbally abused and control children on the Barrier Box task. However, there were many differences when these children were in the teaching task with their mothers. The abused children's interactions with their mothers were characterized by negativity, noncompliance, a lack of affection, and a high degree of avoidance; they were also less persistent and less enthusiastic about the task.

Effects of Psychological Unavailability

By 18 months of age, *all* of the infants whose mothers were psychologically unavailable were anxiously attached. At 24 months, these children exhibited more anger, frustration, noncompliance, and negative affect than children in the control group. All maltreatment groups and the control group showed declines on the BSID between 9 and 24 months; however, the decline for the psychologically unavailable group was the largest. At 9 months, the BSID Mental Development Index score for the children in the psychologically unavailable group was 118, and by 24 months their score was 87. At 42 months, these children were less persistent and enthusiastic in the teaching task. They were noncompliant, negativistic, and avoidant with their mothers. In preschool, the psychologically unavailable children obtained higher scores on the Preschool Behavior Questionnaire and were rated lower on compliance and higher on dependency and negative emotional tone than controls.

Effect of Neglect

Significantly more neglected children than children in the control group were anxiously attached at 12 and 18 months. At 24 months, these children were angry, frustrated, and noncompliant. In the Barrier Box task at 42 months, neglected children showed low agency and flexibility and were apathetic and hyperactive in comparison to controls. They also had low self-esteem and poor ego control, and they displaced little positive but much negative affect. Similarly, in the teaching tasks, neglected children were less persistent and enthusiastic and more negativistic and noncompliant than control children. In preschool, neglected children were dependent, had poor ego control, and had many adjustment problems on the Preschool Behavior Questionnaire.

Summary

In sum, these results indicate that other types of abuse besides the physical variety have very damaging consequences. Unfortunately, these other types of abuse are difficult to prove and nearly impossible to take action against on behalf of a child. While all of the maltreatment groups were functioning poorly, there were some differences between the groups. Physically abused children were the most distractible and noncompliant and the least persistent and enthusiastic. Children of psychologically unavailable mothers exhibited the largest number of pathological behaviors on the various rating scales and checklists at the different ages, and they displayed progressively more maladaptive development at each period of assessment. The major decline in functioning between 12 months and preschool indicates that the caretakers' lack of emotional responsiveness is a devastating form of abuse. The effects of psychological unavailability on a child's development are as serious as the effects of physical abuse and neglect. Neglected children had difficulty organizing their behavior to cope with the environment. They seemed to be most unhappy, displaying the least positive and the most negative affect of all the groups (Egeland et al., 1984).

Positive Outcomes within the Abused Group

An examination of the development between 12 months and preschool age of the 44 maltreated children clearly indicates that, on the average, they were not functioning as well as the controls at each assessment interval. However, within the maltreated group there was considerable variability; there were abused children who appeared competent. Of critical importance is whether or not we can account for these positive outcomes. Unfortunately, children who were competent at one age often were not competent by the next assessment period. As can be seen from Table 10-1, there was a decrease in the percentage of abused children who were competent between 12 months and preschool. There was also a decrease in the percentage of nonmaltreated control children in the competent groups at succeeding assessments; however, the decrease was not as great as the decrease for the abused group. Among the maltreated children, 53.7% and 53.8% were securely attached at 12 and 18 months, respectively, compared to 65.9% and 71.4% for the control group. By preschool age, only 22.2% of the maltreated children were in the competent group, whereas 45.5% of the nonmaltreated controls selected from our total at-risk sample were competent. *None* of the maltreated children were consistently competent—that is, in the competent groups at 12, 18, 24, and 42 months (both the Barrier Box and the teaching task) and preschool. One maltreated child did approach this ideal. She was securely attached at 12 months (not securely attached at 18 months) and fell in the competent group at the 24-month and preschool assessments. At 42 months she was in the competent group only for the teaching task, not for the Barrier Box.

The relationship between secure attachments and later competent functioning was quite high for the control group, as it was in the studies previously cited (Arend *et al.*, 1979; Waters *et al.*, 1979). Most of the abused children who were competent at 24 months, 42 months, and preschool had a history of secure attachments; however, most securely attached abused children were incompetent by the time they reached preschool. A past history of competence, particularly secure attachment, appears to make an abused child less vulnerable to the effects of

Table 10-1. Number and Percentage of Abused and Control Children Who Were Competent at Each Assessment

	12-month attachment	18-month attachment	24-month problem solving	42-month Barrier Box	42-month teaching task	Preschool
Abused						
Competent	22	21	14	3	9	4
Tested	41	39	35	41	40	18
%	53.7	53.8	40.0	7.3	22.5	22.2
Control						
Competent	58	60	39	30	39	20
Tested	88	84	73	79	83	44
%	65.9	71.4	53.4	37.9	46.9	45.5

abuse. Unfortunately for most abused children, however, a past history of secure attachment is not enough to make a child invulnerable to the effects of abuse.

Table 10-2 reports the number and percentage of children in the competent groups at 24 months, 42 months, and preschool who were securely attached at 12 and/or 18 months. Slightly over 50% of both the maltreated and control children who were securely attached at 12 and/ or 18 months were functioning in a competent fashion at 24 months. By 42 months, only 11.1% and 18.5% of the securely attached abused children were classified as competent in the Barrier Box and the teaching task, respectively. Many studies of vulnerability and the effects of abuse on development report only final outcomes. Among our abused children, we have found maltreatment to have a cumulative negative effect on development; this indicates that it is important to consider the effects of abuse within a developmental framework.

In the rest of this section, we examine the abused children who were functioning in a competent fashion at each developmental assessment. We compare these competent children to the abused children who were incompetent, in an attempt to identify the factors that make abused children less vulnerable to the effects of abuse. We have already described the measures used to assess adaptation; we now describe the variables used to account for the quality of adaptation among the abused children.

Data Used to Account for Positive Outcomes

Starting before birth and at regularly scheduled intervals from birth through preschool, we collected detailed and comprehensive data in the areas of infant temperament and behavior; parental characteristics and understanding of child rearing; parent–child interaction; and life stress and life circumstances. These data were used in an attempt to account for competent functioning among the maltreated children.

Infant characteristics and temperament were assessed using several different procedures. Naturalistic observation ratings were obtained by having the nurses in the newborn nursery rate each infant on such behaviors as activity level, alertness, and soothability; the nurses also rated the mother's skill with and interest in the baby.

The Neonatal Behavioral Assessment Scale (NBAS; Brazelton, 1973) was administered to each infant at home on two separate occasions. The NBAS consists of 26 behavioral items and 21 reflex items. The behavioral items examine habituation to repeated stimuli, orientation to inanimate and animate stimuli, motor maturity, state control, and physiological regulation. The first administration of the NBAS was

Table 10-2. Number and Percentage of Abused and Control Children Judged Competent at 12 or 18 Months Who Were Competent, Noncompetent, or Not Tested at Each Subsequent Assessment Age

	24-month problem solving			42-month teaching task			42-month Barrier Box			Preschool		
	Competent	Non-competent	Not tested	Competent	Non-competent	Not tested	Competent	Non-competent	Not tested	Competent	Non-competent	Not tested
Abused												
n	12	11	6	5	22	2	3	24	2	3	7	19
% of total	52.2	47.8	—	18.5	81.5	—	11.1	88.9	—	30.0	70.0	—
Control												
n	34	29	9	33	34	5	27	33	6	18	20	34
% of total	54.0	46.0	—	49.2	50.7	—	45.0	55.0	—	47.4	52.6	—

scheduled for the second day after release from the hospital, usually the infant's seventh day of life. The second administration was usually on the infant's 10th day of life.

At 3 and 6 months after each child's birth, the parents were asked to complete the Carey Infant Temperament Questionnaire (Carey, 1970), which assesses nine dimensions of temperament. Infant characteristics were also rated in feeding and play situations observed at 3 and 6 months.

Maternal characteristics were assessed at approximately 36 weeks of pregnancy and 3 months after delivery, using a battery of tests to measure the following personality characteristics: intellectual level (Shipley, 1946); aggression, defendence, impulsivity, succorance, and social desirability (Personality Research Form—Jackson, 1967); anxiety (the Institute for Personality and Ability Testing [IPAT] Anxiety Scale—Cattell & Scheier, 1963); locus of control (Egeland, Hunt, & Hardt, 1970; Rotter, 1966); and feelings and perceptions of pregnancy, delivery, and the expected child (Maternal Attitude Scale—Cohler, Weiss, & Grunebaum, 1970; Pregnancy Research Questionnaire— Schaefer & Manheimer, 1960). The Maternal Attitude Scale measures attitudes and feelings toward controlling the child's aggression (Scale 1), maternal understanding of the need to encourage reciprocity (Scale 2), and maternal feelings of competence in meeting the baby's needs (Scale 3). The mothers were also given the Wechsler Adult Intelligence Scale (WAIS) during the 48-month assessment, along with the Profile of Mood States (McNair, Lorr, & Droppleman, 1971) and the Center for Epidemiologic Studies Depression Scale (Radloff, 1977).

Mother–infant interaction was assessed at 3 and 6 months in a feeding situation. After watching a feeding, the observer rated a variety of maternal behaviors, infant behaviors, and interactions between the mother and the baby. A total of 33 items were rated, including expressiveness, facility in caretaking, synchrony, positive regard, and negative regard. Ainsworth's scales of Sensitivity and Cooperation (Ainsworth et al., 1978) were also used to rate the mothers at 6 months. In addition, the mothers and babies were observed in a standardized play situation at 6 months and rated on 12 items. Further observations of mothers' behaviors were obtained during the 24-month tool-using situation and the 42-month teaching situation.

A life stress scale was given at the 12-, 18-, 30-, 42-, and 48-month assessments. At the same times, an interview was used to obtain detailed information about the families' life circumstances. Of particular interest were the families' living arrangements and the degree of emotional support the mothers received from their husbands or boyfriends and other family members.

Accounting for Secure Infant Attachments within the
Maltreatment Groups

The data were analyzed separately for the 12- and 18-month attachment classifications. Abused infants who were securely attached at 12 months were compared to those who were anxiously attached on baby behaviors and temperament, parental characteristics, interactional factors, and life circumstances. The same comparisons were made between the abused infants classified as securely and anxiously attached at 18 months.

Despite the relatively large number of infants classified as securely attached at 12 months (53.7%), there were few significant findings to account for competent functioning at this age. There were no differences between the securely and anxiously attached infants on measures of infant characteristics and temperament or parental characteristics, except for Scale 3 of the Maternal Attitude Scale—acceptance versus denial of emotional complexity in child care. There were no differences on mothers' age and education, severity of maltreatment, or life stress. There was only one significant difference based on the feeding and play factor scores: Mothers of infants classified as securely attached at 12 months were more sensitive to their infants' cues, compared to mothers of anxiously attached infants.

The family living patterns were highly related to attachment outcomes. In the intact families, 72% of the abused infants were securely attached and 28% were anxiously attached. Conversely, in the one-parent families, 33% of the abused infants were securely attached and 67% were anxiously attached. Ratings of the quality of emotional support the mothers received from husbands/boyfriends and family members also differentiated the two groups: Mothers of securely attached abused children received more emotional support than did mothers of anxiously attached infants.

The results were similar at 18 months, in that there were very few significant differences between maltreated infants classified as anxiously or securely attached. Mothers of securely attached infants obtained a lower score on the hostility scale and a higher score on Scale 1 of the Maternal Attitude Scale, indicating more appropriate control of the child's aggression. The effects of family living arrangements were not as dramatic at 18 months as they were at 12 months. In two-parent families, 66% of the abused infants were securely attached at 18 months and 33% were anxiously attached. In single-parent families, 48% of the abused infants were securely attached.

In sum, there is no clear explanation for the secure attachments among the abused infants. Among the large number of variables examined, only a few differentiated securely from anxiously attached infants. Stable two-parent families, maternal sensitivity, and mothers' understanding of the psychological complexity of their relationship with her infants seem to have made the abused infants less vulnerable to the development of an anxious pattern of attachment. The two scales of the Maternal Attitude Scale that differentiated the two groups reflect the extent to which the mothers had the psychological maturity and sophistication necessary for establishing a relationship with their children, and the ability to deal effectively with the ambivalent feelings inherent in a first pregnancy.

Each of the variables that differentiated between the abused infants classified as securely or anxiously attached were also found to be highly related to attachment for the entire risk sample (Egeland & Farber, 1984). However, for the entire risk sample, we found a number of additional infant, parental, and interactional factors as well as life circumstances related to attachment outcomes. It is difficult to understand why these same factors were not related to the quality of attachment for the maltreated subsample. For the maltreated group, the range of parental and interactional scores were restricted, and averages were usually quite low compared to the total sample. Since the scores were low for the maltreated sample, it would be expected that a larger percentage of the infants would be anxiously attached. Despite the poor-quality care, approximately 50% of the infants were securely attached.

A closer examination of individual test scores, anecdotal data, and case studies provides some further information to account for secure attachments within the maltreated sample. It is obviously impossible to draw any definite conclusions or make any generalizations from examination of individual cases, however. Our conclusions must be considered highly tentative and are offered only as hypotheses to be tested with a sample of adequate size.

As infants, some of the securely attached abused children were described as especially robust and able to elicit support from their mothers as well as others. They were alert, easy to soothe, and socially responsive. There were some instances where secure attachments were associated with the presence of a supportive family member, usually the grandmother. In a few cases of neglect, the mother's warmth came through to the infant even though the external appearance was one of neglect.

It is noteworthy that the quality of the attachment relationship for the maltreated infants was highly unstable. Only 9 of the 21 securely attached infants at 12 months (43%) were securely attached at 18 months. The stability of secure attachment classifications between 12 and 18 months for our entire risk sample was 74%. In the control group, 90% of the securely attached infants at 12 months remained securely attached at 18 months. For our at-risk sample in general and our abuse subsample in particular, there was considerable instability in quality of attachment. Waters (1978) found 96% stability between 12 and 18 months for a middle-class sample. It appears that the stability in attachment patterns between 12 and 18 months is highly related to the amount of chaos and disruption in the home.

Adaptation among Toddlers

To assess adaptation at 24 months, the children were compared on seven global behavioral ratings obtained in the problem-solving situation. The children were placed in groups based on the results of a statistical cluster analysis using the ratings. (A cluster analysis provides a behavioral configuration or pattern that is used to place individuals in groups.) With the 24-month problem-solving data, the cluster analysis resulted in a four-group solution. The most competent group was lowest on dependency, noncompliance, anger, and frustration, and highest on persistence, coping, and enthusiasm. Only four abused children were placed in the most competent group. In order to create enough statistical leverage, the four abused children in the most competent group were combined with the 10 children in the next most competent group. The children of this group were rated low on dependency, average on ratings of anger and frustration, and slightly above average on persistence, coping, enthusiasm, and noncompliance.

Of the abused children, 40% were placed in the first two cluster groups (i.e., were competent), and 53% of the nonabused controls from the total risk sample were competent at 24 months. Of the abused children who were securely attached at 12 and/or 18 months, only 52% continued to function in a competent fashion at 24 months (see Table 10-2). This decrease in the number of securely attached abused children who were placed in the two competent groups at 24 months is similar to the decrease noted for the control group. This indicates that high-risk children in general, regardless of whether or not they are abused, show a decline in the quality of adaptation between infancy and 24 months of age. Resolution of the struggle for autonomous functioning, the significant developmental task at 24 months, may be especially difficult for at-risk families, particularly abusing mothers and their children.

In an attempt to determine the factors related to invulnerability at 24 months, the 14 abused children who were placed in the two competent groups were compared to the 21 abused children who displayed maladaptive patterns of development. Perhaps the most striking finding is that 12 of the 14 competent children at 24 months had been securely attached at 12 and/or 18 months. Clearly, a prior history of developmental adaptation makes a child less vulnerable to the negative effects of abuse and other forms of maltreatment.

Except for a prior history of competent functioning, there were few factors that accounted for competence among the abused children at 24 months. Severity and type of maltreatment were not significantly related to competent–incompetent functioning. The competent abused toddlers had been rated higher on orientation, alertness, and physiological response to stress when they were newborns, compared to the incompetent abused children. None of the maternal characteristics of personality variables were related to invulnerability. There was only a tendency for certain interaction variables to be related. Mothers' caretaking skills in both the 6-month feeding and play situations, and their affective behavior in play, tended to differenetiate between the competent and incompetent abused children at 24 months. Maternal behavior, quality of instruction, and emotional support were also rated in the 24-month problem-solving situation. Surprisingly, neither of these variables were related to adaptation at 24 months for the maltreated children. They were highly related for the mother–child pairs in the total risk sample. Maltreating mothers of both competent and incompetent children were well below average, compared to the total risk sample, on the ratings of mothers' skill and emotional responsiveness at 24 months.

An examination of the interviews and anecdotal information for the competent children indicates that in some cases a grandmother or another family member was assuming greater responsibility in the care of a toddler. Some of the mothers were returning to work and/or school and were leaving babysitting responsibilities to the grandmothers. In each of these instances, the assessment of the child at 24 months included the grandmother rather than the mother.

In sum, very few of the statistical analyses identified infant, mother, interactional, or environmental factors that accounted for competent functioning at 24 months for children who had a history of maltreatment. Many of the factors related to adaptation for the total risk sample were not related to competent functioning for the abused subsample. The most important factor related to competent functioning for the abused children at 24 months was a prior history of competence. Of the 14 competent children at 24 months, 12 were securely attached at 12 and/or 18 months. The 2 infants who were anxiously attached but appeared competent at 24 months displayed maladaptive patterns of development at each later assessment. Thus, they cannot be considered invulnerable. It should be noted that had assessment only occurred at this point in time, a very different picture of these children would have resulted.

Adaptation at 42 Months

Only 3 (7.3%) of the 44 abused children approached the frustrating situation of the Barrier Box in a competent fashion, and only 9 (22.5%) children fell in the competent group on the teaching task. The percentages of maltreated children classified as competent on the Barrier Box and the teaching task were considerably lower than the percentages of nonabused control children (38.0% and 47.0%, respectively). It is somewhat surprising that more of the maltreated children were functioning well in the teaching task, where the mothers were present, than in the Barrier Box, where the mother was absent. While one might think that the children behaved well from fear of maternal retribution, the children in this group were more than just compliant. They were enthusiastic, creative, and persistent, and in general were able to work well with their mothers.

Because of the small number of competent children in the Barrier Box and the teaching task, the two groups were combined in order to test for statistically significant differences between the competent and incompetent abused groups. Only one child was competent in both tasks. The behavioral profile of the competent group in the Barrier Box was as follows: high on ratings of self-esteem, positive affect, and clarity of help seeking; moderately high on flexibility, agency, creativity, and persistence; moderate on ego control, dependency, and intensity of help seeking; and low on negative affect and withdrawal. In the teaching task, the competent group was described as follows: high on persistence, enthusiasm, compliance, experience in the session, and affection toward mother; and low on negativism, reliance on mother, and avoidance of mother.

It would appear that the major factor related to good developmental outcomes at 42 months was a prior history of developmental adaptation. The abused children who were securely attached and competent at 24 months were less vulnerable to the effects of abuse by the time they were 42 months of age. All three competent children in the Barrier Box had been securely attached at 12 and 18 months. Five of the nine abused children who were competent in the teaching task had been securely attached.

For the first time, severity of maltreatment was related to developmental outcome. The children judged to be mildly abused were more likely to be competent at 42 months than the children who were severely abused. We have already seen the negative cumulative effects of abuse between infancy and the toddler period. By 42 months of age, only one severely abused child was in the competent group.

There were no differences in family intactness between the two groups; however, the stability of the family situation (intact or nonintact) was important. Of the stable families in the abuse group, 52% had competent children. It is noteworthy that 29% of the abusive mothers of incompetent children were themselves abused by their husbands or boyfriends, compared to 0% of the abusive mothers of the competent children.

There was only one baby variable that differentiated between the competent and incompetent abused children at 42 months: The competent children were rated as more alert and attentive as newborns. There were no differences between groups on the mother variables, except for age and education. Abusing mothers who had competent children at 42 months were older (21.8 years vs. 19.1), and they were better educated (11.9 vs. 11.1 years in school). Age and education were not reflected in higher scores on any of the measures of maternal understanding and expectation. There was, however, a large difference in IQ: Abusing mothers of competent children scored higher on the WAIS than mothers of incompetent children. Since one set of tasks at 42 months required that the mothers teach the children, it is not surprising that the older, better-educated, and more intelligent mothers were more successful with their children in this situation. For the children, there were no differences between groups on IQ, but there was a difference on a measure of verbal comprehension and expression. It appears that the competent abused children, as compared to the incompetent group, had better communication skills and thus were more likely to be successful in the teaching tasks.

Observations of the abusing mothers in the teaching task highlighted a number of differences between the two groups. Maltreating mothers of the competent children were rated as providing better-quality instruction, giving more emotional support, and showing greater respect for the children's autonomy, compared to mothers of the incompetent children. They were also better at structuring the situation and setting limits, and were more confident in dealing with the situation. Except for the emotional support dimension, high ratings on the other dimensions required that the mothers have an understanding of the situation, flexibility, the ability to communicate, and other skills related to intelligence. It is important to point out that the ratings of the mothers were not involved in the placement of the children in the cluster groups. In this situation, the children's success to a large extent depended on the mothers' skills. The more skillful and flexible the mothers were in the teaching situation, the more likely it was that they would be able to avoid conflict and frustration with the children. The mothers' skills at teaching, however, do not explain the competent children's enthusiasm and positive affect. The mothers' role in the teaching task was highly structured, and the tasks were quite easy for the children. Perhaps if the teaching tasks were more difficult and less structured, the mother–child pairs would have become disorganized, and the children would have received less positive ratings.

An earlier history of positive mother–child interaction was also related to positive outcomes at 42 months. Abusing mothers of competent children were more cooperative in feeding and play at 6 months than were mothers of incompetent children. The central issue in the cooperation dimension was the extent to which a mother's activities broke into her infant's ongoing activities. Interfering mothers were inconsiderate of their infant's wishes and activities, and they appeared to have no respect for the infants as autonomous persons. The interfering mothers tried to direct and control their babies' behavior, rather than gearing their interventions to the babies' state, mood, and interests. The cooperative mothers did not act upon their infants; instead, they interacted with them.

In sum, a prior history of developmental adaptation appears to make an abused child less vulnerable to the negative affects of abuse. For the abused children, one variable that was related to secure attachments and competent functioning at 24 months was an early history of maternal emotional responsivity. Mothers' affective behavior did not seem to be related to competence at 42 months. We would not conclude that maternal emotional responsivity is no longer important at this age. The failure to find a relationship was probably due to the nature of the teaching situation, one of the tasks used to assess competence at 42 months.

As would be expected, children whose mothers were "good teachers" appeared competent. The socialization of the child, which is the central developmental task at 42 months, involves a process of "teaching." Unfortunately, we do not have data at this point to say that success of the mother–child pairs in our structured teaching situation was predictive of the children's actual social behavior. Our preliminary analyses for the total at-risk sample indicate that there was a relationship between the children's behavior in the 42-month teaching task and social behavior and peer acceptance in preschool.

Before examining the adjustment of our abused children in preschool, we briefly describe the backgrounds of the four abused children who, in the teaching task at 42 months, were in the competent group for the first time. As we have noted, a major factor related to competence for abused children is a prior history of competence. We examined the interview and anecdotal data in order to determine whether there was anything in the background of the four children that could explain why, with a history of maladaptive development, they appeared competent for the first time at 42 months. In three of the four cases, there was a noticeable improvement in caretaking skills and a decrease in the severity of maltreatment.

CASE 1

R. J. was 17 when she had Richie, and she lived at home with her parents until Richie was about 2. R. J. then married Jack, an older man with five children by an earlier marriage, whom she had met while traveling with the circus in the summertime. At the end of the summer they returned home penniless, several hours before she had her second baby. The four of them moved in with Jack's ex-wife and her five children. Due to severe neglect, the children, prior to the 42-month visit, were removed from the home and placed in foster homes. The foster mother was interested in Richie and provided good-quality care, which was reflected in the smooth interaction observed between the two in the teaching task. Unfortunately, the child was only in that placement for 9 months, after which time R. J. regained custody. About the same time, Jack was arrested for sexually abusing his children, and the home situation deteriorated even more. R. J. and her children were placed in therapy, but after a few sessions she refused to continue. Subsequent assessments of Richie in preschool indicated a return to a maladaptive pattern of development. At approximately 60 months, Richie was placed in another foster home, and this time his adjustment did not improve. At the time of our 64-month assessment, Richie was extremely withdrawn and displayed a number of behavior problems. The temporary foster home placement prior to our 42-month visit seemed to have a positive effect, but the child's return home and subsequent placement in another foster home reversed the trend toward competent functioning.

CASE 2

In the second case, the mother, H. B., had a history of hospitalization for schizophrenia during the first 3 years of the child's life. The child was placed in a foster home between the 12- and 18-month assessments because of the extremely depriving environment and the mother's inadequate care. She was told by the Child Protection Agency that after she bought a crib and other provisions, the child would be returned. The child was returned, but the situation did not improve. Prior to the 42-month assessment, H. B. got a cleaning job and the child started day care. The child responded positively to day care, and the mother seemed to be functioning in a more competent fashion. Unfortunately, the mother stopped work, and the child was removed from day care. Since the child was not in preschool, we are uncertain as to his current functioning.

CASE 3

J. D., who came from a small town, was raised by strict parents who had very high expectations for their daughter. At 18, she left home and became a student at a small liberal arts church-affiliated school. During her second year at college, she met Bob in the bus depot when returning from a visit home. She moved in with him, and he convinced her to become a prostitute. Although he originally intended to send her to New York, some semblance of a relationship evolved, and they ended up getting married. Shortly after their marriage, Bob started physically abusing her. Each time it occurred, he would swear that it would never happen again; she would believe him, but the abuse continued. Three years after they were married, J. D. had a child. She tried to leave prostitution, but Bob would pressure her to continue because they needed the money. The child was neglected both physically and emotionally, beginning shortly after birth, and at times was physically abused. The maltreatment was not severe. The major problem seemed to be that the mother's emotional energy was spent in trying to cope with her relationship with Bob and the conflicts arising from prostitution. Caring for the baby seemed to give J. D. a feeling of confidence and control over her life. She became more independent, and eventually she refused to return to prostitution. When her baby was 12 months old, J. D. took a job as a legal secretary, which gave her more confidence and self-respect. She was obviously intelligent and introspective. She had thought about how she wanted to raise her child and what to do about her relationship with Bob, which was becoming increasingly difficult. It was clear that she cared for her child, but the circumstances of her life prevented her from providing adequate care and attention.

By the time the child was 18 months of age, J. D. and Bob had separated, and by 30 months they were divorced. During their separation, he raped and beat her on two occasions. One of the rapes resulted in a pregnancy, which ended in a miscarriage. At about the time of the 30-month visit, J. D. went into therapy, and she seemed to greatly profit from the experience. At about the same time, she met another man, whom she married. He provided her with needed support and stability; as a result, she continued to gain confidence and feel in control of her life. Her child was also seen in therapy, which J. D. felt had a very positive effect. Not long after her remarriage, they moved out of the area. J. D.'s child looked good for the first time at the 42-month assessment. We do not know whether the child attended preschool or how he is adjusting to kindergarten, but we are confident in predicting that as long as J. D.'s life is reasonably stable, the child will continue to function in a competent fashion. This mother had the skills to take care of her child, and she loved him. Her chaotic life style and bad relationship overwhelmed her to the point where she was unable to provide care for her child. A change in life style and a supportive relationship made a tremendous difference in her attitude about herself and in her ability to care for her child.

CASE 4

D. C. has a history of severe depression and received outpatient treatment that included medication. She openly rejected her son and let it be known to everyone that she disliked the child. The home was described as extremely chaotic; the mother drank heavily, and she would physically attack her son as well as her friends and family. The one experience in the child's life that may have accounted for his competent functioning at 42 months was his placement in a day care center at age 30 months. The child enjoyed the day care experience, and the day care workers were interested in him. This may have also provided some respite for the mother.

SUMMARY

Even though it is not possible to draw any generalizable conclusions from the four case studies, one trend is apparent. These abused children who had a history of maladaptive development but were competent at 42 months all had experienced major changes in their lives, in the form of either a more stable home environment, foster home placement, or enrollment in good-quality day care. The day care finding is an interesting one. We found in an earlier investigation of the entire risk sample that children placed in "out-of-home settings" were more likely to be anxiously attached than were children whose mothers remained at home (Vaughn, Gove, & Egeland, 1980). In general, mothers did not have high-quality day care available to them. They made arrangements based on what was available and affordable on a day-to-day basis. This inconsistent and poor-quality care may have been one reason for the anxious attachments. The evidence from two of the case studies of the abused children who were competent at 42 months suggests that good-quality day care for abused children may have a positive effect on development. It is unfortunate that the majority of our children from impoverished homes, particularly those who were maltreated, did not have such care available to them on a consistent basis.

Adaptation in Preschool

Altogether, 18 of the abused children were in preschool; 4 of these (22%) were classified as competent. By comparison, 46% of the children in the control group were in the competent group. It was not possible to conduct statistical analyses with the small number of abused children who were in preschool. Our attempt to determine the factors that make an abused child less vulnerable to the effects of abuse at this stage involved an examination of the interview and anecdotal information.

None of the four abused children who were competent were severely maltreated. Children with a history of chronic and severe maltreatment were observed to have serious behavior and adjustment problems by the time they reached preschool age. We did not find any invulnerable children among this group. Even though some of the moderately maltreated children were competent, we are pessimistic about their future. We have already seen that between 12 months and preschool, an increasing number of abused children showed maladaptive patterns of development. Those children who experienced the most severe and chronic abuse were incompetent at an early age, and unless major changes occur in their later lives, this maladaptive behavior is not likely to be reversed. Although the children who were less severely abused showed more nearly normal patterns of development on the variables we studied, we anticipate that the cumulative effects of abuse will eventually result in developmental maladaptation for them as well.

Of the four abused children who were competent in preschool, three had a history of secure attachments and competent functioning at other assessment periods. The child who did not have a history of a secure attachment was classified as competent in the teaching task at 42 months. It was clear at the preschool assessment, as was also true for earlier developmental assessments, that a major factor in "invulnerability" was a prior history of competence. Following is a brief description of the four cases.

CASE 5

D. C. described in the preceding section as Case 4, became pregnant at about the time of the 42-month assessment. She was the only mother of the four competent preschool children who was not living with a male. The pregnancy and birth of a baby girl seemed to change the mother's life. She stopped drinking and fighting, and her life became less chaotic and disruptive. D. C. had always wanted a baby girl, and was pleased at finally having one. Her interest in her baby seemed to carry over and have a positive effect on her relationship with her son. This child remained in day care until approximately age 4, at which time he was enrolled in preschool. Good-quality day care and preschool situations, along with the mother's changing attitude toward her son, seemed to be the key factors related to competent functioning for this abused child.

CASE 6

During the first few years of her life, Alicia was frequently bruised, and there was strong evidence of sexual abuse. The father had a history of mental illness; he physically beat Alicia's mother, S. T.; and he had been in jail for sexual abuse of his other children by a previous marriage. An interview with S. T. when her daughter was 5 indicated that the home situation remained chaotic. However, there were no obvious examples of physical abuse at ages 4 and 5, and it appeared that the mother was more relaxed.

Alicia and her younger sister were involved in long-term therapy, which may have had a positive effect on Alicia's development. The parents refused to be involved in therapy, although they had been in various Child Protection

Agency programs. In addition to therapy, Alicia attended a full-time day care/ preschool program for children with special needs, starting prior to her third birthday and continuing until she started kindergarten. This program was run by Child Protection for the purpose of providing intervention for children and relief for parents who were unable to cope with their children 24 hours of every day. At the time we observed Alicia in the special-needs preschool, she had attended it for 2 years. Her familiarity with the setting, teachers, and other children may explain, in part, her competent functioning in this milieu. In addition, the family lived in the same building with aunts, uncles, grandmother, and stepgrandmother, all of whom provided support and child care. Therapy, good-quality day care, and the extended-family support seemed to be the important factors in accounting for Alicia's competent functioning in preschool, despite a long history of chronic maltreatment.

CASE 7

T. J. had a history of being emotionally detached from, rejecting of, and psycho- logically unavailable to her son, Jamie. There were no indications of physical abuse. As we have reported earlier (Egeland et al., 1984), children who are raised by psychologically unavailable parents suffer severe maladjustment. Jamie's parents had been married since before his birth, and the relationship was considered highly stable. Jamie had a history of competent development. This may have been due to his early placement in high-quality day care when he was 1 year old and the care he received from his father. It appeared that Jamie received much-needed emotional support from his father. The mother came from an educated background and was highly rejecting of her own parents.

CASE 8

The case of N. D. was very similar to that of T. J. N. D. was well educated, came from an intact middle-class family, and clearly rejected her own parents. She provided for intellectual stimulation of her son, Johnny, but was rejecting, hostile, and psychologically and emotionally unavailable. She had high expecta- tions for her child and considered obedience to be the most important charac- teristic of a young child. She seemed to have an "approach–avoidance" conflict with Johnny. She wanted to be a good mother and to have him develop normally, but she was unable to relate to the child emotionally. N. D. was married, and the relationship was stable. The husband shared in the caretaking responsibilities and provided some emotional support for the child.

SUMMARY

Three of the women described here seemed very angry and rebellious as young mothers. These mothers were, however, typically well edu- cated, and they seemed to gain control of their anger as they became older. Their confidence in caring for their children and coping with life also seemed to improve with age. In addition, the mothers who had been raised in stable two-parent families were able to fall back on their experiential knowledge of good parenting. Finally, in two of these cases, the father or father figure was able to provide emotional support for the child.

In sum, it is impossible to draw any definite conclusions from the case studies of the four abused children who were competent in preschool. Unfortunately, the majority of the abused children did not attend preschool. A prior history of competence, a stable and intact family (both currently and in the mother's past), and mild as opposed to severe maltreatment are among some of the factors that seem to make a preschool child less vulnerable to the effects of chronic abuse.

Discussion

When trying to account for the effects of child maltreatment, other researchers have noted that it is important to consider "the invulnerable child" (e.g., Martin, 1980). However, to our knowledge, no one has presented data indicating that there are children who function competently despite an ongoing exposure to abuse. We have attempted to find such data in a comprehensive exploration of the first 5 years of abused children's lives. Not surprisingly, results of this study indicate that there are few competent survivors among physically or emotionally neglected children. We are convinced that the few competent preschool children will display maladaptive patterns of development in the early school years if their home situation remains abusive. It is highly unlikely that *any* children remain unscathed if they experience chronic maltreatment during the early years of their life.

Our study found that there was a significant decline in competence over the first 5 years of life for abused children. This decline was greater than that for children at risk who were not abused. While few children remained competent, those who did were more likely to have had a history of secure attachment. Earlier in this chapter, we have pointed out that both middle- and lower-class children with secure attachment histories are more likely to be functioning in a competent fashion several years later than are anxiously attached children. This result seemed to be replicated in our abuse sample, despite the small number of competent children.

There was little evidence that constitutional factors were important in making children less vulnerable. Only in a few cases did infant temperament and behavior play a role in adjustment. Abused children who were competent at 24 months were more alert, had better physiological control, and oriented better as newborns than the incompetent abused children. Environmental factors were more important than constitutional variables. Two of the most important environmental factors were the presence of a male partner in the home and the mother's emotional support of the child. In the majority of the cases where there was a male living in the home on a stable basis, he provided both the child and the mother with support. Of course, there were families, such as Cases 3 and 6, where the father's presence was detrimental to the mother's emotional and physical health and subsequently the child's as well. At each age, it was noted that the emotional support provided by the mother made the child less vulnerable to the effects of maltreatment. In general, even though the children were maltreated, they were more likely to be competent where there was some indication of maternal interest in them and where the mothers were able to respond to them emotionally. Few of those children whose mothers were in the psychologically unavailable group were competent. The exceptions were the children who had grandmothers or fathers who provided them with emotional support. Clearly, the lack of emotional support has devastating consequences on a child's development. For children who are physically abused and neglected, emotional support and responsiveness are major factors in making them less vulnerable to maltreatment.

Several of our findings are similar to those presented by Werner and Smith (1982). Although they were not studying abused children, resilient children in their sample were likely to have received more attention from their primary caretakers in infancy, and their mothers had more alternate caretakers available to them. While their ratings were quantitative (amount of attention) rather than qualitative, their findings also highlight the importance of the first year of life and of a supportive network in developing competence.

Given our findings, what does invulnerability mean from a developmental perspective? If children are well adapted at one age, are they invulnerable? Do they need to be competent at every age, or do we have to wait until the long-term data are in to make a judgment? Several ideas are relevant in considering these questions.

Assessing children only once ignores the facts that as they grow, they change, and that their development is a function of their history and current environment. Half of our abused children were securely attached as infants, but less than one-fourth were competent 3 years later. No child was consistently competent in the 5 years that our assessments covered. Our results would have been deceptive, had we assessed adjustment and determined invulnerability at only one point in time.

The issue of reliability in measurement is another reason for assessing outcomes at numerous points in time. Despite the fact that we used instruments that are reliable, there is always some imprecision in measurement. Numerous assessments insure that one is less likely to reach a false conclusion.

It is also important to collect a variety of data from multiple sources that address all aspects of a child's functioning, and to have long-term outcome data. The use of laboratory assessments, interview data, and home and school observations gave us a fairly complete picture of each child's functioning. It is now necessary to follow these children through to adulthood to determine whether they are truly resilient—whether they have the capacity for mature, intimate relationships, for adequate parenting, and so on.

Furthermore, to fully understand invulnerability, one must distinguish among adaptation, competence, and emotional health. Some children develop coping strategies that enable them to adapt over time to the situation they are in, and thus to appear competent. However, they may not be emotionally healthy. For example, Alicia (Case 6) spent the first 2 weeks of preschool silently curled up in a corner by herself. Her approach was to protect herself, yet to be vigilant and learn everything she could about her new environment; in the past, her environments had been very unpredictable. After 2 weeks of this behavior, Alicia's vigilance was discovered when she overheard a teacher looking for another child, and Alicia volunteered the child's whereabouts. Gradually, Alicia left her "safety corner" and began participating in class. When classroom observations were made after several months, she was rated as competent. She had made a remarkable adjustment over time to the preschool situation, but would anyone knowing the sequence of events believe she was healthy, and would she appear competent in a new and unfamiliar situation?

It should also be noted that most of the research on invulnerability has dealt with children of psychiatrically ill parents. In these cases (e.g., where a parent has schizophrenia), there is a genetic predisposition as well as an occasionally disruptive environment (e.g., parental hospitalizations) that may precipitate the disorder in the child. With child abuse there is no clear genetic contribution, but the environment is often chronically bad. Under these circumstances, children have very little opportunity to develop competence. The concept of invulnerability has to be used cautiously when evaluating risk situations with only an environmental component.

One hope behind invulnerability research is that, by studying the good outcomes along with the bad, investigators may find factors that will be useful in prevention and/or intervention. The results of our study indicate that resources for prevention should be directed toward helping at-risk mothers in the first year of life. An important focus of any intervention will be these mothers' emotional relationship with their children, not just their caretaking skills (Egeland & Farber, 1982b). Helping these mothers to become more sensitive and responsive to their children's needs can help the children to develop secure attachments. This will then give the children a greater chance to negotiate other important developmental issues successfully. It may also help the mothers to continue to be more sensitive to their children as they grow, despite their own chaotic lives.

We have presented a rather dismal but accurate picture of the effects of abuse; however, we do not believe that they are absolutely irreversible. Children do respond in predictable ways to environmental changes. With serious intervention, children can survive and even reverse the pattern of decreasing competence. Several of the children in our study benefited greatly from environmental interventions, including high-quality day care and therapeutic foster placement. It is, of course, too early to know whether and how the trauma of their first few years will ultimately affect their development.

Finally, there is an ethical issue to consider when spreading the notion that there are children who are invulnerable to abuse. A decade ago, child abuse became a popular topic, and money was channeled for research, prevention, and intervention. Unfortunately, the interest in abuse seems to have peaked, and currently the public seems less concerned about the problem. Social scientists have to be responsible in discussing invulnerability, lest policy makers come to harbor the idea that if children are only strong enough, they will survive. We do not believe that many children can develop coping skills *and* be emotionally healthy in a chronically abusive or neglectful environment.

REFERENCES

Ainsworth, M., Blehar, M., Waters, E., & Wall, S. (1978). *Patterns of attachment.* Hillsdale, NJ: Erlbaum.

Ainsworth, M., & Wittig, B. (1969). Attachment and exploratory behavior of one-year-olds in a strange situation. In B. Foss (Ed.), *Determinants of infant behavior* (Vol. 4). New York: Barnes & Noble.

Alvy, K. (1975). Preventing child abuse. *American Psychologist, 30,* 921–928.

Arend, R., Gove, F., & Sroufe, L. A. (1979). Continuity of individual adaptation from infancy to kindergarten: A predictive study of ego resiliency and curiosity in preschoolers. *Child Development, 50,* 950–959.

Barahal, R. M., Waterman, J., & Martin, H. P. (1981). The social cognitive development of abused children. *Journal of Consulting and Clinical Psychology, 49,* 508–516.

Behar, L., & Stringfield, S. (1974). A behavior rating scale for the preschool child. *Developmental Psychology, 10*(5), 601–610.

Bowlby, J. (1969). *Attachment and loss* (Vol. 1). New York: Basic Books.

Brazelton, T. B. (1973). *Neonatal Behavioral Assessment Scale.* Philadelphia: J. B. Lippincott.

Carey, W. (1970). A simplified method for measuring infant temperament. *Journal of Pediatrics, 70,* 188–194.

Cattell, R., & Scheier, I. (1963). *Handbook for the IPAT Anxiety Scale.* Champaign, IL: Institute for Personality and Ability Testing.

Cohler, B., Weiss, J., & Grunebaum, H. (1970). Child care attitudes and emotional disturbance among mothers of young children. *Genetic Psychology Monograph, 82,* 3–47.

Egeland, B., & Brunnquell, D. (1979). An at-risk approach to the study of child abuse: Some preliminary findings. *Journal of the American Academy of Child Psychiatry, 18,* 219–236.

Egeland, B., & Farber, E. (1982). What can we learn from recent research findings? In *Proceeding Highlights of the Fifth National Conference on Child Abuse and Neglect, Milwaukee, Wisconsin, April 1981.*

Egeland, B., & Farber, E. (1984). Infant–mother attachment: Factors related to its development and change over time. *Child Development, 55,* 753–771.

Egeland, B., Hunt, D., & Hardt, R. (1970). College enrollment of Upward Bound students as a function of attitude and motivation. *Journal of Educational Psychology, 61,* 375–379.

Egeland, B., & Sroufe, L. A. (1981). Developmental sequelae of maltreatment in infancy. In R. Rizley & D. Cicchetti (Eds.), *New directions for child development: Developmental perspectives in child maltreatment.* San Francisco: Jossey-Bass.

Egeland, B., Sroufe, L. A., & Erickson, M. (1984). The developmental consequences of different patterns of maltreatment. *International Journal of Child Abuse, 7,* 459–469.

Elmer, E., & Gregg, G. (1967). Developmental characteristics of abused children. *Pediatrics, 40,* 596–602.

Erikson, E. (1963). *Childhood and society* (2nd ed.). New York: Norton.

Garbarino, J. (1976). A preliminary study of some ecological correlates of child abuse: The impact of socioeconomic stress on mothers. *Child Development, 47,* 178–185.

Garmezy, N., & Devine, V. (1975). *Longitudinal versus cross-sectional research in the study of children at risk for psychopathology.* Paper presented at a conference on Methods of Longitudinal Research in Psychopathology, Rochester, NY.

Garmezy, N., & Neuchterlein, K. (1972). *Invulnerable children.* Paper presented at the meeting of the American Orthopsychiatric Association, Detroit.

Gelles, R. (1973). Child abuse as psychopathology: A sociological critique and reformulation. *American Journal of Orthopsychiatry, 43,* 611–621.

George, C., & Main, M. (1979). Social interactions of young abused children: Approach, avoidance, and aggression. *Child Development, 50,* 306–318.

Jackson, D. (1967). *Personality Research Form manual.* New York: Research Psychologists Press.

Kagan, J. (1971). *Change and continuity in infancy.* New York: Wiley.

Kempe, C. (1962). The battered child syndrome. *Journal of the American Medical Association, 181,* 17–24.

Kempe, R., & Kempe, C. (1978). *Child abuse.* London: Fontana/Open Books.

Kinard, E. M. (1980). Emotional development in physically abused children. *American Journal of Orthopsychiatry, 50,* 686–696.

Martin, H. (1972). The child and his development. In C. H. Kempe & R. E. Helfer (Eds.), *Helping the battered child and his family.* Philadelphia: J. B. Lippincott.

Martin, H. (1980). The consequences of being abused and neglected: How the child fares. In C. Kempe & R. Helfer (Eds.), *The battered child* (3rd ed.). Chicago: University of Chicago Press.

Martin, H., & Beezley, P. (1977). Behavioral observations of abused children. *Developmental Medicine and Child Neurology, 19,* 373–387.

Martin, H., Beezley, P., Conway, E., & Kempe, C. (1974). The development of abused children. *Advances in Pediatrics, 21,* 25–73.

Matas, L., Arend, R., & Sroufe, L. A. (1978). Continuity of adaptation in the second year:

The relationship between quality of attachment and later competence. *Child Development, 49,* 547–556.

McNair, D., Lorr, M., & Droppleman, L. (1971). *Profile of Mood States.* San Diego: Educational and Industrial Testing Service.

Mischel, W. (1968). *Personality and assessment.* New York: Wiley.

Morse, C. W., Sahler, O., & Friedman, S. (1970). A three-year follow-up study of abused and neglected children. *American Journal of Diseases of Children, 120,* 439–446.

Parker, R., & Collmer, C. (1976). Child abuse: An interdisciplinary analysis. In E. Hetherington (Ed.), *Review of child development research* (Vol. 5). Chicago: University of Chicago Press.

Radloff, L. (1977). The CES-D Scale. A self-report depression scale for research in the general population. *Applied Psychological Measurement, 1,* 385–401.

Rotter, J. (1966). Generalized expectancies for internal versus external control of reinforcement. *Psychological Monographs, 80*(1, Whole No. 609).

Sameroff, A., & Chandler, M. (1975). Reproductive risk and the continuum of caretaking casualty. In F. Horowitz (Ed.), *Review of child development research* (Vol. 4). Chicago: University of Chicago Press.

Sandgrund, A., Gaines, R., & Green, A. (1974). Child abuse and mental retardation: A problem of cause and effect. *American Journal of Mental Deficiency, 79,* 327–330.

Schaefer, M., & Manheimer, H. (1960). *Dimensions of parental adjustment.* Paper presented at the meeting of the Eastern Psychological Association, New York.

Shipley, W. (1946). *The Shipley–Hartford Vocabulary Test. Shipley Institute of Living Scale.*

Sroufe, L. A. (1978). Attachment and the roots of competence. *Human Nature,* 50–57.

Sroufe, L. A. (1979a). The coherence of individual development: Early care, attachment, and subsequent developmental issues. *American Psychologist, 34,* 834–841.

Sroufe, L. A. (1979b). Socioemotional development. In J. Osofsky (Ed.), *Handbook of infant development.* New York: Wiley.

Sroufe, L. A. (1983). Patterns of individual adaptation from infancy to preschool. In M. Perlmutter (Ed.), *Minnesota Symposium in Child Psychology* (Vol. 16). Hillsdale, NJ: Erlbaum.

Sroufe, L. A., & Waters, E. (1977). Attachment as an organizational construct. *Child Development, 48,* 1184–1199.

Terr, L. (1970). A family study of child abuse. *American Journal of Psychiatry, 127,* 665–671.

Vaughn, B., Gove, F., & Egeland, B. (1980). The relationship between out-of-home care and the quality of infant–mother attachment in an economically disadvantaged population. *Child Development, 51,* 1203–1214.

Waters, E. (1978). The reliability and stability of individual differences in infant–mother attachment. *Child Development, 49,* 483–494.

Waters, E., Wippman, J., & Sroufe, L. (1979). Attachment, positive affect, and competence in the peer group: Two studies in construct validation. *Child Development, 50,* 821–829.

Werner, E. E., & Smith, R. S. (1982). *Vulnerable but invincible: A study of resistant children.* New York: McGraw-Hill.

11

Resilient Children as Adults: A 40-Year Study

J. KIRK FELSMAN
GEORGE E. VAILLANT
Dartmouth Medical School

Joe looked again at the little gurgling girl in her improvised playpen and thought, as many have before him, what wonderful children sometimes come out of such places as this.—William Carlos Williams, *White Mule* (1937)

Introduction

Working as a gifted pediatric clinician, the poet and novelist William Carlos Williams spent countless hours in the homes of poor, hard-pressed immigrant families struggling to "make it" in America during the early decades of this century. He implanted his resulting anger, confusion, awe, and virtually his entire spirit into the soul of Joe Stecher, protagonist of *White Mule* (1937). Through Joe's eyes, Williams observed the signs of human strength and resiliency that sometimes emerge amidst stark, relentless, and seemingly unforgiving social conditions.

The passage quoted above captures the spirit of shared irony that lies at the base of the growing inquiry into so-called "invulnerability," a tradition of testimony to the enormous human capacity to face, endure, and master the arbitrariness of fate and circumstance. Moreover, Joe Stecher's world serves as a near-perfect backdrop for introducing the Study of Adult Development at the Harvard Medical School, upon which this chapter is based. The men of its Core City sample are Joe's children and his children's children. Thus far, the study has documented 40 years of their individual and collective struggles—histories of recovery and triumph, as well as of resignation and defeat.

This chapter is presented in three parts. First, we provide an overview of the study's methodology and offer relevant findings on the entire sample. Next, we turn to our preliminary findings on the midlife outcome of a subsample of men determined to have been, as children, at "high risk" for psychopathology. Finally, we discuss our observations as they relate to the central topic, "invulnerability."

The Core City Sample

The Study of Adult Development at Harvard Medical School has followed a Core City sample of 456 men from early adolescence into late middle life. Attrition due to the men's withdrawing or becoming lost to the follow-up has been held to 6%. In the United States, only the Terman Study (Terman & Oden, 1959) and the Berkeley Growth Studies (Block, 1971; Eichorn, Clausen, Haan, Honzik, & Mussen, 1981) have followed adults longer. In contrast to most investigations of adult development, all three of these longitudinal studies have had the advantage of observing their samples at multiple points in time. This process yields a more dynamic view of change than that reflected through the limited time frame of a cross-sectional design. Admittedly, all these longitudinal studies are distorted by reflecting a single historical cohort.

Originally, the men of the Core City sample were selected by Sheldon and Eleanor Glueck as a control group for their prospective study, described in their book *Unraveling Juvenile Delinquency* (Glueck & Glueck, 1950). From 1940 to 1944, nondelinquent boys of an average age of 14 (±2 years) were chosen from Boston inner-city schools and paired with a cohort of 500 youths who had been remanded to reform school. The boys in the two groups were matched on the basis of four variables: age, intelligence, neighborhood crime rate, and ethnicity. Within the control group, the portraits of these boys' lives have been compiled through a careful systematic investigation that now spans four decades. Sampling bias included the exclusion of the severely delinquent, the intellectually gifted, and, more importantly, blacks and women. Within the limitations of sampling bias and "historical moment," the accumulated data's richest yield is the comparisons of the men with one another over the life span.

As a whole, the Core City men were materially disadvantaged. Half of them lived in clearly blighted slum neighborhoods in families known to five or more social agencies; 61% of all their parents were foreign-born; 31% of their parents were in class V according to the socioeconomic status (SES) criteria of Hollingshead and Redlich (1958). Over two-thirds of their families had recently been on welfare. Prosperity was a goal few families had achieved when the study was initiated, and the struggle toward it was to continue to dominate their lives and those of their children.

How They Were Studied

The Gluecks' original study methodology involved two parallel investigations of each boy and his family by a multidisciplinary team of physicians, psychologists, psychiatrists, social investigators, and physical anthropologists. Findings obtained from interviews with the boy, his school, and his family were compared and integrated with data obtained from an exhaustive search of public probation, mental health, and social agency records—a search that allowed documentation of familial delinquency, alcoholism, mental illness, and mental retardation. The difficult judgments on such factors as parental affection and supervision were often accomplished by triangulation, based upon documentation from several observers at multiple points in time.

About five-sixths of the surviving 456 Core City men were reinterviewed at ages 25 (ca. 1955), 31 (ca. 1962), and 47 (ca. 1977). Since 1974 they have been sent biennial questionnaires by the Study of Adult Development.

We now present a brief discussion of the five "early life" ratings and five "adulthood" ratings most relevant to this chapter. The entire study and its methodology are described in detail elsewhere (Vaillant, 1982; Vaillant & Milofsky, 1980; Vaillant & Vaillant, 1981).

Early Life Ratings

Clinicians blind to all postadolescent information rated the men on the basis of a search of all social service records and detailed interviews with each subject, his parent(s), and his teacher. The following subsections are brief descriptions of the five childhood ratings: the Childhood Environmental Strengths scale, the Childhood Environmental Weaknesses scale, intelligence, parents' SES, and the Boyhood Competence scale.

CHILDHOOD ENVIRONMENTAL STRENGTHS

The 20-point Childhood Environmental Strengths scale, described in detail elsewhere (Vaillant, 1974, 1977) rated the men by a clinical judgment of childhood environmental strengths. Points were assigned for the absence of childhood problems with physical, social, and mental health and for the presence of parental relationships and a home atmosphere conducive to the "development of basic trust, autonomy, and initiative" (Erikson's [1963] terms). The intent of the scale was to focus on what went right rather than what went wrong.

Childhood Environmental Strengths included the following sub-scales, scored from 0 to 2: childhood emotional problems, childhood physical health, home atmosphere, mother–child relationship, father–child relationship, sibling relationships, school/social adjustment, and global impression. The childhoods of those men whose scores fell in the top quartile were characterized as "warm," while the childhoods of those men whose scores fell in the bottom quartile were characterized as "bleak." Interrater reliability (three raters) ranged from .70 to .89.

The childhood emotional problems subscale was used as an independent variable. A child received 0 points if there were clear problems of any kind; 1 point if his was a not particularly problem-filled childhood; and 2 points if there were no known problems, and the child seemed good-natured and social.

CHILDHOOD ENVIRONMENTAL WEAKNESSES

The 50-point Childhood Environmental Weaknesses scale was based on 25 specific items that encompassed the Gluecks' more subjectively defined Delinquency Prediction Table (Glueck & Glueck, 1950). The scale included 5 items reflecting gross lack of family cohesion (e.g., nine or more social agency contacts, raised for more than 6 months apart from both parents); 10 items reflecting lack of maternal affection and supervision (e.g., mother delinquent; mother mentally retarded; mother failed to provide supervision when absent from home; multiple observers described maternal affection as inadequate); and 10 items reflecting inadequate paternal supervision and affection (e.g., father alcoholic, delinquent, or cruel to boy; multiple observers described paternal affection as inadequate). Interrater reliability was .94.

INTELLIGENCE

IQ was assessed by means of the Wechsler–Bellevue, administered by a research psychologist. A third of the men had IQs of less than 90. However, a cautionary note is necessary regarding this assessment. As a whole, the intelligence of the subjects in the Core City sample was most likely underestimated. The reliability of the early Wechsler–Bellevue may have been affected by verbal and cultural biases, due to the fact that the majority of the boys were from first- or second-generation immigrant families living under materially disadvantaged circumstances. Nevertheless, the same instrument was administered to all subjects, and thus it retains its validity for within-sample comparisons. The block design subtest was singled out for special attention.

PARENTS' SES

Parental SES was evaluated by the 5-point classification devised by Hollingshead and Redlich (1958), which is derived from assigning separate weights to scales for education, residence, and prestige of occupation, then summing up the three scores. In general, SES class I included managers and professionals with a college degree who owned their own house in prosperous suburbs. SES class V included unskilled laborers with less than 10 grades of schooling who lived in deteriorating rented housing. SES class III included skilled blue-collar workers with a high school education who owned a house in a working-class neighborhood, but class III could also include men with a year of college who owned a little store and lived in an apartment in a middle-class suburb.

BOYHOOD COMPETENCE

The 8-point Boyhood Competence scale (see Table 11-1) was an effort to quantify Erikson's (1963) fourth stage in the life cycle, "industry versus inferiority." Erikson described the dominant virtue of this stage as "competence." He later went on to define this period in the life cycle as follows: "Industriousness involves doing things beside and with others, a first sense of the division of labor. Competence, then, is the free exercise of dexterity and intelligence in the completion of serious tasks. It is the basis for cooperative participation in some segment of the culture" (1968, pp. 289–290).

Clearly, translating Erikson's conceptual framework to a numerical score risked reductionism. Yet, this scale, defined more fully elsewhere (Vaillant & Vaillant, 1981), was based on what the boys did—not what they said or felt. The items reflected an assessment of systematically

Table 11-1. Boyhood Competence Scale

Measure	Points assigned
Regular part-time job	0–1
Regular household chores	0–1
Participation in extracurricular clubs/sports	0–1
School grades relative to IQ	0–2
Good participation in school activities	0–1
"Coping capacity": planfulness, making the best of the environment	0–2
Total	0–8

recorded observations made when the boys were between 11 and 16 years of age. (Their average age was 14 ± 1.) The scale included these objective measures: regular part-time job; regular household chores; participation in extracurricular clubs/sports; school grades relative to IQ; regular school participation in activities; and "coping capacity." Common sense was used in making the Boyhood Competence ratings. For example, the requirements for receiving credit for a part-time job were more stringent for older boys, and such jobs reflected both after-school and vacation employment. The most subjective item measured was "coping capacity." The purpose of this item was to give special credit to boys who, in spite of very disorganized homes, were coping particularly well. The rater took into account available data from psychiatric interviews with the boy and with his mother, as well as multiple reports from social service agencies. (Twenty-five men were assessed by all three raters; the Pearson correlation coefficients for the ratings of the three possible pairs of judges were .78, .79, and .91.)

Adulthood Ratings

Clinicians blind to all information collected before subjects reached age 30 rated the men primarily on the basis of a semistructured 2-hour interview conducted when the men were age 47 (ca. 1977). The following subsections are brief descriptions of the five adult ratings most relevant to this chapter: the Adult Life Stage ratings, the Health–Sickness Rating Scale (HSRS), the Object Relations scale, the Maturity of Defenses scale, and adult SES.

ADULT LIFE STAGE

The Adult Life Stage ratings were made on a 5-point scale based on the Eriksonian model (1 = less than Stage 5; 2 = Stage 5; 3 = Stage 6; 4 = Stage 6a—a stage called "career consolidation" and intermediate to Erikson's stage of Intimacy [6] and Generativity [7]; and 5 = Stage 7). (See Vaillant & Milofsky, 1980, for a more detailed discussion). In the clinical assignment of a 47-year-old subject to a given stage, raters adhered to the spirit rather than the letter of Erikson's model, and the exceptional circumstances of a man's full life were taken into account. For example, if a man now functioned at a lower stage than previously, he was assigned to the highest stage achieved. Similarly, a deeply committed Catholic priest who became a successful parochial high school principal was rated as generative, although he never married.

These ratings were a consensus judgment of two clinicians who were familiar with all data about the subjects after age 30 (interrater reliability not determined).

HEALTH-SICKNESS RATING SCALE

Luborsky's (1962) HSRS was the instrument used to assess global mental health. Two raters used 34 case illustrations as guides to place each subject on a 100-point continuum that ranged from total institutional dependency (rating of 0–25) to no psychological dysfunctions and multiple manifestations of positive mental health (rating of 90–100). The reliability and validity of the HSRS have been summarized by Luborsky and Bachrach (1974). Our interrater reliability was .89.

OBJECT RELATIONS

The 9-point Object Relations scale summarized each individual's relative success in accomplishing eight different tasks of adult object relations (excluding marriage) over the last 10 years. One task reflected each of the following: enjoyment of children, family of origin, and workmates. Three tasks reflected friendship networks; two tasks reflected participation in group activities. Because stable marriage is thought by many to reflect 20th-century middle-class morality rather than to reflect an enduring fact of mental health, marital success or disaster was not included in the scale of social competence, but was treated as a separate variable.

MATURITY OF DEFENSES

The Core City sample was assessed on a 9-point Maturity of Defenses scale on the basis of the 2-hour interview at age 47. To quantify clinical impressions, the following procedure was observed: From 1 to 5 points were assigned for the tendency to deploy each of three groups of defenses—mature (sublimation, suppression, anticipation, altruism, and humor), neurotic or intermediate (displacement, repression, isolation, obsession, and reaction formation), and immature (projection, schizoid fantasy, masochism, acting out, hypochondriases, and neurotic denial/dissociation). It was required that all three ratings sum to 8. Relative maturity of overall defensive style was estimated by subtracting the rating for immature defenses (rating of 1–5) from the rating for mature defenses (rating of 1–5), giving a 9-point range. (For a more detailed discussion of defenses, see Vaillant, 1977.) Interrater reliability was .83.

The rating of adult SES was calculated using Hollingshead and Red-lich's (1958) classification, exactly as it was used for the assessment of the subjects' parents.

Interrelationship of Early Life Ratings and Midlife Outcome

When, at age 47, the midlife outcomes of men in the top and bottom quartiles of global mental health (HSRS) were compared, there was an almost complete distinction between them—both in terms of *lieben* (achievement of social competence and happy marriages), and in terms of *arbeiten* (regularity of employment and income—Vaillant & Milofsky, 1980). Perhaps what is most striking, and of most relevance to this chapter, is that of all the childhood measures chosen, the Boyhood Competence scale (see Table 11-1), reflecting success at Erikson's Stage 4 tasks, correlated most strongly with all facets of adult adjust-ment (Vaillant & Vaillant, 1981). Of the youths, 45 received very high scores (7 or 8) on this scale, and 67 received very low scores (0–2). At age 47, the men who were most successful at Stage 4 tasks of industry were twice as likely to be rated as generative (Erikson's Stage 7), were twice as likely to have warm relations with a wide variety of people, and were 16 times *less* likely to have experienced significant unemployment. As children, they were dramatically more likely to have come from family environments that seemed to have many positive attributes. They were also far less likely to have been seen as afflicted with emotional problems (i.e., to have been phobic or dissocial, or to have manifested other clearly rated psychological difficulties).

The 67 men who had been least successful at Stage 4 tasks in childhood were far more likely 30 years later to manifest sociopathic behavior, and 10 times more likely to be rated as emotionally disabled on the HSRS. As children, they were more likely to have come from multiproblem families.

While we found that IQ powerfully affected educational attain-ment and itself appeared to be enhanced by childhood environmental strengths (especially factors of adequate maternal affection and super-vision), intelligence and parental SES appeared relatively unimportant in overall midlife outcome. For example, 7% of men with IQs under 80 were unemployed for 10 or more years, but so were 7% of the men with IQs over 100. Also of interest was the fact that the two groups of men did not differ in parental SES and differed only modestly in subsequent educational opportunity. In this sample, then, Boyhood Competence results could neither be attributed to intelligence nor to social opportunity per se. Thus, the Boyhood Competence scale appeared to be a measure of "ego strength," an indicator more of emotional well-being then of intellectual endowment or social good fortune.

In reviewing the midlife outcome of the men in the Core City sample, it remains unclear to what extent subsequent adult positive mental health depends upon innate childhood strengths and/or the absence of childhood problems. What Table 11-2 does suggest, however, it that what goes right (e.g., Boyhood Competence and Childhood Environmental Strengths) is more important than what goes wrong. Thus, parental SES, IQ, and membership in a multiproblem family predicted the future only weakly. Such variables may be more important in cross-sectional studies than in those with a life span perspective. Clearly, it is the prospective longitudinal method that offers the most dynamic view of human development.

In addition, the seemingly collective yearning for images of continuity encompassed in an invariant sequence of developmental stages may find less confirmation in prospective studies than in those of cross-sectional or retrospective design. Life portraits drawn from men of the Core City sample reveal enormous discontinuity—periods of growth and mastery, interwoven with periods of limitation and regression. Certainly, the more that sustained social and historical events impinge on the life of an individual, the more complex, more heterogeneous, and less predictable that individual's development becomes. Ultimately, the understanding of any individual is to be found in the unique config-

Table 11-2. Relation of Childhood Variables to Adult Outcome

Childhood variables	Object Relations	SES (age 47)	Adult Life Stage	Sociopathy (Robins & Lewis, 1966)	Mental health (HSRS)	Maturity of Defenses
Boyhood Competence	.23	.28	.27	−.22	.24	.16
Childhood Environmental Strengths	.12	.21	.24	−.19	.21	*
Childhood emotional problems subscale	−.20	−.19	−.23	.13	−.19	.13
IQ	.13	.35	.17	*a	.13	.15
Childhood Environmental Weaknesses	*	−.13	*	.18	*	*
Parental SES	*	.14	*	*	*	*

Note. The Pearson product–moment correlation coefficient was the statistic used. Correlations greater than .15 are significant at $p < .001$, and those greater than .12 are significant at $p > .01$. Since hundreds of correlations were obtained, many by chance would have been significant at $p = .05$.

[a]Asterisks indicate

uration of internal and external forces that coalesce to embody that particular life. However, general observations can be made.

While the development of psychosocial maturity is no more a foregone conclusion than is the development of Piagetian formal operations, such maturation, when achieved by men in our study, supports Erikson's extraordinary generalization that "the human personality, in principle, develops according to steps predetermined in the growing person's readiness to be driven toward, to be aware of, and to interact with a widening social radius" (1963, p. 2). The men's lives revealed ever-increasing maturation, yet we found no fixed chronological age at which interpersonal or occupational competence was established. Perhaps what is most encouraging in the collective portrait of these men's lives is their enormous capacity for recovery—evidence that the things that go right in our lives do predict future successes and the events that go wrong in our lives do not forever damn us.

Observations of childhood strength and resiliency naturally generate a companion question of adult outcome and concerns over continuity and predictability. Does resiliency witnessed in childhood hold up over time, and if so, what is its natural history? Most prospective studies now under way in the United States are patiently straining for the accumulation of sufficient longitudinal data for analysis. The men of the Core City sample, however, are now in their 50s, and have passed the generally accepted period of vulnerability for a wide range of psychopathology. Thus, with the previously mentioned limitations of the Core City sample in mind, analysis of the midlife outcome of these men may shed some light on the issues of continuity and predictability in the study of childhood risk and resiliency.

A Pilot Study of the Antecedents of "Invulnerability"

While remaining at the level of informed speculation, the following observations are of particular relevance to the topic of "invulnerability." They are drawn from preliminary findings of a study now in progress—a consideration of the "best" and "worst" outcomes of men, who, as children, were considered to be at high risk for developing psychopathology. A thorough report on our findings will follow the completion of the project.

A high-risk subsample of 75 men was drawn from the Core City sample. Risk was assessed on the basis of the Childhood Environmental Weaknesses scale. In defining this subsample, we must restate that the ratings were performed by clinicians blind to all postadolescent information, and the interrater reliability was .94. For the entire Core City sample, the mean score on the 25-item scale of Childhood

Environmental Weaknesses was 5.4. The childhoods of 25% of these men manifested two or fewer "weaknesses" and clearly did not fit the criteria of membership in a multiproblem urban family. In contrast, the 75 high-risk men manifested 10 or more family "weaknesses."

The social investigator's notes drawn from a representative multiproblem family went as follows: The walk-up apartment was located in a multifamily dwelling in the midst of a "factory neighborhood with a high crime rate, and the presence of gangs, barrooms and alleyways." She documented the apartment's lack of space with the observation, "four children in one bed"; she added that "the apartment had no hot water and the toilet was located outside, down the hall." Both parents were illiterate, and the father was an illegal alien with a history that included problems with alcohol, arrests, and irregular employment. The family's economic situation was described as "marginal—from hand to mouth." As for possessions, there was an old radio present in the kitchen, but there were "no toys for the children." The mother did "day work and cleaning," and the family's average weekly income, divided by its members, was $7.14 per person. Despite this bleak portrait, the investigator was sensitive to evidence of soundness and strength. The home was described as "orderly and clean"; the children were "well disciplined"; and there appeared to be a strong "'we' feeling" in the family. If the Childhood Environmental Weaknesses score was one of the lowest in the study, the Childhood Environmental Strengths score fell squarely in the midrange.

Certainly, an assessment of "risk" ought to be multidetermined. Our ratings have been based largely on environmental criteria. Thus, such factors as genetic predisposition, early birth history, and childhood temperament have not been given their full weight. However, measures of family discord, parental deviance, social disadvantage, and residence in high-crime neighborhoods have long been associated with increased levels of childhood psychopathology (Robins & Lewis, 1966; Rutter et al., 1975). Moreover, Rutter (1970; Wolkind & Rutter, 1973) has suggested that boys may be particularly vulnerable to factors of family discord.

On the one hand, the men in the Core City sample were environmentally at increased risk for becoming delinquent. On the other hand, they had been selected at age 14 for not being delinquent. Thus, based upon objective criteria, the men from multiproblem families constituted a "high-risk" group, but a group who by early adolescence had resisted overt antisocial behavior.

Inclusion in the Core City high-risk group, however, had very real consequences. These men have by far been the most difficult to follow. Whereas attrition in the overall sample has been held to 6%, the attrition rate from the multiproblem family sample has been 29%. Much of the attrition was due to early mortality; the excess deaths were from suicide or violence (Vaillant & Vaillant, 1981).

Out of the 75 youths from "multiproblem" households, we compared the 13 "best" outcomes with the 13 "worst" outcomes to see what, if any, premorbid variables would separate the two groups. Given the high correlation of Boyhood Competence scores with adult outcome in our earlier studies, we were particularly interested to see whether these ratings would hold positive predictive validity for the high-risk group. Again, as in the overall study, the men were assessed by the following early life ratings: Childhood Environmental Strengths, Childhood Environmental Weaknesses, parental SES, IQ, and Boyhood Competence. Special attention was paid to the block design subtest of the Wechsler–Bellevue. The interrelated adulthood ratings were Adult Life Stage, HSRS, SES, Object Relations, and Maturity of Defenses. Elsewhere (Vaillant & Milofsky, 1980) it has been shown that the Adult Life Stage ratings are highly correlated with ratings of HSRS, SES, Object Relations, and Maturity of Defenses.

Having been judged to have attained "generativity," the men with the "best" (the "invulnerable") outcomes all had received scores of 5 on the Adult Life Stage scale. By clinical judgment, men who had achieved generativity demonstrated a clear capacity for "care," "productivity," and "establishing and guiding the next generation" (Erikson's terms). They had assumed sustained responsibility for the growth, well-being, and leadership of others.

In contrast, the men from multiproblem families who had fared worst in adult life had a mean score of 1.5 on the Adult Life Stage scale. Not only had these men not achieved intimacy or stable career identities, but also few had achieved at midlife a capacity to live independently.

Preliminary data regarding premorbid variables of these two outcome groups from multiproblem families are consistent with the findings obtained in the larger study. First, Table 11-3 reveals no significant difference in mean scores between the two groups on the Childhood Environmental Weaknesses scale, the Childhood Environmental Strengths scale, and parental SES.

What did separate the two groups were the scores on the scale of Boyhood Competence, a subscale of Childhood Environmental Strengths (childhood emotional problems), and though less significantly, IQ. Generative adult outcome was most highly correlated with the ratings of Boyhood Competence. The two outcome groups were also separated by at least one standard deviation on score of the subscale of childhood emotional problems. That is, the men with the "best" adult outcomes were less likely to have exhibited evidence of emotional problems as children. Although these are preliminary findings, they do

Table 11-3. Comparison of Men from Multiproblem Families Who Experienced the Best and the Worst Adult Outcomes

	Total Core City sample $(n = 456)^a$	Multiproblem family sample	
		Best outcomes $(n = 13)$	Worst outcomes $(n = 13)$
Premorbid variables			
Childhood Environmental Weaknesses[b]	5 ± 4	11.2	11.8
Parental SES	4.2 ± .6	4.4	4.5
Childhood Environmental Strengths	9 ± 5	5.7	4.0
Childhood emotional problems subscale	2.1 ± .6	1.7	2.3
Boyhood Competence	4.9 ± 1.9	4.9	2.8
WAIS IQ	95 ± 13	101	88
Block design subtest	8.9 ± 3.0	11.2	7.5
Outcome Variables			
Adult Life Stage[c]	6.6 ± 1.2	5.0	1.5
HSRS	75 ± 13	85	52
Adult SES	3.4 ± 0.8	2.9	4.2
Maturity of Defenses[d]	5.2 ± 2.4	2.6	8.3

[a]Data on all variables were not available for all subjects.

[b]This was the variable used to select the multiproblem family sample. All had scores of 9.5 or higher.

[c]This was the variable used to distinguish the outcome groups.

[d]1 = "most mature"; 9 = "least mature."

add weight to the observations that Boyhood Competence is tied to "ego strength," and that, as an indicator of childhood resiliency, it holds some continuity and predictive power for long-term adult outcome.

On Invulnerability

The issue of "invulnerability" has, in part, emerged out of the timely convergence of two complimentary areas of investigation—the field of risk research (Garmezy, 1974; Mednick & Schulsinger, 1973; Rutter, 1970; Rutter *et al.*, 1975) and the very different realm of developmental ego psychology (Erikson, 1963; Freud, 1937; Loevinger, 1976; Murphy, 1962; Murphy & Moriarty, 1976).

At the heart of this growing inquiry is its emphasis on health; it is no longer defined simply by the absence of illness. In the early pages of

The Widening World of Childhood (1962), Lois Murphy called attention to the serious problem posed by the use of clinical terminology. Indeed, clinical language is severely limited and oriented to encompass only what is most immediate and pressing in the realm of psychopathology. Clinical language rarely includes the process of healthy adaptation. What is healthy and going well is often overlooked and obscured in the shadow of illness. Thus, there is a failure to respond to the duality of tension that *is* illness—a tendency to focus only on one dimension of the disequilibrium that the fuels struggle. Clinically, this orientation has biased the approach to the individual patient and has overweighted attention to weakness and pathology, at the expense of attention to strength and resiliency.

First, the diverse and ever-widening field of developmental ego psychology has contributed to an improvement in clinical vision. The landmark work of Anna Freud (1937) set a theoretical turning point. Her elaboration of the workings of the unconscious defense mechanisms of the ego emphasized its healthy, adaptive qualities. Erik Erikson (1963) formulated his epigenetic stages of development upon this foundation. Erikson's view provides insight into the social, cultural, and historical forces that mediate between internal and external demands as they impinge upon the sequential tasks of individual development.

Of critical importance, too, is Jean Piaget's (1929, 1952) massive contribution to the field of cognitive development. His interactionist view—the child as an active agent engaged with the environment—is at the heart of this shift in orientation. Within this framework, development hinges upon the internal workings of maturation and the external forces of experience.

Emphasis on healthy adaptation continued in the diverse theoretical work of such people as Harry Stack Sullivan, Heinz Hartmann, and Robert White. Sullivan (1953) insisted upon the critical importance of interpersonal relationships to personality development. He paid particular attention to the adaptive nature of what he termed "security operations" and to the possible ameliorating impact of "corrective emotional experiences." Hartmann's (1958) conceptualization of a "conflict-free" sphere of ego development also stressed the ego's healthy adaptive capacity. White's (1959, 1960) concepts of "competence" and "effectance motivation" centralized the role of active mastery and the natural human propensity for healthy adaptation.

More recently, major theoretical insights have been augmented by Loevinger's (1976) work on ego development and the conceptualization of a hierarchy of ego defense mechanisms by Semrad (1967), Norma Haan (1977), and others. Finally, Lois Murphy's (1962; Murphy & Moriarty, 1976) work on the "coping styles" of vulnerable children serves as a theoretical and methodological forerunner for much of the current research on invulnerability.

The second major theoretical underpinning of the inquiry on invulnerable children is the field of "high-risk" research. Concerned with the identification and study of particular individuals or populations determined to be vulnerable or generally predisposed for specific psychopathology, it traces its origins back to the early work of Barbara Fish (1957, 1959) and to the work of Mednick and Schulsinger (1971, 1973) in Denmark in the 1960s. Their work and much of what soon followed it (Anthony, 1968; Garmezy, 1974) was concerned with the longitudinal study of schizophrenics and their offspring. Gradually, this orientation and its prospective methodology have been broadened and applied to groups of individuals determined to be vulnerable to a range of psychopathology.

Great literature has always provided a balance to the lopsided preoccupation of psychological science with pathology. Novels offer portraits of individuals who have been maimed or spiritually crushed, having undergone what Freud referred to as "too searching a fate," as well as of those who have survived and even thrived against seemingly overwhelming odds. We are left, then, with the essential and enduring mystery of how to account for the broad range of human capacity to cope, adapt, and get along in a problem-filled world.

The Myth of Invulnerability

Certainly, such irony, mystery, and ambiguity fuel natural human curiosity. However, the quick embrace of the term "invulnerability" by both clinicians and researchers deserves—even requires—a pause. Uncritical attempts to give some children such a label may reflect a vulnerability shared by diverse professional observers. In contrast to the reductionism of science, the model of great literature often enlists an interactionist, longitudinal perspective and seeks to illuminate the myriad forces at work within and without an individual. A novelist would never diminish his protagonist with a finite label. Continuing to sift and weight evidence as it settles and accumulates, the novelist will seldom risk explaining away the individual character in order to hastily resolve a larger collective mystery. Herein lies a message for researchers and clinicians alike.

As Anthony (1974) has pointed out, concerns with invulnerability are linked to underlying preoccupations with immortality. The contrasting forms of invulnerability and their etiology as embodied in the myths of Hercules and Achilles are perhaps models for further inquiry—the unfolding of innate strengths, real or fabricated, as they are pressed and formed by supports in and demands of the environment. Moreover, Anthony has, if indirectly, suggested the importance of myth in our contemporary lives. Once embraced, myths become real as part of the internal imagery that informs our values and helps fuel our behavior.

Reliance on myths, however, can be misleading. While the term "invulnerability" as metaphor captures much of the enthusiasm and spirit of this inquiry, it is all to easily seized upon as myth, especially by the popular press. One repeatedly reads and hears misguided reports of "superkids" and references to "invulnerability." The term "invulnerability" is antithetical to the human condition. Kierkegaard was right when he said, "Fear and annihilation dwell next door to every man." Perhaps it is this inner knowing that adds to our eager, even blind embrace of the myth of invulnerability, and, in turn, increases our propensity for exaggeration and misinterpretation. If unqualified, our vision becomes myopic; human vulnerability is equated with weakness and invulnerability equated with strength. In bearing witness to the resilient behavior of high-risk children everywhere, a truer effort would be to understand, in form and by degree, the shared human qualities at work. As Freud illuminated the shadows of psychopathology as it exists in everyday life, so might studies of resilient children reveal how much all children are like one another, rather than to place great distance between them.

The image of invulnerability holds a prominent position, especially in American mythology. In a sense, it is the Horatio Alger theme—that one is solely and necessarily responsible for one's own progress—for "making it" in America. The traditional American hero generally manages to triumph over all obstacles that fate has placed before him. Sadly, the often deep psychological pain to the character and those to whom he is connected (family, friends, community) is accepted as simply the ways things are—the inevitable consequence of individual triumph and achievement.

These solitary characters, however, are pseudoheroes; they travel alone in a driven manner, possessing a distorted sense of "survivorship." Like Achilles, they wage their battles externally, and they fail to draw strength, insight, and understanding from past wounds. Their achievements are formed of displacement and reaction formation, not of sublimation and altruism. This pseudoinvulnerability does not provide the spiritual tempering and insight that yields more intimate contact with one's internal life. It is, instead, a model of unconscious conflict.

Thus, a critical question for "invulnerability" research becomes this: Are we all talking about the same qualities and individuals? The pictures that have emerged from the preliminary work of the Study of Adult Development and in other work (Felsman, 1981) are not rare, isolated portraits of "superkids" or "geniuses." On the contrary, we are finding courageous individuals who have demonstrated long-term patterns (including periods of limitation and setback) of continued mastery and competence, despite the multiple factors working against them. It is the sustained maintenance of these characteristics in the face of enormous odds that distinguishes them from their peers.

One of our most important preliminary findings on the "high-risk" group from the Core City sample is based on the correlation of Boyhood Competence with positive adult outcome and the substantial data gathered on the men's object relations. These men are not alone. Most are married, reflect genuine enjoyment of their children (and grandchildren), and have friendships that reach beyond family ties. Nor were they solitary or isolated as children. Criteria for Boyhood Competence included participation in group activities (e.g., clubs, sports, church and school activities, etc.). Thus, our observations lend no support to speculations that childhood resiliency will necessarily come at the expense of impaired object relations later in life.

Bleuler (1978) has studied the long-term outcome of the children of schizophrenics and has noted his impression of a "steeling—a hardening—effect on the personalities of some children, making them capable of mastering their lives with all its obstacles, in defiance of all their disadvantages" (p. 409). He also says of such children, however, that those "who are successful in life can never fully free themselves of the pressure imposed on them by memories of their schizophrenic parents and their childhoods" (p. 401). Our preliminary indications are that the "successful" men in our high-risk group are likewise not free of their difficult early memories. We would speculate that it is the style of their remembering *and* feeling that is important—ultimately either adaptive or maladaptive. In short, these men seem to rely more on suppression than repression. Most do have access to their pasts and are able to bear that pain and sorrow, and in so doing, to draw upon it as a source of strength. It should also be noted that their memories are by no means exclusively bleak and painful. They possess perspective and can differentiate between extremes. They take satisfaction in what they have achieved and secured for themselves and their loved ones. A critically important distinction is the genuine capacity of these men for "empathy." Based upon the broad range of positive attributes present in their outcomes at midlife, it is our firm impression that these men can remember and do feel; it seems to inform that "generative" quality in the way they live.

As reported, the Boyhood Competence scale was the variable most highly correlated with positive adult outcome in both the entire sample and the high-risk subsample. Of all the indices we used, Boyhood Competence is perhaps the closest to the elusive concept of "ego strength." Viewed as a mediator or executor, the "ego," with varying degrees of success and efficiency, marshals the individual's cognitive, affective, and physical resources to meet internal and environmental challenges. For Loevinger (1969), "the striving to master, to integrate, to make sense of experience is not one ego function among many but the essence of the ego" (p. 85). An important and most difficult task is that of unraveling the inner logic of ego development—the natural history of individual innate capacities as they interact with the supports and demands of a particular environment. As only the exceptional case ever proves the rule, the pursuit of broader, more generalized traits must be tempered with the recognition that ultimately a coalescence of factors, in manner and by degree, represents a unique configuration in each individual.

To aid our discussion, we have drawn two statements from the original interviews concerning the boy from the multiproblem family we described earlier. One remark was made by the boy himself; the other was made about him by his teacher. Both touch upon theoretical issues germane to the topic of invulnerability.

In a discussion concerning the family's poverty and amount of delinquent activity in his neighborhood, the subject, whom we here call Bill, was asked why he didn't steal when so many other boys did. His straight response was "I don't have to. I can earn what I need." Indeed, he was earning money and had been for some time. Bill was one of those boys who, on the basis of multiple reports, had been credited with possessing "coping capacity"—that is, being planful and making the most of a difficult, disorganized home. His competent behavior at school, with peers, and at work embodied what Robert White (1959) called "effectance." One aim and consequence of such behavior is the *feeling* of "efficacy," a subjective, affective satisfaction derived from competent involvement with one's environment. Certainly, effectance is tied to self-esteem, to Grinker's (1968) reference to "expecting well," and to what Van der Waals (1962) spoke of as "healthy narcissism." Mary Engel's (1967) research on working children focused on young, inner-city kids, especially shoeshine and newspaper boys. Her analysis of their backgrounds, behavior, and expressed attitudes yields rich illustrations of the character traits mentioned above.

Particularly for boys in the high-risk group, goals and challenges in the environment were immediate and abundantly clear. Success brought tangible reward and satisfaction. It did not rest upon the hollow praise children so easily see through when being showered with compliments for success at tasks that are of no major challenge. Certainly, the "press" of the environment was a major contributing factor here; yet it was the self-starting, self-directing capacities of these children that were most noteworthy. Flexibility, determination, and persistence were called forth in this active accommodation to and assimilation of the environment, all of which was reflected in mastery of an ever-widening scope of both cognitive and social skills.

This view of competent behavior in a high-risk environment requires consideration of Ernst Kris's (1950) discussion of "optimal stress"—that is, the notion stress can promote as well as hinder development. The two-part Chinese symbol for "crisis" is represented by "danger" and "opportunity," suggesting that recovery from the threat of defeat and resignation can deepen an individual's wisdom and resolve. However, it is important to distinguish between the impact of the isolated "crisis" and multiple, long-term stress factors.

One of the most intriguing qualities of the men with the "best" outcomes in the high-risk group was (and is) their apparent capacity to bear up to and endure multiple stresses. It stands in direct contradiction to much of what we know about the determination of risk and subsequent outcome. It is sustained emotional trauma, not sudden insult, that does lasting damage to the human spirit. Rutter's (1978, 1979; Rutter *et al.*, 1975) comparative studies of children of inner-city London and the Isle of Wight indicate that it is multiplicity of stress factors that most determines a child's psychiatric risk. With only one major stress factor present (even if chronic), a child's psychiatric risk remained at the same level as that of the control group. However, with two or three stress factors operating simultaneously, the level of psychiatric risk increased fourfold. Each additional stress factor continued to increase the risk of psychiatric disorder dramatically. Similarly, Langner and Michael (1963) found in the Midtown Manhattan Study that it was the sheer number of risk factors alone that best predicted adult mental health problems.

A phrase Bill's teacher used in describing him suggests an area for further inquiry. In providing an overall assessment, she chose to highlight one asset: "He draws people to him." Unfortunately, she did not go on to speculate about the characteristics she believed accounted for this quality. However, we are aware that some children are particularly adept at seeking out, identifying, engaging, and drawing upon the supports that do exist, even in a bleak environment.

Vygotsky (1978) has suggested that the "zone of proximal development" is perhaps the most important, yet overlooked factor in the assessment of children's intelligence. His concern is not with knowledge possessed. Rather, it is with the child's capacity to make use of additional clues—to engage and manipulate them in an effort to solve the problem at hand. Certainly, Vygotsky's conceptualization of this cognitive capacity is multidetermined, including factors of attention, flexibility, persistence, and so on. However, clues emanate from the environment at large, and we suggest that the term not be limited to cognitive tasks alone, but include the realm of social interaction as well. Bill's observed capacity to "draw people to him" and his ability to "earn what I need" seemed to reside at the heart of his social competence.

Bill's resilient behavior in the midst of a most difficult environment suggests another factor in the assessment of individual risk. It speaks to Erikson's (1964) distinction between "actuality" and "reality." "Actuality" is concerned with objective facts, while "reality" deals with how the individual *feels* about the actuality and what it *means* to him or her. Drawing upon the foundation of child therapy, this distinction necessitates a shared search for meaning, a critical effort to obtain a child's-eye view. In Bill's case, the assessment of material poverty was straightforward. However, interviews and projective tests revealed no indication that he experienced himself as "impoverished" (materially or emotionally), or that his "disadvantaged" position was somehow deserved and his own fault. On the contrary, he was clear about the fact that he could make what he needed, and he had every expectation that there was more to come. These attributes, whether of perception and/or belief, affect a child's understanding of causality of past events, notions of responsibility in the present, and expectations for the future. In turn, they inform his behavior. The growing research on "cognitive style" (Witkin & Goodenough, 1977; Witkin, Goodenough, & Oltman, 1979) and on "locus of control" (Phares, 1976; Rotter, 1966) focuses on these specific variables and may well make major contributions to our understanding of individual strength and resiliency as it is witnessed in childhood.

Bill's tough, competent stance toward the world and active mastery of his environment was representative of the resilient children in our high-risk group. Assessing and quantifying these attributes on the scale of Boyhood Competence and demonstrating its actuarial, predictive validity for long-term adult outcome have been important steps. Yet in raising this powerful necessary abstraction," ego strength," we remain better equipped to describe it than to explain what underlies it. To what extent is its individual composition innate, learned, and/or absorbed?

Our findings on Boyhood Competence add weight to the contention that a significant dimension of "ego strength" rests upon innate factors. In underscoring the role of innate capacities, however, we are not saying "in place of" social factors; we are saying "in addition to." A person's internal psychological resources can never be extricated from his social–environmental context.

A specific example is the issue of temperament. In describing the delinquent boys in the original study, Glueck and Glueck (1968) observed that "such characteristics as a tendency to act out their difficulties (extroversion), greater freedom from fear of failure and defeat, and less dependence on others, might under proper circumstances and influential guidance, be assets rather than liabilities" (p. 27). In recent years, much attention has been paid to the interactionist model of temperament—a particular child with particular caregivers in a particular environment (Rutter, Quinton, & Yule, 1977; Thomas, Chess, & Birch, 1968). The apt phrase "goodness of fit" (Thomas & Chess, 1980) captures the contextual significance of individual temperament.

Moreover, dimensions of intelligence, competence, and mastery are also most accurately appreciated contextually. The skills and behavior that are competent and adaptive in one environment (or at one developmental stage) may be quite maladaptive in another. Recently, a clinician accustomed to working with children in Boston's wealthy suburbs was a guest visiting an inner-city guidance clinic. While participating in a team evaluation of a family, he had the opportunity to speak with a 10-year-old boy who was reportedly having trouble with fighting in school. The clinician listened to the boy describe a specific incident and then wondered out loud if he had ever "just tried to talk his way out of such a difficult situation." The boy's unhesitating reply was "That don't work. You try that round my way and you be gettin' your head busted, quick." It is a statement as indicative of the way environmental actuality impinges upon psychological reality as it is of individual predisposition or defensive style.

Indications for Further Research

Though retrospective, cross-sectional, and short-term follow-up studies will certainly play a role in the growing inquiry on resiliency in high-risk children, it is the prospective longitudinal method that is best able to address the natural question of long-term outcome. That is, how will these resilient children fare as adults? The limitations and shortcomings of the longitudinal method have been addressed by Baekland, Lundwall, and Kissin (1975), Baltes (1968), Garmezy (1977), Robins and Smith (1980), and Vaillant (1983).

However, while the refinement of methodological problems continues, the promising but relatively overlooked area of cross-cultural studies deserves attention. Field work conducted among high-risk children in natural environments, or in settings that lack traditional familial and institutional supports, may yield points of triangulation for cross-cultural validation as well as fresh avenues for inquiry. The field work of Felsman (1981) and the ongoing work of Boothby (1982) are specific examples.

The study by Felsman (1981) focused on the "gamins" or street urchins of Cali, Columbia. Darting in and out of traffic, begging in open-air restaurants, singing for change on city buses, bathing in public fountains, or curled up sleeping together beneath the shelter of an overhanging roof, these young waifs managed the often tangled course of human growth and development with little help from the traditional institutional supports of family, school, church, or state. An atypical self-selecting group of children, they stood at the intersection of human strength and vulnerability. On the basis of environmental factors alone, they were at high risk for psychopathology. Indeed, many of these children did succumb to the perils and stresses of this harsh environment, as evidenced through physical ills and psychopathology. More striking, however, was the clear evidence of physical and psychological health they individually and collectively demonstrated despite such circumstances.

Felsman's (1981, 1984) examination of these children's competent behavior and active mastery in a high-risk environment suggests a coalescence of individual, internal factors with elements of external support secured from the environment. Specifically, elements of physiology, temperament, cognitive style, locus of control, and individual level of cognitive–psychosocial development are considered as they merge with external dimensions of peer support and intervention efforts. A descriptive overview of the gamins' daily life, as well as specific clinical case studies, illustrates the theoretical positions taken.

Boothby's (1983, in press) current work on Southeast Asian refugee children provides a sustained, detailed clinical observation of children separated from their families under the stress of war. His analysis of resilient behavior in these children is followed through the sequential phases of initial separation, camp internment, and resettlement, all shedding light on the changing nature of risk and vulnerability as it coincides with the internal maturation and evolving capacities of the individual child. The real-life setting of this work dramatically raises the difficult moral and ethical social policy issues of intervention and long-term follow-up of high-risk children.

Conclusions

What is most important about the nascent study of competence and resiliency in high-risk children as its orientation toward health—a posture that necessitates valuing strengths and assets as highly as signs of illness and vulnerability. Such a stance holds promise for concerns of primary prevention, but is unlikely to conform to a model of immunology and provide the vaccine of invulnerability. In the myth, Achilles was rendered invulnerable by a moments' immersion in a magic bath, but myths are poor science. If the term "invulnerability" is to be useful, it must be a metaphor for a lifelong process of adaptation. The study of high-risk children necessitates an interactionist effort. Disciplined attention must be given to the unique matrix of internal and external factors at work in the individual child.

Garmezy (1980) has drawn upon a quote attributed to Robert Louis Stevenson as an analogy for stress resistance: "Life is not a matter of holding good cards but of playing a poor hand well." Certainly, the randomness of cards dealt is reflective of the awesome arbitrariness that marks every child's entry into this world. Indeed, we all must work with what fate and circumstance continue to provide or deny us. Yet the cards dealt (i.e., innate capacities) are critically important, as is the specific game (i.e., the environmental context) being "played." It is the unique coalescence of the two that constitutes the individual's "playing." We would emphasize that the living of a life is not realized in the playing of a single hand. On the contrary, the weight and value of cards change, as do both the ability *and* opportunity to play and replay them.

In the finale of *Middlemarch*, George Eliot wrote,

> Every limit is a beginning as well as an ending. Who can quit young lives after being long in company with them, and not desire to know what befell them in their after years? *For the fragment of a life, however typical, is not the sample of an even web;* promises may not be kept, and an ardent outset may be followed by declension; latent powers may find a long-waited opportunity; a past error may urge a grand retrieval. (1872; italics added)

The findings of the Study of Adult Development have confirmed a novelist's expressed need (personal and analytical) for the longitudinal/ life span perspective. Over the life span, the discontinuities are enormous, and in the development of psychosocial maturity we found no fixed chronological age at which interpersonal or occupational competence was established.

In addition, our preliminary findings on a specific group of resilient, high-risk children who have achieved "generativity" as adults reveal similar longitudinal lessons. As children, they were not "geniuses" or "superkids," nor do they represent lone individuals. Most importantly, their lives do not reveal any invariant, linear sequence of repeated success and triumph. The portraits of their individual and collective lives contain periods of limitation and regression, while reflecting traits of mastery and competence possessed by the vast majority of everyday people. What, if anything, sets them apart is that despite enormous odds, their lives reveal a clear pattern of recovery, restoration, and gradual mastery.

REFERENCES

Anthony, E. J. (1968). The developmental precursors of adult schizophrenia. In D. Rosenthal & S. Kety (Eds.), *The transmission of schizophrenia*. Oxford: Pergamon Press.

Anthony, E. J. (1974). The syndrome of the psychologically invulnerable child. In E. J. Anthony & C. Koupernik (Eds.), *The child in his family: Children at psychiatric risk* (International yearbook, Vol. 3). New York: Wiley.

Baekland, F., Lundwall, L., & Kissin, B. (1975). Methods for the treatment of chronic alcoholism. In R. Gibbons, Y. Israel, H. Kalant, R. Popham, W. Schmidt, & R. Smart (Eds.), *A critical appraisal in research advances in alcohol and drug problems* (Vol. 6). New York: Wiley.

Baltes, P. (1968). Longitudinal and cross-sectional sequences in the study of age and generation effects. *Human Development, 11*, 145.

Bleuler, M. (1978). *The schizophrenic mental disorders in the light of long-term patient and family histories*. New Haven, CT: Yale University Press.

Block, J. (1971). *Lives through time*. Berkeley, CA: Bancroft.

Boothby, N. (1983). The horror: The hope. *Natural History, 92*, 64–71.

Boothby, N., Ressler, E., & Steinbock, D. (in press). *Unaccompanied children in emergencies: Their care and protection in wars, natural disasters and refugee movements*. New York: Oxford University Press.

Eichorn, D., Clausen, J., Haan, N., Honzik, M., & Mussen, P. (1981). (Eds.). *Present and past in middle life*. New York: Academic Press.

Eliot, G. [M. A. Evans]. (1872). *Middlemarch*. Cambridge, MA: Riverside Press, 1956.

Engel, M. (1967). Children who work. *Archives of General Psychiatry, 17*, 291–297.

Erikson, E. (1963). *Childhood and society* (2nd ed.). New York: Norton.

Erikson, E. (1964). *Insight and responsibility*. New York: Norton.

Erikson, E. (1968). The life cycle. In *International encyclopedia of the social sciences* (Vol. 9). New York: Macmillan.

Felsman, J. K. (1981). *Street urchins of Cali: On risk, resiliencyy and adaptation in childhood*. Unpublished doctoral dissertation, Harvard University.

Felsman, J. K. (1984). Abandoned children: A reconsideration. *Children Today, 13*, 13–18.

Fish, B. (1957). The detection of schizophrenia in infancy. *Journal of Nervous and Mental Disease, 125*, 1–24.

Fish, B. (1959). Longitudinal observations of biological deviation in a schizophrenic infant. *American Journal of Psychiatry, 116*, 25–31.

Freud, A. (1937). *The ego and the mechanisms of defense*. London: Hogarth Press.

Garmezy, N. (1974). Children at risk: The search for the antecedents of schizophrenia. Part II: Ongoing research programs, issues and intervention. *Schizophrenia Bulletin, 9*, 55–125.

Garmezy, N. (1977). On some risks of risk research. *Psychological Medicine, 7*, 7–10.

Garmezy, N. (1980). Children under stress: Perspectives or antecedents and correlates of vulnerability and resistance to psychopathology. In A. Robin, J. Arnoff, A. Barclay, & R. Zucker (Eds.), *Further explorations in personality*. New York: Wiley.

Glueck, S., & Glueck, E. (1950). *Unraveling juvenile delinquency*. New York: The Commonwealth Fund.

Glueck, S., & Glueck, E. (1968). *Delinquents and nondelinquents in perspective*. Cambridge, MA: Harvard University Press.

Grinker, R. (1968). Psychiatry and our dangerous world. In *Psychiatric research in our changing world: Proceedings of an international symposium, Montreal* (Excerpta Medical International Congress Series No. 187). Amsterdam: Excerpta Medica, 1968.

Haan, N. (1977). *Coping and defending*. New York: Academic Press.

Hartmann, H. (1958). *Ego psychology and the problem of adaptation*. New York: International Universities Press.

Hollingshead, A., & Redlich, F. *Social class and mental illness*. New York: Wiley.

Kris, E. (1950). Notes on development and on some current problems of psychoanalytic child psychology. *Psychoanalytic Study of the Child, 5*, 24–46.

Langner, T., & Michael, S. (1963). *Life stress and mental health*. New York: Free Press.

Loevinger, J. (1969). Theories of ego development. In L. Berger (Ed.), *Clinical cognitive psychology: Models and integrations*. Englewood Cliffs, NJ: Prentice-Hall.

Loevinger, J. (1976). *Ego development*. San Francisco: Jossey-Bass.

Luborsky, L. (1962). Clinicians' judgments of mental health. *Archives of General Psychiatry, 7*, 407–417.

Luborsky, L., & Bachrach, H. (1974). Factors influencing clinicians' judgments of mental health: Eighteen experiences with the Health–Sickness Rating Scale. *Archives of General Psychiatry, 31*, 292–299.

Mednick, S., & Schulsinger, F. (1971). Perinatal conditions and infant development in children with schizophrenic parents. *Social Biology, 8*, 103–113.

Mednick, S., & Schulsinger, F. (1973). Studies of children at high risk for schizophrenia. In S. R. Dean (Ed.), *Schizophrenia: The first ten Dean Award Lectures*. New York: MSS Information Corp.

Murphy, L. (1962). *The widening world of childhood: Paths toward mastery*. New York: Basic Books.

Murphy, L., & Moriarty, A. (1976). *Vulnerability, coping and growth: From infancy to adolescence*. New Haven, CT: Yale University Press.

Phares, E. J. (1976). *Locus of control in personality*. Morristown, NJ: General Learning Press.

Piaget, J. (1929). *The child's conception of the world*. New York: Harcourt, Brace.

Piaget, J. (1952). *The origins of intelligence in children*. New York: Norton.

Robins, L., & Lewis, R. (1966). The role of the antisocial family in school completion and delinquency: A three generation study. *Sociology Quarterly, 7*, 500–514.

Robins, L., & Smith, E. (1980). Longitudinal studies of alcohol and drug problems: Sex differences. In J. Kalant (Ed.), *Alcohol and drug problems in women*. New York: Plenum Press.

Rotter, J. (1966). Generalized expectancies for internal versus external control of reinforcement. *Psychological Monographs, 80* (1, Whole No. 609).

Rutter, M. (1970). Sex difference in children's responses to family stress. In E. J. Anthony & C. Koupernik (Eds.), *The child in his family* (International yearbook, Vol. 1). New York: Wiley.

Rutter, M. (1978). Early sources of security and competence. In J. Brunner & A. Gaston (Eds.), *Human growth and development*. Oxford: Clarendon Press.

Rutter, M. (1979). Protective factors in children's responses to stress and disadvantage. In M. Kent & J. Rolf (Eds.), *Primary prevention of psychopathology: Social competence in children*. Hanover, NH: University Press of New England.

Rutter, M., Quinton, D., & Yule, B. (1977). *Family pathology and disorder in children*. Chichester: Wiley.

Rutter, M., Yule, B., Quinton, D., Rowlands, O., Yule, W., & Berger, M. (1975). Attainment and adjustment in two geographical areas: III. Some factors accounting for area differences. *British Journal of Psychiatry, 126*, 520–533.

Semrad, E. (1967). The organization of ego defenses and object loss. In D. M. Moriarity (Ed.), *The loss of loved ones*. Springfield, IL: Charles C Thomas.

Sullivan, H. S. (1953). *Interpersonal theory of psychiatry*. New York: Norton.

Terman, H., & Oden, M. H. (1959). *The gifted group at midlife*. Stanford, CA: Stanford University Press.

Thomas, A., & Chess, S. (1980). *The dynamics of psychological development*. New York: Brunner/Mazel.

Thomas, A., Chess, S., & Birch, H. (1968). *Temperament and behavior disorder in children*. New York: New York University Press.

Vaillant, G. (1974). The natural history of male psychological health: II. Some antecedents of healthy adult adjustment. *Archives of General Psychiatry, 31*, 15–22.

Vaillant, G. (1977). *Adaptation to life.* Boston: Little, Brown.

Vaillant, G. (1983). *Natural history of alcoholism.* Cambridge, MA: Harvard University Press.

Vaillant, G., & Milofsky, E. (1980). Natural history of male psychological health: IX. Empirical evidence for Erikson's model of the life cycle. *American Journal of Psychiatry, 137*, 1348–1359.

Vaillant, G., & Vaillant, C. (1981). Natural history of male psychological health: X. Work as a predictor of positive mental health. *American Journal of Psychiatry, 138*, 1433–1440.

Van der Waals, H. (1962). *Lectures on narcissism.* Topeka, KS: Topeka Psychoanalytic Institute.

Vygotsky, L. S. (1978). *Mind in society.* Cambridge, MA: Harvard University Press.

White, R. (1959). Motivation reconsidered: The concept of competence. *Psychological Review, 66*, 297–333.

White, R. (1960). Competence and the psychosexual stages of development. *Nebraska Symposium on Motivation.* 97–144.

Williams, W. C. (1937). *White mule.* New York: New Directions.

Witkin, H., & Goodenough, P. (1977, July). *Origins of field dependence–independence.* Princeton, NJ: Education Testing Service.

Witkin, H., Goodenough, P., & Oltman, P. (1979). Psychological differentiation: Current status. *Journal of Personality and Social Psychology, 37*, 1127–1145.

Wolkind, S., & Rutter, M. (1973). Children who have been "in care"—an epidemiological study. *Journal of Child Psychology and Psychiatry, 14*, 97–105.

12

The Traits of True Invulnerability and Posttraumatic Stress in Psychoanalyzed Men of Action

EDWIN C. PECK, JR.
Southern California Psychoanalytic Institute

Introduction

Much of the study of invulnerability to date has been focused upon children's personalities and the characteristics of the families in which they grew up. Most notably, Anthony (1974, 1978) has succinctly described the personality patterns of true invulnerables growing up in family settings with one psychotic parent.

Invulnerables' exposures to such high-risk developmental experiences as a psychotic parent, or violence, or both, are the sorts of stressors defined as criteria for posttraumatic stress disorder in the *Diagnostic and Statistical Manual of Mental Disorders*, third edition (DSM-III). With current developments in studies of both invulnerability and posttraumatic stress disorder, I think we are at the point where some observations and models in each of these subspecialties can be woven together and applied to psychoanalytic case material, thus enhancing each field and pertinent cases.

The cases to be explored in this chapter I call "adult invulnerable characters." The case data, I believe, support my preliminary thesis that the invulnerable's prominent drive to mastery is an adaptive complex subvariant of the phenomena of re-enactment in posttraumatic stress disorders. I have found that these mastery patterns of the adult invulnerables are laid down during overwhelming traumas encountered in the first 20 years of life. Complicating these re-enactment patterns seems to be a parallel process of identifying with the parent or parent surrogate in grappling with the overwhelming trauma.

Recent studies of posttraumatic stress disorder recommend, first, that we go beyond the current DSM-III definition. My own experience and recent summary studies indicate that we need to do so by focusing our symptom categories on the patient's traumatic imagery, his related affective and somatic states, and his defenses against them (Brett & Ostroff, 1985; Van Der Kolk, 1984).

Second, we need to attend more fully to details of patients' imagery, re-enactment behavior, and related traumatic events. In so doing, I think we can go beyond our current understanding of the repetition compulsion and a phenomenon for which it can be mistaken: re-enactment. I think our clinical work is furthered by asking this question: "Repetition (or re-enactment) of what, to what degree, and for how long?" The cases presented here begin to show how, by exploring answers to these questions and the connections among re-enactment, traumatic events, affects, and underlying dynamics, the repetitions can be ceased or constructively modified.

Because Anthony's explorations of patients' patterns of mastery and related issues of invulnerability, detachment, and immunity are so fruitful and so apt for the cases I present, I use his terms for the character traits in question. I pause at the start to further explore connections between current research on posttraumatic stress disorder and Anthony's work. For example, with my cases, I hope to demonstrate this sequence emerging from major trauma experiences:

1. Major trauma overwhelms sensory and affect-regulating mechanisms.
2. Waves of affect storms and numbing defenses against these are linked to traumatic imaging and nightmares.
3. Defenses become rigidified and thought patterns become more concrete.
4. Re-enactments (main patterns of re-enactment formed with great precision by traumatic events and subsequent imaging) are initiated as the patient's traumatic images mold and are molded by (a) pre-existing fantasies; (b) defensive structures; (c) ego skills; (d) physical qualities; (e) object relationships; and (f) the patient's social contact and traditions.

Now the reader sees the viewpoint into which I fit Anthony's crucial term of "mastery," the force leading a person to test his strength even against overwhelming odds. Combining the sequence described above with my case presentations, I wish to demonstrate how the invulnerable's other key traits of detachment and immunity are mainly consequences of his enormous investment of psychic energy and concentration in the structural axis of his traumatic imagery, affects, and re-enactments.

Anthony lays down the gauntlet of a central challenge in invulnerability therapy and research when he wonders "whether, having helped him [the invulnerable] one could follow him closely, over time, to learn his secret" (1974, p. 534). He goes on to note that if this is possible, one can claim that a crucial advance has been made in the field of psychiatric prevention.

The following set of research questions to which this chapter's psychoanalytic study provides some preliminary answers have been posed by Anthony (1974, pp. 533–534).

1. Is there a point in life when a "natural selection" begins to operate, permitting the fittest to survive and the unfit to succumb, or does a coat of invulnerability gradually build up from repeatedly successful adjustments?
2. Is there such an entity as psychological immunity; is it ever complete? The corollary of this question would be this: Is the Achilles heel always present in some part of the makeup?
3. If there is immunity, is it permanent, or does the wear and tear of everyday existence eventually reduce its efficacy?
4. Is the immunity paid for out of the store of good human characteristics, with the subsequent development of insensitivity, detachment, and self-absorption?
5. Does the individual really master fate, or is he especially fortunate in being treated benignly by the world in which he lives?
6. Is it possible to distinguish between the early and late invulnerables, and between the true and false invulnerables?

Considering such questions while grappling with the 6-year psychoanalysis of a homicide detective patient named Jim, I repeatedly observed traits of invulnerability. He not only survived multiple, devastating losses and assaults, but responded to them by mastering new career challenges through driven work, new skill development, and effective planning. While he manifested such defensive structures as reaction formation and compulsive working, identifying these defenses and their sources did not much clarify his characterological pattern of mastering high risk and challenge at work. Many patients with compulsions and reaction formations do not show Jim's pattern of mastering risk.

At this point, Anthony's studies of invulnerable children helped elucidate my analysand's pattern of mastery. I decided that the uniquely intimate observational setting of an adult psychoanalysis provides some especially advantageous data describing transference responses and long-term character patterns, with associated answers to some research questions posed by Anthony, myself, and others.

In addition, one of our richest, most enduring elucidations of a childhood fantasy and phobic–obsessional structure was taken by Freud from his analysis of the adult Wolf Man. It seems time once again to follow this neglected precedent and to further explore the childhood fantasy and character structure of a true invulnerable who was analyzed in his adulthood.

Before describing the psychoanalysis of my patient, Jim, and two related cases, it is useful to present the central definitions of "invulnerability" and "mastery" that guide and focus the following case presentation. Anthony (1974) writes: "Invulnerability (and vulnerability) are states of mind induced in the child by exposure to risks. . . . Mastery is a force that leads one to test his strength constantly against the environment and to assert himself, even against overwhelming odds" (p. 537).

Jim and His Analysis

This is the story of an analysand's exposure to multiple great risks in all developmental epochs. The subplot describes his repeatedly testing himself against overwhelming, sometimes hair-raising, odds.

Presenting Complaints and Background Data

Jim was an intelligent, witty, 42-year-old homicide detective who began a 6-year psychoanalysis for treatment of severe tension, abdominal pain, vomiting, recently increased drinking, identity diffusion, and panic. He had just concluded a highly successful 17-year detective career when he came to me. Before becoming a detective, he had been equally successful as a team leader both in the aerospace field and in Korean War cryptography. Often during treatment, Jim said he felt driven to master tasks that his bosses and colleagues considered impossible. His preoccupations with reorganizing and mastering his work experiences were associated with a concomitant disengagement from family and friends.

Jim's descriptions, in his first year of analysis, of how he handled various risks involved in homicide detection began to reveal some of the mechanisms involved in his development of mastery in this area. It was only in later treatment years that Jim described preoedipal and oedipal childhood experiences and fantasies that also contributed to his drive for mastery in his high-risk work. Periodically in early treatment, Jim mentioned his pride at never firing a shot at another person. He had worked in high-crime districts, and had had numerous hand-to-hand fights with homicidal individuals, disarming them without injury. He saw his success in such fights as coming from his absolute determination and concentration; his total belief in his willingness to move without hesitation against any and all life-threatening situations and individuals; and his total belief in his greater quickness, determination, and strength. The accuracy of Jim's views of mechanisms involved in his work success was soon to be documented by his transference behaviors, demonstrating remarkable levels of commitment and determination as he dealt with outer and inner obstacles. In sum, Jim had a marked sense of invulnerability when undertaking tasks. Coupled with his invulnerable sense were high-level intellectual and athletic skills honed by extremely well-disciplined practice.

Far from living in a benign world, Jim was suffering from a number of stresses that had begun 2 months before the analysis. (1) His stepfather died. (2) His second wife, who was going blind, insisted they move from their hillside house and filed for divorce. (3) At work, there were increasing numbers of murder cases for him to handle; in addition, corrupted, disorganized city officials were dismantling the police department. (These data were confirmed and elaborated in local newspapers.) (4) Also, at work, his boss was pushing him to take a higher-ranking administrative position. In sum, unmanageable disappointments were occurring to a person who, throughout his life, had carried a sense of an invulnerable self.

At the start of his analysis, Jim precisely described the pathological disorganization and corruption in his city's government. His observations concerning abusive treatment of victims of crime and ineffectual dealing with many perpetrators of cirme were borne out, point by point, in works by leading social critics and veteran judges. For our purposes, it becomes striking that after about 4 years of psychoanalysis and the lifting of considerable childhood amnesia (experiences of neglect and physical and mental abuse, as well as sexual fantasies), Jim manifested his powerful curiosity about and knowledge of the psychiatric diagnoses involved with the highly abusive and disruptive behavior of his parents.

This curiosity brings to mind that Anthony found the same traits in invulnerable children. A specific example of Jim's applying these traits to parent figures in his environment just before treatment is as follows. His last homicide case before the end of his career involved a city's leading high school all-American athlete and scholar, who had had his heart carved out during a gangland attack on a party. Jim told how for months he had advised the murderer's father that his son had violently knifed other individuals and was likely to repeat the act with disastrous effects unless steps were taken to remove him from the activities of his gang group. The father ignored Jim. He went on to describe the criminal justice system that hounded and harmed the victim's family and let the murderer off with 2 years in prison.

The main points of Jim's childhood history of deprivation, neglect, and assault are given in this summary, for the reader's orientation. Years of analytic work were needed to lift amnesia and reveal these traumatic memories (later cross-checked and validated by family members). First, oedipal and latency memories of unique beatings and coercions were recalled; then, with 1 to 2 years more of analysis, preoedipal experiences of extreme loss and neglect emerged. In infancy, he experienced life-threatening starvation, exposure to winter in an unheated, freezing home, and repeated severe infections. His mother and father often had intense arguments, and his father was unavailable for long stretches of time, all before he was 2½ years old.

At age 2½ Jim suffered a striking series of losses. First, his father left the home completely to become a hard-drinking wanderer. Second, a surrogate mother figure, a great-aunt who had been comforting and teaching Jim, developed bone cancer with rapid deterioration over a few months. Also, at this time, his maternal grandmother had a long-term psychiatric hospitalization; during this confinement his mother experienced increased amounts of anxiety, depression, and withdrawal, for which she did not have psychiatric evaluation or treatment.

Throughout his childhood, Jim's family changed homes yearly for real estate profits. Jim's stepfather entered the family when Jim was 4. The stepfather was, in early treatment, described as a prince of a fellow; by contrast, a year into psychoanalysis while Jim was working with a series of traumatic dreams, it became clear that the stepfather would violently beat Jim, as often as twice weekly. These beatings began when Jim was about 5 and continued until he was 15 years old. Between the second and seventh grades, Jim had repeated bouts of pneumonia and ear infections, which often forced him to miss school. With all this, his childhood was isolated.

When he was 8 and 10 years old, his mother neglected his care to concentrate on his newborn half-sister and half-brother, respectively. His sister grew up to be an attractive girl and a good student. He described his brother as completely lacking in ambition and always following the rules. His early memory of his sister was this: "As a child, I pushed her too fast in a wagon, and the wagon tongue cut her deep. After this, I felt depressed."

From age 10 onward, Jim worked at part-time jobs, some involving long hours cleaning chicken coops and stables; he thus substantially contributed to the family finances while still going to school. His parents did not acknowledge his straight-A grades in school or his financial contributions, nor did they attend his sports and music events, at which he excelled.

In sum, Jim came from a extremely abusive environment in which he developed a character trait of working furiously to overcome whatever tasks or challenges placed before him. The mechanisms involved in this character trait development are explored in the subsequent presentation of transference developments in Jim's psychoanalysis. In any case, it is clear from these summary data that, in answer to Anthony's fifth question, Jim was mastering a fate quite the opposite of benign. Two additional cases that I present later in this chapter provide a similar answer to this question.

Pertinent background data in Jim's case indicated that his sexual activities were characterized in part by their having a quality of driven work. Specifically, he recalled beginning masturbation in eary latency. He reported scattered memories and dreams of being injured, suggestive of high levels of castration and annihilation anxieties. His associations, discussions of sexual life, and direct questions from me produced no memories or outside information indicating he was exposed to parents' or other family members' sexual activities. Starting at age 10, he would usually masturbate several times daily. He concentrated on physical pleasure and denied having associated fantasies. His stepfather once saw him masturbating and calmly cautioned that doing anything in excess was not a good idea. Sex, like other personal topics, was not discussed with him by his parents.

In his mid-teens, Jim initiated heterosexual activity. (He also had a long-time girlfriend in his teens with whom he did not have sex.) In these years and afterward, he had several lovers, mostly women about 10 years older with whom he had frequent, mutually gratifying sexual intercourse. He married for the first time at age 19 and for the second time at age 32. In both instances, the women he married were intensely needy and suffering from serious levels of anxiety and depression. Nevertheless, his sexual life in both his marriages was highly satisfying for both partners. It was typical that he was conscious mainly of furthering his partner's sexual satisfaction in each case. He spoke on this to the exclusion of discussing or thinking of his own satisfaction, fantasies, or emotional experiences. He would not fantasize during sex, and he strongly felt it important and correct not to do so.

Delineating his driven work approach to sex was Jim's report that before analysis and during the early months of analysis, he looked upon lovemaking as a competitive act wherein it was his duty to wear the woman out. It was in his preadolescent period that Jim began experiencing a repetitive nightmare that haunted him for about 3 years and intermittently thereafter. He described the nightmare as follows: "This real ugly woman, like a witch, was after me. She walked toward me. I backed up. I would be at the top of a cliff. She would come forward, and I would start falling off the cliff. Then I awoke before hitting bottom. Sometimes I would fall out of bed." Jim's immediate associations after first describing the nightmare were these: "We were moving around a lot then. My folks were buying and selling homes." (It turned out that Jim's mother had launched an intensive push for real estate profits and was uprooting the family from one home to another.) "I would not want to go to sleep after that dream. That witch would never touch me. She was so damn ugly and grotesque. It scared the hell out of me."

Next, addressing Anthony's second and fourth research questions, I can now elucidate Jim's characteristic invulnerable's Achilles heel as the need to maintain distance in intimate relationships. At the 1-year point in analysis, as I was going on vacation, the transference situation took on a maternal cast. Jim was controlled and unable to identify direct feelings toward me, while at the same time, in his associations, he again recalled the witch nightmare and spoke at length of his first feelings of hurt and anger when his homes were uprooted and he left school friends. Jim said that after a year or so of these reactions, he developed a habit of limiting his emotional contact by "keeping his personal bags packed when entering new schools." During this period, his parents' pressure and his own perfectionistic competitiveness forced him to work long hours at jobs he could barely tolerate. One of his jobs was to help his father pluck feathers from chickens and clean up the bloody remains. Another job that he did between the ages of 10 and 16 was to maintain his parents' apartment house lawns. He repeatedly described the endless drudgery of pushing a hand mower around the yards, only to start again when he finished the circuit. He felt these yards were his prison.

Full consideration of Jim's childhood adversity is oppressive and fatiguing. Acknowledging these realities while maintaining analytic balance is an important treatment challenge in such cases. As noted earlier, after presenting the psychoanalysis of Jim, I turn to the summaries of two related cases, illustrating main themes of the adult character and their backgrounds of great adversity in varying phases of childhood and adolescence.

Opening-Phase, First-Segment Transference Developments in Jim's Psychoanalysis

I now return to the beginning of Jim's psychoanalysis. He manifested unique and prominent traits of rigid control over his thoughts, feelings, behavior, and immediate environment. Still, to have a correct picture of this man, the reader must understand from the start that interspersed among expressions of his uniquely controlling traits were periodic expressions of direct personal warmth and compassion, and, on other occasions, rage handled with massive amounts of projection and denial. The warmth and rage came across to me as distinctly split apart, not integrated aspects of his personality. While such positive expressions occurred in early sessions, they were by no means the main theme; they would commonly be denied, and Jim lamented his declining capacity to make such expressions to his wife and children.

To illustrate Jim's controlled behavior, I have never met a patient or anyone else as punctual as he was. I could set my watch to the second by his entrance, knowing that he always arrived 10 minutes before the scheduled hour. During the first treatment year, Jim's total resistance to any interpretations of this behavior were as rigid as his habit. When lying on the couch, Jim maintained a rigid neck posture, keeping his head on a stiff couch edge, avoiding a pillow, and keeping his shoulders a bit off the couch. Confrontations of this unique posture were met by Jim's ridicule. In the early months of analysis, Jim revealed that he carefully counted the steps from his car to this or any location. Like Sherlock Holmes, Jim periodically revealed his disciplined capacity for observation, noting details like a drop of oil near my car, a scratch on the wall, or a bit of dust on my shoe. Like Holmes, Jim told stories using notably clear and to-the-point language.

These traits, combined with his patterns of imagination and his ego ideals, reveal someone who kept objective distance from whatever he was dealing with within himself or within others. He was a systematic student and was excessively self-reliant and autonomous.

These traits answer Anthony's fourth research question: Yes, the immunity (invulnerability) is paid for in the coin of fixed detachment. However, while Jim, when most depressed, could be insensitive and self-absorbed, he did not manifest these traits with the fixed regularity characteristic of his detachment.

The ego ideal's formation makes important contributions to the above-described character traits, as is demonstrated by this analysis of Jim and related analyses. Specifically, there is consistent evidence of fixed and extreme ego ideal formations. In Jim's case, the creation of fantasy heroes on his own, or the incorporation of radio broadcast figures, furthered his development of ego skills and such integration as he was able to achieve. Such fantasies, while aiding his development, also helped fill his many lonely hours. For example, Jim recalled in the early and middle phases of analysis his use of a fantasy hero detective, beginning at age 5. His favorite heroes included Sherlock Holmes (whose stories he had read by his middle teens), the Lone Ranger, and some soap opera heroes. His heroes shared the common traits of near-perfect performance and self-denial. In school studies and in sports, Jim's habit was to work mainly alone and then imaginatively inquire of his own heroic ideals what would constitute a perfect, self-denying performance in the case at hand. Deciding this, he would proceed accordingly.

For example, it was at about age 5, 6, or 7 that Jim had gone off to a swimming hole with some boys and had been humiliated by his inability to swim. In response to this, Jim read and learned from books and successful swimmers, and then developed and carried out his own training program, becoming the town's best young swimmer. In fact, during the late opening phases of analysis, Jim responded to a vacation break and disappointment with his girlfriend by repeating a driven sports program, this time with racquetball. He responded repeatedly with originality and resourcefulness to lift himself out of predicaments into new worlds of functioning.

In sum, at age 6, Jim had developed an early childhood prototype pattern of ego ideal formation and character traits with which he adapted to severe trauma, and to his related terrors and fantasies of the terrifying, phallic "witch woman." His childhood pattern formed the basis for his adulthood pattern for dealing with such traumatic personal life disruptions. Central to Jim's adaptation was the formation, by compensating identifications, of an ego ideal figure of an invulnerable superdetective. He then molded his behavior, striving to act like this hero.

Unique to these particular ego ideal formations were a certain fixedness and rigidness in holding on to, and being guided by, this ego ideal. In addition, data from later phases of Jim's psychoanalysis provide evidence from his moods and transference responses of an extremely harsh and rigid superego into which the ego ideal hero was fit.

Jim chose to enter detective work just after sustaining one of his life's numerous severe traumas. Just after he had been laid off from his job, his second child was born with a life-threatening brain tumor. Serious disease again invading his life as it had in early childhood, Jim felt intense tension and panic. After learning of the near-lethal tumor, he began, with a vengeance, his career as a detective. During his psychoanalysis, Jim repeatedly stated that in his career, he guided his most successful investigations by imagining what the perfect observing, analyzing detective would do and proceeding accordingly. Again, the ego ideal, the companion of his childhood, had developed into an important guiding vehicle for his adult productivity. His driven work approach contributed to wearing down his adaptive capacities and energy, and to keeping him increasingly lonely. There are some challenging correlations between patterns of Jim's ego ideal formation and similar patterns manifested by some detective story writers and their heroes, such as Agatha Christie's Hercule Poirot and Sir Arthur Conan Doyle's Sherlock Holmes.

Consistent with the character of Jim's ego ideal figure, Holmes, were Jim's pronounced manifestations of depression, lowered self-esteem, and anxiety seen in the early and middle phases of Jim's psychoanalysis.

Aggravating his depression, additional loss and illness invaded Jim's life in the early months of his analysis: His second ex-wife had back surgery and suffered from near-psychotic depression; his mother had bladder trouble; a friend was killed.

Early in treatment, when he was most depressed, Jim's gallows-humor quips were at their most bleak as he made such comments as "I'm the kind of guy who'd complain because he's not getting hung by a new rope." As the transference neurosis unfolded and was interpreted, and the patient's rigidity and depression significantly lifted, his humor became more imaginative and lively.

Destructive, impulsive actions were conspicuously absent from most of Jim's life. Two exceptional episodes occurred in his first treatment year. These, I think, are examples of what Terr (1981, 1983) has called "re-enactment phemonena," repetitions in action of highly traumatic childhood experiences.

The first such action occurred at the 4-month stage. While feeling depressed and lonely with the finalizing of his divorce, Jim moved in with a past girlfriend who was recovering from drug abuse associated with serious schizoaffective schizophrenic illness. My efforts of confronting and interpreting this action were met by his denial and repetitive ridicule. By midanalysis, interpretations of this action were accepted, and met with excellent analytic results.

The second episode occurred a month later, before a week's treatment break. Jim left on a 200-mile trip in a racing car. His mistress got drunk, grabbed the steering wheel, and yanked them off the road, nearly overturning the car. A police car approached and a chase ensued, during which Jim finally outraced his pursuers. Immediately afterwards, Jim called me, and we discussed the self-destructive nature of his actions and those of his mistress. Jim established some affective understanding of the connection between this car race and his unbearable levels of depression and tension.

Jim's later psychoanalytic work has much to teach us about sources of desperate actions of physical escape from harsh superego figures. Data were later obtained (and cross-checked with family members) that revealed that in the late preoedipal period, between the ages of 1½ and 2½, Jim had undergone the trauma of being confined to a small room and bed with a beloved surrogate parent—the great-aunt who was dying of bone cancer. While the recovery of memory traces for this experience and related reconstructive work were naturally not possible at the time Jim engaged in the car race re-enactment, related reconstructions were successfuly made later in the analysis.

Finally, characteristic of Jim (and many other severely traumatized patients) was his psychosomatic abdominal pain, which, like his re-enactment responses, was initially resistant to interpretive intervention. In the midphase of the analysis, with interpretation, this pain complaint was resolved entirely except for a brief, mild recurrence in the termination phase.

A dream of Jim's, described just after he first lay down on the couch, well illustrates the early mixed transference. "I was in a canyon in heavy woods, near a vet's hospital, with a nice-looking blond. We were looking for a place to make love. A woman said, 'Here.' A doctor said, 'No.' We never found a place. Frustrating!" Associating, Jim said, "I've been in a lot of hospitals looking for victims. I pass an animal hospital on a boulevard near my ex-wife's home." I later observed that Jim was working with his concerns over whether the analyst would be a restrictive or permissive figure. He partly confirmed this.

In this early phase, the combined effects of Jim's tightly obsessed traits, his traumatic developmental history, and the manifestations of his split-off expressions of warmth and rage, in addition to my own countertransference responses of feeling tightly controlled and frustrated, all led me to suspect that there would be some highly stormy and intense unfolding of later, more fully formed, maternal and paternal transference phases. It did not take long for this expectation to be fulfilled.

Opening-Phase, Second-Segment Transference Developments

A few sessions later, Jim dreamed of John Wayne dancing in a TV benefit with a flower on his head. Associating, he mentioned his feeling foolish and hurt with his dependence upon me, which did not fit with his self-image of rough masculinity. Obviously, at this point, the livelier side of his humor and imagination were beginning to emerge.

Unfortunately, a few sessions later, it was learned that a close police friend of Jim's had died of a heart attack and that his mistress had attempted suicide. Following these events, the transference was one of bleak despair, with worsening of his psychosomatic symptoms and reverting back to his more controlled style of associations. Jim's massive loss experiences elicited a countertransference experience of great fatigue akin to that encountered with concentration camp victims (DeWind, 1984). Recognizing and coping with this are crucial for successful working through.

Two months after these setbacks, Jim described a dream of running all day on an oval track. "There was a coach there who said I ran 33 miles. After the dream, I felt like I had run that far." Jim's first associations described his habit of counting steps and distances. I interpreted that he was letting go of his controlling habit of counting, and was letting the coach (i.e., me) help keep track of things; I observed that recently he had listened to my comments and dropped his mocking style. Jim responded with confirming associations. He also indicated that he felt some increased comfort and trust.

In earlier sessions, Jim often had described the following screen memory: He was an 8-year-old Cub Scout out on a hike. A rock was dislodged by careless companions, just missing Jim and injuring another hiker. The den mother on the scene was ineffectual, and Jim took charge, obtaining help for the injured boy. This screen memory had faded away and had not been brought in for many sessions. I was impressed by the shift in the transference and countertransference feelings, and by findings of Greenacre (1949) and Glover (1929) delineating a subgroup of screen memories that accurately described recent overwhelming experiences and earlier severe traumas. It seemed that important new material was about to break through.

While Jim was regularly describing variations of the screen memory, he spoke of his parents, idealizing them. Once the screen memory had faded, a grossly different picture emerged. One week after the coach dream, Jim brought in a set of dreams, the associations to which included important new memories of his stepfather, mother, and early childhood severe traumas. For the first time, Jim actively expressed resentment toward his biological father for his desertion and abusive ways. I confronted and clarified this anger, interpreting Jim's need to control both the analytic setting and me, whom he felt to be influencing the emergence of the anger.

In these five dreams, there were unique episodes of violent acts. Precisely describing such acts, Jim felt a sense of immediacy of the dream events and a strong sense of actual physical exhaustion from participating in the dream violence. In experience and that of many analysts, this sense of immediacy combined with precisely detailed description, accurately indicates that violent acts have actually been experienced by the patient. Superimposed upon and modifying the usual childhood fantasies, fusing together violence and parental sexual activity, are memories of patients' actual involvement in violent situations. Concomitantly, in such patients, one finds trends such as Jim's toward literal actions and interpretations of situations, and a sensing of pressing immediate threats.

This dream set contained two separate cycles, both containing a man doing violence to another man, and subsequently a dream of denigrating a woman. In the third dream of the set, Jim described a dream of giving a vicious beating with a belt to another man who was himself beating a small child with a belt. The physical, postural transference communications were an important part of this dream description. Jim's tense body posture was even more rigid during and just after describing the dream. For the first time in analysis, Jim talked of his stepfather's actual habit of whipping him with a belt. Jim told how every few weeks during his childhood, from ages 5 to 15, his stepfather would unpredictably fly into a rage, lock Jim in a bathroom, and whip him with a belt until he was too exhausted to continue.

Describing a lifelong pattern of physical activity involving what appeared to be re-enactment phenomena, Jim went on to tell how, during these beatings, while terrified, he learned to be hyperalert and to develop various quick moves to protect himself. He observed that the skills he developed in these episodes were a major source of his ability to triumph in a fight with a criminal, with neither party being seriously injured. Jim described how being hyperalert to the earliest sign of physical attack enabled him to control and diffuse fights.

I made a transference observation that he expected sudden attacks from me as he did from his stepfather. Jim's response included a sudden start and turning of his head toward me. He commented, "You wouldn't stand a chance." The physical reflex level of these responses, involving Jim's physical learning to cope with the literal physical engagement during the oedipal struggle with his stepfather, was thus demonstrated. This mastering of the art of successful defensive physical fighting during the oedipal and latency age served him throughout his detective career. It also appeared to have made its contribution to his characteristic detachment in his intimate life. In addition, this transference material revealed another experience from which Jim escaped into the world of his ego ideal; his companion heroes were often individuals who had successfully mastered such physical fighting.

Another part of these beating episodes that was discovered during successive months of analysis was the pre- and postbeating family experience. After the whippings, the stepfather would stagger out of the bathroom complaining of a severe headache and partial loss of sight. He would then wander out into the neighborhood, losing himself sometimes for days. Jim would find him and guide him safely back home. Jim and his mother would then nurse the stepfather back to health until the next attack. Later, it came to light how commonly, before these attacks, Jim's mother would express her displeasure with Jim, implying that the stepfather should provide him with discipline. It was only after 2 more years of work, developing the gradual lifting of amnesia and resistances, that Jim was able to connect these events with the obviously phallic, threatening "witch" of his childhood nightmares.

Repeatedly, Jim traced his own hyperresponsible dedication to attending to the details of caring for disabled criminals, colleagues, or family members to these early experiences. Also, it was repeatedly delineated how Jim expended great effort and skill to avoid the beatings and related disruptions that he had experienced in the past, and that he anticipated in his present life and in the transference. It was only with much gradual re-examination of these experiences as they presented themselves in treatment that Jim slowly was able to partly let go of his physical hyperpreparedness, and his associated fantasy of imminent physical attack coming from me.

Working through and slowly reconstructing the pre-, during-, and postbeating scenes, Jim gradually experienced the resulting humiliation, rage, and hurt. He was then able to recognize the self-destructive, driven, caretaking efforts involved in some hopeless episodes in his current family life, and gradually to disentangle himself from these. For instance, in the transference setting, he would introduce such observations as noting a drop of oil under my car, thus bringing up his meticulous skills used in caring for his stepfather. Repeating such transference experiences over many months, Jim underwent a gradual affective shift from his state of highly anxious alertness to a state of severe depression with some continued alertness.

As I have already noted, Jim's traits of sharp observation, quick and thoughtful action, meticulous caring, preference for working alone, and periodic bouts of depression bring to mind the enduring, popular fictional detectives, such as Poirot and Holmes. In my work, evaluating and doing therapy with police detectives, I have found a good correlation between the degree to which these four character traits are present and the degree of success at work. It seems to me that particularly in the area of dedication to systematic, close observation, there is something of a tradition passed back and forth between some fictional figures and some leading actual detectives. Indications of this have come from statements by the first modern detective, Eugene Vidocq; Edgar Allan Poe; Holmes's creator, Doyle; the director of the Lyon, France, police force; and the Washington (State) police chief, who, after helping break the Hillside Strangler case, reported that he was a dedicated student of Holmes and a member of a local Sherlock Holmes society. Kenneth Millar, creator (under the pseudonym of Ross Macdonald) of Lew Archer and Harper, has made similar reflections on cross-influences between fictional and working detectives (Millar, personal communication).

The beating dream brought up so many issues of long-standing periodic, major traumas, with mastery of these, and subsequent reenactment fighting behaviors (and their career significance), that I have jumped ahead in the story of Jim's analysis. Let us now back up to the rest of the unique dream series.

The next dream in the series was a fragment about which Jim stated that the dreaming of it was an exhausting experience. He said, "I had a hell of a dream last night. I can't remember much of it. It was a nightmare about my stepdad. It was about something I could have prevented. Something I could have done to stop him from dying, that I didn't do." Jim's first associations were about going to visit his stepsister the following day. He next thought of his mother, whom he had been visiting more often. He spoke of how his mother, grandmother, sister, and in fact all his family members had dark hair and angular features. This brought, both to his mind and mine, the nightmare of the "witch." Jim went on to express his own painful sense of being a lonely outsider in the family, since he was the only one with blond hair and lighter features.

The final dream in the series was a brief one of the patient's recently divorced wife "taking silencers" (putting a gun with a silencer into her mouth). Jim associated this with grisly police scenes of suicides, and interpretation was made of his experiencing my recent comments as those of a nagging mother, which infuriated him. His responses in this and subsequent sessions confirmed this observation.

After the analysis entered into this phase of dreams, associations, and interpretations, there were notable, overall treatment shifts. As indicated, there was a marked reduction in Jim's distant mocking responses to interpretations, with a shift toward initiating interpretive work of his own. His stiff posture on the couch very slowly relaxed, and even more slowly, his rigid punctuality varied somewhat.

Late-Opening to Midphase Transference Phenomena

Three months later, Jim's dependency feelings were more fully and directly explored, using the following dream report and interpretive work: "I dreamed there were three people, two men and a woman, who wanted to drain blood out of my stepdad, who was in this hospital bed. They wanted to take his body and drain blood with a machine. I kept the people in the closet." Associating, Jim spoke first of his days by his dying stepfather's bed more than 2 years ago. He had thought his stepfather wanted to ask him for an overdose of medication to relieve his misery, although he never asked. I noted the closeting of the threatening characters, indicating extra-powerful feelings with which he was struggling. Following this observation, Jim said, "It would be a relief to quit fighting and let someone take over and completely care for me. I'm afraid I'd never make it back again if I did that." This first expression of Jim's profound dependency wishes and fears was accompanied by his first statement of resentment toward his mother, as he recalled being left alone for days in his sickroom during his late oedipal and latency years.

In the next session, Jim described a hallucination, or vivid memory, of the smell of burning human flesh. He next spoke of how, as a detective, he was under constant pressure to make right decisions. He was also aware that he generated the bulk of the pressure himself by pushing for perfect decisions. He commented that the only negative work report ever made on him was one about his being seen with a mistress. Following these comments, I observed that he could be wondering what I might have in the way of negative notes about him in my notebook. Jim responded immediately with one of his old black-humor comments, confirming my observation.

In the same session, for the first time, Jim mentioned three episodes of severe abuse and neglect suffered at the hands of his mother, the first before he was 2 years of age. He had received electric shocks when he had been allowed to wander unsupervised into dangerous areas. These experiences were later confirmed by family members. At this point, there emerged from behind the screen memory of the woman and small boy hurt by the arguing father, new memories of the mother attacking her son. He told of how she would goad the step-father into conducting the belt beatings. In addition, his mother had obtained a successful business from her first husband, leaving him in a bad way. Clever property management had made her considerable money while she persisted in keeping her family living at poverty level, sometimes literally eating table scraps.

As this picture of his mother unfolded, Jim experienced monumental levels of depression and resentment. Working through these insights, Jim began to see that his leaving home for work duty had been his shield against depression. I noted that Jim had unraveled community crimes with success but very little satisfaction; now he was unraveling family crimes committed against him and in so doing, he was experiencing satisfaction and relief along with his depression. During more than a year of this treatment work, analytic reconstructions were commonly made, restating the actuality of Jim's mother's consistent neglect, abuse, and manipulation. Jim slowly and hesitatingly connected his angry, resentful affect with his mother, and with me in the transference setting, in more full and effective ways. As this work went on, a clearer sense was obtained of the interaction between the patient's fantasy of the phallic "witch" and his repeated experiences with his mother's mean actions, which served to intensify and fix the fantasy/nightmare of the threatening witch.

Midphase Psychoanalytic Transference Interpretations, Documenting Preoedipal Presence and Development of Invulnerable's Drive to Master High Risk

Continuing the maternal (though now mixed) transference stage, Jim extended and deepened his contact with his great fears and desires involving dependency upon a maternal figure. Talking with his mother, he learned for the first time that it had been his great-aunt who had provided most mothering functions in the first 2½ years of his life. In the family circle, this aunt had had some renown for her child care skills, such as knowing what a baby needed before it cried. Relatives found that children thrived under her care. She also taught Jim how to read before he was 3.

This great-aunt/surrogate mother, as noted earlier, had died of bone cancer when he was 2½. Jim further learned from his mother that while his aunt was bedridden, Jim, sick himself, would curl up in bed next to her as they read stories to each other. This information helped to make sense out of the compelling power contained in Jim's stories, fantasies, and obsessions dealing with death.

Over 3 weeks of treatment, Jim reported another series of nightmares, the first of which involved a baby with a tube draining black fluid out of its chest and rectum, and the last of which involved a woman with a garbage-disposal vagina. Prominent among his associations were feelings of dread, as he thought how every person in his life who gave him things ended up dying.

Responding, I introduced the interpretation that was to be confirmed and extended often in the analysis. I said that with the development of intimacy and related feelings, Jim feared the destruction of his partner and himself. He responded without hesitation, saying, "Yes, I've watched people I've been close to deteriorate much of my life. That was also my job." During a several-month period, when interpretation often returned to this theme of the annihilating force of intimacy, Jim experienced a severe depression. He also slowly became more involved with his children and more socialized than ever before, developing a successful, intimate life with an able woman whose caring he could accept (and continue accepting after the termination of psychoanalysis 3½ years later).

This interpretation and Jim's responses introduce the first of two related conflicts on which the midphase of analysis focused during the third and fourth treatment years. Jim sought, with tremendous motivation, the reliable intimacy of the treatment relationship. At the same time, he was terribly afraid of the sought-after intimacy. He demonstrated the strength of his motivation by driving over 100 miles each way to his treatment during a temporary move in the third year of analysis. His coexisting terror of the intimacy has been described above and will be seen more later.

The next conflict focused on Jim's struggle to tightly control his feelings and actions, as earlier described. He had felt that such control was vital to his survival. With this case's two major sets of nightmares and related expression of feelings and interpretive work, we now have a fuller sense of the feelings, memories, and fantasies that Jim struggled to keep controlled and was now able to release.

The treatment history of Jim's conflict over intimacy was one of dramatic change and improvement. As noted earlier, when my first vacation came up, Jim's re-enactment and/or acting-out response was manifested in the sports car chase. After a year of analysis, at a similar treatment break, Jim experienced abdominal cramping, which was then only in part connected with disrupted contact with the analyst. More than 2 years into analysis, when Jim's capacity to articulate a range of feelings had grown, another treatment disruption occurred. At this time, Jim reported a dream of a lonely poor boy at a market; he then cried intensely while expressing his own painful sense of aloneness and disturbing strong need for contact with me, and his associated affectionate feelings for me.

SURVIVING GREAT RISK IN FIRST YEAR OF LIFE

In the following session, Jim described the dream of the baby with the tubes draining its black secretions. Two sessions later, Jim mentioned the dream again, emphasizing that it had occurred during the holiday season, when he was feeling intense sadness. He reworked the theme that those to whom he was close would up being destroyed by disease or bullets, or disappearing. I interpreted that he was again fearing that, with our closeness, I would be destroyed. Jim responded by indicating that in his early childhood, he had repeatedly asked to have the fairy tale "The Little Match Girl" told to him. At this point, Jim brought in the new information that during his second year of life, he had experienced starvation, freezing, and multiple infections. He observed, "My mother told me she tried to breast-feed me and I couldn't get any milk from her. I was starving nearly to death for 2 weeks. She told me I had a tube in my mouth when I was a year and a half old. I had bronchial pneumonia and tubes to drain my lungs shortly after that. That screwed up my lungs for a long time afterwards."

An uncle later confirmed that there was great poverty and deprivation in Jim's first year, further indicating that these risks had been mastered by the baby Jim. Here is evidence that genetic factors generating a resilient physiology with high tolerance for cold and infection contributed to Jim's invulnerability, and to his related drive and capacity to master high risk. For a while, molding and aiding in the development of Jim's verbal and imaginative capacities was the surrogate mothering of the great-aunt. This is evidence for the contribution of the preoedipal great-aunt experiences to the underpinnings of Jim's ego ideal development. The great-aunt encouraged the development of his existing imaginative capacity to make constructive use of ego ideal figures. When she died, the event further honed Jim's fantasy and pattern of dreaded expectation that his intimate contact destroyed loved ones.

The following treatment week, Jim described a nightmare of two black worms oozing out of his penis. Associating, he first said, "That's the scariest dream I've even had. That really upset me. I felt sick and rotten inside during that dream. It was like dying or rotting away. It was a hopeless feeling. Nothing I could do about it. I have felt that way since the dream." Jim went on to discuss his caring for his sick step-father, and noted that he had been close to decaying bodies of parents a lot. In a subsequent session he spoke of his great-aunt, who was a very strict teacher, and associated the worms to whips.

A week later, Jim brought in the nightmare of a woman with a garbage-disposal vagina, which he described as follows: "She was lying on the bed and her vagina looked like a garbage disposal. There was spaghetti and junk coming out of it and it had a metal ring around it." His first association was to the repulsiveness he felt with the dream. I interpreted that he felt and thought about the vagina as a damaging place, to which he quickly responded, "Yes, I have thought that. It has not been productive for me. It has produced children and cost me a fortune. I still have a lot of women relying on me and I resent it." I interpreted that Jim was relying on me and was acutely aware of this, to which he gave this graphic confirmation: "Yes, before this I never relied on anybody. Yes, now I notice I'm attached to you, and it's a hopeless feeling."

Toward the end of the third year of analysis, my summer vacation was announced in advance to Jim. Ten days later, he dreamed of fixing two race cars, a line of work he had since stopped. At first, he focused on his many constructive activities with his two boys. After minimizing his feelings concerning the disruption, Jim expressed thoughts of leaving first. However, this time he called and rearranged one session so he could help his son get his driver's license. He went on to speak directly, although with reluctance, of his wishes for help and sadness with the disruption.

NEW MEANING FOR A FAMOUS OLD RAYMOND CHANDLER PHRASE:
"DOWN THESE MEAN STREETS A MAN MUST GO"

The progress of Jim's struggle to control his feelings stirred up by the intimacy of treatment and its disruption could be summed up by the roles he assigned to race cars. Early in his analysis, besieged by deaths in his family and feelings only recently discussed in an intimate situation, Jim literally risked death in a race car. A year later, struggling to find his way in stormy relationships, he was rebuilding race cars. Later, at a point of desolation, he in fact dreamed of a race car from which the smell of death could not be removed. At the end of his third year of analysis, he openly discussed his need to get away from his soon-to-be-disrupted treatment. At this time, he had given up contact with race cars. His dream of the cars carried with it thoughts of his increasingly close contact with his sons, from whom he had previously been alien-ated.

This detective had worked a beat of California streets and cars throughout his career. This California beat formed the backdrop for the emergence of Sam Spade and heroes like him, who were to add the "tough guy" trademark to the previously more genteel English detective stories. Spade, Philip Marlowe, and Lew Archer tracked down their fictional criminals on California streets. As Marlowe's creator Raymond Chandler put it, "Down these mean streets a man must go" (Chandler, 1944). While Chandler's essay addresses other matters, that particular phrase beautifully captures Jim's driven crime search.

We can use the phrase differently, speaking of character traits, fantasy structure, and psychoanalytic work with patterns of a true invulnerable's personality. Passing down the "mean streets" of ruthless exposure of life-threatening risks, Jim developed the driven pattern of visualizing mastery over high-risk situations and honing it through practice. Concomitantly, his repeated experiences with the death and deterioration of loved ones created a uniquely intense and fixed fantasy modification of the usual oedipal and preoedipal fantasies. This is a pattern I have seen in other analysands exposed to sustained close experiences with untimely deaths of loved ones. Grimly, our current society can barely bring itself to address the physical needs of the impoverished; by and large, it totally ignores the emotional torture inflicted upon those with multiple losses encountered in severely deprived environments.

Later, in Jim's fourth treatment year, marked shifts in his defensive structure became evident when I announced another upcoming vacation. Responding with his characteristic, terse precision, Jim said, "I feel depressed. It creates an inner void. My mind just doesn't feel as active." After the vacation break, Jim described a dream of a stickup occurring in a store he owned. He dreamed he was shot in the right side. Associating, he was reminded of his hurt feelings at the disruption of analysis when I was not at his usual place, his right side.

As Jim more precisely identified his feelings toward me and better understood the associated conflicts, he was also making major changes in his object relationships. In the third and fourth years of analysis, as earlier noted, Jim met and moved in with a new woman, Alice. In contrast to his former partners, Alice was highly capable both financially and socially. She was a first-rate sculptress, amateur actress, and businesswoman. They were a mutually caring and thoughtful couple. She was sexually vigorous and regularly orgasmic. In this new relationship, a gradual shift occurred in Jim's sexual functioning. He slowly dropped his emphasis on wearing out his lover. His preferences for intercourse and for cunnilingus and fellatio during foreplay were not remarkable or troublesome and did not change during the course of analysis. As Jim became more involved with Alice, he spoke of their lovemaking episodes as lasting for an hour or less, rather than being bouts to exhaust the woman, as had previously been the case.

Noting this shift in the pattern of Jim's sexual functioning and the analytic lifting of his amnesia for severely traumatic relationships, I had some evidence that his need to sexually exhaust women was a symbolic equivalent of keeping the destructive phallic "witch" of his nightmares at bay. However, Jim's sexual functioning was so gratifying to both partners, and his most pressing conflicts were in the areas of aggression and intimacy, there was not sufficient treatment exploration of this earlier need to exhaust women. At any rate, with this sexual pattern as with Jim's patterns of conducting many of the basic functions in his life, there was evidence of Jim's achieving mastery over what were initially highly risky situations and then proceeding to apply his mastery overvigorously and overrigidly. This approach would help him achieve such goals as exhausting a woman, winning a contest, and the like, but it would also keep him at a detached distance from his partner.

CURRENT LIFE EFFECTS OF LOOSENING PREVIOUSLY RIGID TRAITS OF INVULNERABILITY

Not surprisingly, in view of his background and early treatment transference experiences, Jim had a rough struggle toward establishing intimate involvement with his new, positive girlfriend, Alice. Jim realistically acknowledged Alice's assets of a caring personality, sexual responsiveness, and working capacities. Jim did, however, have a pattern of periodically criticizing Alice for allegedly showing an authoritarian streak by asking him to help with the housework. He proceeded to talk of this as an excuse for breaking up with her.

When I interpreted his pattern with Alice as acting toward her as though she were his disappointing and exploitive mother, Jim dropped his plan of action and dealt with his depressed and angry feelings relating to his mother and me. While struggling with his involvement with Alice, Jim continued, with less conflict, to deepen his highly productive relationship with his sons. Their recent life together had now continued for 2 years, and Jim expressed much pride and satisfaction at his sons' personality development and academic and work productivity.

Termination Phase of Analysis, Emphasizing Alterations in Main Traits of Invulnerability

Due to Jim's impressive background of losses, disruptions, and abusive violence, termination of his case seemed a particularly challenging and sensitive issue. While with any case I would avoid unilateral suggestion of termination, with Jim it seemed particularly challenging to master transference and countertransference and to scrupulously avoid being drawn into any comments or responses that would even remotely imply that I would set a termination date. When Jim began treatment, he had, by his prominent traits of overwork, hypercritical comments, and rigid withdrawal, greatly influenced his wives and children to pull back from or completely leave him. When his second wife did leave, there was a pathological recreation of his multiple early traumas, which aggravated both his pathological character traits and anxiety symptoms described at the start of this report. This, I concentrated upon, and succeeded in, avoiding any recreation of this pattern. Jim, with his increasing flexibility of character and deepening of his independent use of insight, demonstrated an increasing readiness to enter a termination phase.

Jim first spoke of terminating analysis about 2 weeks before a preannounced week-long treatment break. This occurred 2 years prior to the actual termination of treatment. When he first brought up the subject of termination, his related ambivalence was unusually great. He began by observing that with his treatment progress, he had been noticing that he was able to directly express his depression and resentment with the disruption. Adding this development to his observed increased involvement with his children and girlfriend, he thought it might be a good time to consider ending treatment. Shortly after making these comments, Jim manifested increased tension, depression, and the recurrence of abdominal pain.

Two sessions later, he brought in a dream about watching some sexual activity and also about being watched. This dream was one indication of his analytic progress in developing a more realistic and less rigid superego. At the same time, the dream gave warning signs of Jim's continued strong inclination to use projection and hostile envy in dealing with feminine internalized objects and with his day-to-day experiences with women in his life.

This first dream after exploration of termination began with a coworker's asking Jim to help him check for a gun in a building restroom. Opening the door, Jim found a woman taking a shower. Next, he walked to the building basement and found two well-dressed secretaries and a couple of men having intercourse on the floor. The man with Jim said he would do something about this illegal activity. Jim said they were having sex and there was nothing wrong with that. After listening to Jim's associations of having sex with a coworker at a Christmas party 20 years ago, and about his long-standing trait of tolerance in dealing with people's sexual habits, I made the following interpretation: I observed that Jim's tolerance toward others' sexuality in his work had, at that time, not extended to his own sexuality; in recent months, however, he was slowly developing more tolerant views toward his own sexual thoughts and fantasies. Jim confirmed this, and also pointed out that the women on the floor were getting dirty and that this might express some of his hostile envy toward women. I interpreted that Jim could feel this envy toward me and my so-called "feminine" role of being a quiet listener. He agreed.

Illustrating Jim's heightened self-awareness of tortured feelings of depending on me, brought to the fore with talk of termination, was dream and associational material described several weeks after the session recounted above. Jim presented a dream that he and police colleagues were seeking to arrest someone. At first, the setting was a deteriorated ghetto, and then it shifted to a pleasant suburb. Toward the end of the dream, there was a scene of an angry black dog pursuing Jim. Jim's initial associations were sprinkled with his customary black humor and insightfulness as he said, "Well, I'm not bothered by a good ass-chewing. I'm at the point where I do feel some hate toward my mother for her miserly stunts." I made a preliminary interpretation that he felt plenty of anger toward me for, among other things, my crime of letting this termination talk continue. Jim commented that he thought there might be something to that. He then insightfully observed that every couple of years, in analysis, he had had dreams of searching out criminals. He associated this theme with being in an unpleasant place and feeling some fatigue and depression with such an experience. He went on to talk about his increased involvement with, and dependent upon, his girlfriend, sons, and particularly me. He observed that his dependence on me seemed like needing a heroin fix, and that he was "pissed off" with this. While he still had some tendency to see great anger coming from elsewhere, his frank associations documented his comfort with owning up to his anger in the transference. Although to a degree he could express some of his anger, at the same time, substantial fear of losing me also emerged in his comments.

Enlarging upon related conflictual feelings were Jim's comments after a brief treatment break occurring a few weeks after these two sessions. After this break, he promptly described his feelings about it and the related discussion of termination, saying, "In recent months, I notice I've dropped much of that tight control I used to have. With this happening, I experience depression in a way I never have before. You know, this office is the nicest place there is for me to be. I feel cared for. It will be a big change not to come here most days during the work week."

During his termination phase, Jim clearly manifested his considerable growth in being able to express his feelings of caring, loss, and anger. However, to round out the portrait, it must be said that as termination approached, Jim would have periods of a week or two when he expressed unremitting bleakness and cynicism that was not leavened by the above-described direct expression of mixed feelings. For instance, during one session, Jim made a long string of comments such as these: "As I'm older, it's harder for people to measure up. I'm dissatisfied. Everything is a bunch of shit. I feel pissed and depressed. I know most of this comes from me and the way I look at people. It's not just the way things are outside. Still, I can't stop feeling like this." Nevertheless, in the midst of repetitive statements further expressing such cynicism, he fortunately retained his capacity for intermittently guiding himself with such comments as these: "This makes me think; I'd say I'm grieving for myself. I feel left out, because I can't get strongly interested in something. That's miserable, but I'm not as isolated as I used to be."

I think that this material, in addition to the data from the midphase of analysis, documents a central dynamic shift in Jim away from taking on high-risk criminal investigations and destructively needy wives or sexual partners, toward the risk of confronting his inner world. With analysis, he increasingly mastered his threatening internalized objects and related superego structures, as well as the tension, depression, and rigid character traits related to these structures. With this new inward-directed drive for mastery, Jim's fuller experience of both depression with his losses and enjoyment of his emerging capacity for involvement continued to grow, although he naturally experienced some partial setbacks along the way. I must add that Jim's attraction for taking on some literal high risks, such as his defenses of projection and denial, never completely disappeared. However, the above-described changes attained in these traits went well beyond what I had initially thought possible. This leads me, in retrospect, to observe that the pattern of invulnerable traits in an individual is a significant, positive prognostic factor.

Timely intervention with reconstruction was an important tool in dealing with the long waves of bleakness and cynicism that emerged much more intensely in the invulnerable Jim's termination phase than in the midphase of treatment. For instance, in the above-cited phase of cynicism, as Jim focused these feelings more on his girlfriend, I intervened with the following reconstruction: During those earliest years when he was in bed with the cancer-ridden great-aunt surrogate mother, and given the evidence of their mutual intense involvement, it seemed likely that they would have embraced. This would have given Jim uniquely intense, touching contact with deterioration and related smells. Jim responded with this reconstruction by a brief episode of crying and the re-emergence of stomach pains. After this reconstructive work, his hostile, cynical criticisms of his girlfriend and distancing, controlled responses gradually diminished. It should be clarified that these characterological improvements naturally required repetitive working through with similar reconstructions and responses from the patient.

The following material illustrates the singularly painful, never-completed, long, slow working-through efforts in the termination phase of Jim's analysis. About a year into termination, after the treatment disruption of a long weekend, Jim described the following anxiety dream; with its associations and interpretations, it expressed his previously insufficiently handled rage with a maternal transference context. The dream was of climbing a mountain. (It is noteworthy that periodically in analysis, Jim dreamed of threatening mountain situations. At the start of treatment, there were sharp spikes sticking out of impossibly steep cliffs. This gradually softened to less threatening cliffs without the spikes.) This time, he dreamed of hiking and boating in the mountains with his girlfriend. They encountered bad snow and glaciers. A man in front of them with a sleeping bag proceeded to jump down a 100-foot chasm into icy water, out of which he successfully swam. Jim thought he had no chance in the world, but would freeze if he stayed where he was or freeze if he stayed in the water. The dream had him jumping into the chasm, figuring he was dead no matter what. In associating, Jim mentioned that his mother was manipulating him by praising his old, destructive mistress and indicating he would be better off without his current girlfriend. Rage at his mother's intrusive, critical comments emerged. He had been holding in his rage and feeling more depressed. He continued to speak of his anger, both at his mother and at my recent absences, which Jim saw as harsh, judgmental rejections. As he continued to work through these themes in this and subsequent sessions, Jim's outrage was impressively direct, as was the gradual lifting of his depression.

The material above partly illustrates the storminess involved in working with the profoundly intense memories, fantasies, and feelings that had been built up during the earliest years of Jim's childhood development. While this work documents some re-emergence of his earlier destructive character traits, such as distancing in close relationships, one must also note that throughout the termination of analysis, there were no episodes of Jim's old literal style of re-enactment wherein he mastered literal physical risk experiences.

To balance the picture, it should be noted that while Jim was working through the largely preoedipal material, he was also working through an increasingly effective resolution of his oedipal-level conflicts. This latter achievement was manifested by his still growing and effective involvement with his sons' social function and well-being. He expressed some competitive feelings toward his sons' sports and academic achievements; these feelings were effectively sublimated as he continued to encourage his sons' accomplishments. He was also periodically competitive toward me, challenging me on my knowledge of business and law. His effective sublimations were manifested by his continued dedication to psychoanalytic work, improving his health maintenance efforts, and increasing his social effectiveness and work development.

Further illustrating the profound intensity of Jim's conflicted feelings over a close involvement is the following treatment material, presented about 3 months after the midpoint in Jim's 2-year termination phase. He said, "I dreamed I had this big artery sticking out of my right arm, running up over the right shoulder." (He was seated on the couch; his right shoulder was closest to me.) He went on to associate, saying, "Well, I relate that to you. The artery is swollen, carrying my life blood. Take it easy. Today, I would not say treatment is life-saving, but I am real grateful for it. This treatment has been something stable in my life. You ask about my feelings with ending it; well, I feel a great curiosity. I would not say it's the old anxiety that I feel. You might say it's a lesser version of that. I'd like to live permanently with a woman in 6 months, when we end. I'm having a hell of a time getting that established. I guess one thing that gives me trouble in that area is that with an intelligent woman, I start feeling a little inferior. That makes me think of when I was a kid and I'd look at my parents. I just could not understand what was going on with my mother." I observed that as he was so much more direct in expressing his feelings and observations to the person with whom he was involved, he was more exposed and vulnerable (like a dangerously exposed artery) than he had been in the past. Apropos of psychoanalytic treatment effects upon the invulnerable's state of mind, Jim noted that he now was aware of his frailties in a way he had not been previously.

Further illustrating his growing termination-phase insightfulness concerning his struggles with attachment, dependence, and related feelings, Jim observed, "This is a unique relationship here. I give you abuse and the relationship is not written off. That's new for me. You know, for a long time, I've had the urge to keep it more like a doctor-patient relationship. But with all this contact, our imperfections come out. It's harder to be attached to someone when imperfections aren't there and acknowledged. I'm troubled by this response of mine, wherein if I feel closely attached, it's hard for me to allow that attachment to persist. I find myself pushing away and the involvement going downhill. . . . You know with my wives and the girlfriends, the easiest way for me to leave was to get thrown out. Now that I talk about it, I can recall that they did say to me that they felt set up to the point where they felt they had to leave." I interpreted that he had a very

difficult-to-control urge to do something similar with me. Jim's confirming response was as follows: "Yes, I'd rather push you into ending
this. There's a certain control if I can get you, or the women, to do that.
That repeats my power fantasy that I'm always the one heave-ho'd.
You know, I could want to be thrown out to avoid responsibilities. Yes,
this kind of thinking hurts. I'm tremendously attached, and sometimes
noticing that makes me feel I don't have balls. If I could provoke you to
set the ending of this, and then if something went wrong, I could blame
you. Yeah, now that we mention this stuff, I can see I do it in lots of
situations. I would rather not do it this time." Another manifestation of
his old invulnerable's unique struggle with attachment was Jim's shift
at this point into making brief, adolescent dating contacts with young
women. I interpreted this by noting that he seemed to be avoiding a
threat to our relationship, which could be posed by his being fully
involved with his girlfriend, Alice. Initially resentful of this confrontation, he proceeded to bring in confirming associations describing his
enormous difficulty setting a termination date. After several episodes
of shifting between his semidetached invulnerable mode and his vulnerable feelings of care and loss, Jim set a date in August, 6 months in
advance.

Termination Dream

Finally, this man who had molded his life by mastering a wide variety of
high-risk situations brought in a termination dream wherein he was
dealing with a risky, though finally successful, mountain climb. I think
both the manifest dream and the associations and interpretive work
illustrate the complex evolution of Jim's character, which, at this point,
manifested his old invulnerable's drive to mastery and periodic detachment, as well as his highly vulnerable attachments and direct expressions of caring and mixed grieving feelings.

Jim's dream was as follows: "I was going to climb a mountain with a
teacher, although I wasn't ready, lacking proper shoes and a sleeping
bag. We were climbing to survey the mountain. Being afraid of falling
and of heights, I did not want to go. We got to the top, and when
coming down, I was with a different guide or teacher. When we were
stopping to eat at places on the way down, the prices kept getting
higher. The others had special spiked shoes for climbing; I just had
tennis shoes. I was afraid I'd break my ass. Still, I did climb up the
mountain and back."

With humor and emotional responsiveness re-emerging after his
earlier waves of bleakness, Jim spontaneously went to work with the

dream, saying, "Let's analyze this one. The mountain is the end of treatment. In some ways, I do not feel equipped. I can't know everything that is coming. From my early life, I get some fears about failing. Still, I do not really fail in the dream. So while I anticipate troubles, I'll handle them even though I feel less equipped than I'd like to be. I do feel fear with termination coming, and I sometimes feel very sad. I also come up with some frustration and anger. Keeping busy with activities and friends will help me to handle it. Sleeping with Alice sure helps a lot." I asked him to associate to special shoes, and Jim first stated that German helmets and violent things came to mind. He next spoke of sex and frequent intercourse, and his associated pride in penile function.

I think that Jim's work with this dream documents his capacity for full engagement in the termination phase, and his relatively balanced observing ego in dealing with his girlfriend and me. I should note that, unlike patients with other character disorders, Jim was inclined to overemphasize his inherent aggressiveness, lust, and oedipal fantasies as being little or not at all molded by his early losses and deprivations. I think that with Jim and some other invulnerable characters, there is as much analytic danger in hurrying toward reconstructions that overemphasize inherent drives and fantasies as there is in hurrying toward reconstructions that overemphasize actual experiences with loss, mental illness, neglet, and/or abuse.

In the few remaining weeks of analysis after this termination dream work, Jim was able to maintain the fairly well-integrated, observing ego functions indicated above. Still, his cynicism could, and did, periodically re-emerge with its associated draining and provocative qualities. The intensity and duration of these cynical phases were impressively reduced, however, compared to earliest treatment levels.

Two Related Cases Illustrating Variations in the Development of the Drive to Master High Risk Repeatedly

The two patients to be described next are currently in treatment with me. These two men share an inner conviction that they are the invulnerable ones and will not be killed in fights with lethal weapons, or in race cars going over 200 miles per hour. They retain this conviction while concomitantly seeing a realistic chance of being killed. These additional cases provide the perspective of patients whose neglect and assault experiences occurred in different developmental epochs and different social settings than in the case of Jim. The first patient experienced episodes of loss and neglect in most of his childhood years after the age of 6, while growing up the son of an heiress in an affluent suburb. The second patient, while still an adolescent, faced and mastered war's worst violence and isolation in Tarawa, and in all the other bloody battles of the Pacific in World War II.

Both these patients are undergoing intensive psychodynamic psychotherapy occurring two and three times weekly, respectively. The treatments are essentially psychoanalytic, at least as Gill (personal communication) uses the term, in that the full focus is upon transference and interpretation, and upon reconstructive efforts made during these sessions.

Case of Sam

The first patient, Sam, is a 40-year-old race car driver, designer, and team leader. This case further illustrates main themes of the adult invulnerable's character and unique adaptiveness to great adversity in early life experiences.

Sam has been in psychoanalytic treatment with me over a 5-year period as of this writing. He was referred by a colleague who knew of my special interest in men of action. Sam was seeking treatment for his recent problems of discouragement and confusion over both his career and family life, as well as a combination of problems with sleep disruption, impaired concentration, and a prominent obsessive rumination about his wife's recent experience of a self-limited major illness. In the year preceding treatment, a close friend and an acquaintance committed suicide. These events were preoccupying and depressing him.

In his stormy 16-year marriage, there had been a relatively high level of sexual compatability and satisfaction of both partners. Husband and wife shared an intense interest in the racing world, and both had strong interest and pride in relative successful (albeit stormy) child-rearing accomplishments. There was commonly insufficient structure in dealing with the children, which took some toll on all family members. After the birth of the last of their three children, about 7 years before the start of treatment, there gradually developed increasing discord and distance between the partners as their family responsibilities grew at a rapid and largely unanticipated rate.

FAMILIAL BACKGROUND

Sam's familial background was in stark contrast to Jim's. At least from the oedipal stage onward, Jim was repeatedly confronted with monumental amounts of adversity. Sam grew up in an affluent suburb of a large Midwestern city, greatly influenced by the fact that his mother was heiress to a fortune. In fact, a literal representation of a prominent separation–individuation conflict in the patient has, through much of his life, been the existence of trusts in his name, which were highly controlled by terms initially set so that the money could only be used for specific expenses, such as child rearing.

Although Sam grew up with some access to wealth, his childhood was anything but protected. During his first 4 or 5 years, his mother, who had been a gifted poet and student at a leading university, manifested at least some responsiveness and satisfaction as a mother. However, when Sam was about 6 years old, and a portion of his mother's inheritance was about to be disbursed to her, his biological father developed a worsening drinking problem. Distance and tension in the marriage grew rapidly, and the parents soon divorced. While Sam was growing up, his mother remarried twice, both times to men who manifested alcoholism and/or drug abuse problems. She divorced each of them in turn. In his early treatment months, Sam was in touch to some degree with feelings of hurt, loss, and anger, which developed at the time of his parents' divorce. The next episode in almost an endless cycle of deterioration was that when Sam was 8 or 9, his mother became an alcoholic. He has memories of his grammar school and high school life wherein he would often return home to find his mother passed out with a bottle. Most pertinent to our considerations are Sam's repeated memories of developing his particular pattern of maintaining tightly controlled distance in his family and close personal relationships from that point forward. The impression emerges that with Sam, this pattern is not quite as rigidly maintained as in the cases of Jim and Alan (described below).

Continuing Sam's massive exposures to deterioration and disillusionment were the facts that both his biological father and his two stepfathers eventually died of end-stage alcoholism when Sam was in his late teens and 20s. When these experiences come up in treatment, they continue to be accompanied by most intense levels of hurt, anger, scorn, and disillusionment.

Amid the gross chaos of Sam's oedipal, latency, and teen years, with his alcoholic parents and stepparents drifting in and out, Sam did experience some consistent, responsive involvement. At about 6 years of age, his great interest and love for mechanical things emerged; when he wanted various parts to assemble bikes and other machines, his mother was encouraging and responsive. By contrast, when Sam manifested some serious learning problems in latency, he recalls his mother's response being one of rejecting, hypercritical comments. Throughout latency and early teens, Sam recalls frequently being taken to educational and clinical psychologists for considerable tests. He felt that his mother and the psychologists commented about him as though he were a freakish individual with some incurable disease. The learning difficulty he manifested was one wherein he would do quite well for a few weeks in a course, and then show a rapid deterioration to nonperformance. His reading was seriously impaired and many grades below level throughout his schooling.

Confirmation of reconstructions made in treatment has indicated that Sam had something of a paradoxical experience with development between the approximate times of the rapprochement and midlatency phases of his childhood. On the negative side, his mother, with her narcissistic preoccupations (mainly expressed in terms of intellectual attainment and financial control), had an impaired capacity for fully giving and responding to young Sam. This block in development particularly occurred when issues of Sam's verbal capacity and his preschool and early elementary school accomplishments arose. By contrast, in dealing with many of Sam's mechanical and outdoor interests, his mother was responsive, admiring, and giving; thus she facilitated and allowed Sam's further successful development beyond rapprochement and into at least a partially attained stronger sense of self, particularly when dealing with things mechanical.

At this writing, it is beginning to emerge that in the midoedipal phase, a substantial and overwhelming traumatic experience occurred involving an older sister and a car.

The obviously deficient, painful, and threatening identifications of Sam with his father seemed to have been somewhat compensated for by the following surrogate fathering experiences. Throughout his latency and early adolescence, Sam had an uncle whose preoccupation was with things mechanical and sports cars. This uncle provided periodic encouragement and interested support for Sam's bike- and car-building efforts. On a closer, day-to-day basis, beginning at age 8, Sam discovered a car repair shop in his neighborhood that was managed by two Japanese-Americans. Sam hung around this shop, admiring the exceptional care and craftsmanship they lavished upon their rebuilding of cars. These men gradually allowed him to participate more and more in the daily work. They proceeded to talk, joke, and share good times in his presence. Eventually, when he was in his midteens, they subsidized and supported his first car-building effort. This pattern of successful re-emergence from a tense, traumatic situation in childhood was repeated when, after he had made progress with his adult life analytic treatment, one of Sam's more successful adult racing ventures was backed by a Japanese consortium.

Again, the case of Sam demonstrates that in the background of the adult invulnerable, there are multiple experiences of exposure to great adversity and related severe traumas undergone at different developmental levels. Concomitantly, there are exposures to parent surrogates. Sam's mother's healthier side, manifesting the pattern of taking and mastering serious amounts of risk, was a pattern of adapting that was identified with Sam as an adult invulnerable.

PERTINENT CAREER HISTORY

Sam began his professional career with cars in his late teens, as a designer and builder of one particular class of vehicle. He gradually developed success in this area, but became increasingly frustrated and dissatisfied with the performance of those driving the cars he designed and built. As a result, he proceeded to race them himself. As time went on, he took on the challenge of three different classes of racing cars.

In his mid-20s, when Sam had just started racing one particularly fast and dangerous class of car, he was involved in a bad accident, sustaining compound spinal fractures. Graphically demonstrating the trend of the adult invulnerable's character (constantly seeking to master risk), Sam, against much advice, took on racing another top-speed car class after recovering from the accident. At the same time, he thoroughly studied car qualities needed to maximize safety and performance. Sharply distinguishing the adult invulnerable's personality from that of the grandiose daredevil is Sam's capacity to take great pains with racing details. For instance, in the week before any race, Sam will mentally drive through the course hundreds of times, reconsidering the techniques and equipment necessary for various track situations.

Sam has demonstrated, in sessions over the years, a thorough knowledge of cars and tracks, enabling him to maximize safety and minimize risk. He has a profound love and interest in the workings of cars in general and of racing cars in particular. This is associated with his highly informed familiarity with the equipment.

Finally, further illuminating one unique aspect of the adult invulnerable's mental state are the following data. Prior to treatment, and in the opening phase of analysis, Sam had the conviction that he would not be killed or seriously injured while racing at speeds of over 200 miles an hour. During the third to fifth treatment year, he had this conviction before and during races, but it wavered between races. Later in treatment, he also expressed fear of injury as he considered giving up driving for design and management work.

Prior to his treatment, Sam had no familiarity or contact with, or bias toward, psychoanalysis. In several sessions, he has spontaneously described an unusual level of consciousness involving his reacting and making decisions while driving at a preconscious or unconscious level. In order to drive most effectively, Sam has said he needs to be in a trance-like state, during which he attains an alert level of relaxation. Specifically, he has emphasized that it is quite important that his responses in driving unfold without conscious thinking, and that he react to situations while in his favored trance-like state.

Case of Alan

The second patient, Alan, is a 61-year-old man who manifested exceptional hunting skills and had much success during 5 years as a Marine in combat, 20 years on high-risk police assignments, and, finally, 20 years as a director of security for a large corporation. He is a once-married father of two children.

Alan presented for evaluation and treatment problems of headaches, dizziness, disruption of sleep by highly specific nightmares, and worsening social withdrawal. He had previously had a wide range of medical consultations, including a prior psychiatric evaluation. These doctors could not locate abnormalities upon physical examination and laboratory studies, and they were unable to assist him with the same presenting symptoms. He particularly wanted help with his nightmares.

Early in life, his mentors had taught Alan that personal distress could be alleviated by trying to understand one's dreams. This, like many invaluable lessons, he had learned while growing up among Cherokee, Seminole, and white Southern rural traditions of teaching, through vivid story telling, the arts and sciences of living off the land.

ALAN'S UNIQUE CHIEF COMPLAINT OF A SPECIFIC
RE-EMERGING NIGHTMARE

Talking about his nightmare, Alan said, "I was a Marine in the battles to take the South Pacific islands from the Japanese." (Alan had lied about his age and joined the Marine Corps at age 16, before the outbreak of World War II. Subsequently, at age 17, he had fought in the bloodiest battles of the Pacific.) "This nightmare has bothered me periodically since the fight for the island of Tarawa. It started up again just 2 weeks ago and disturbed me a lot. It goes like this: 'We had a hard time getting ashore on Tarawa. [This landing was one of the bloodiest ever made by U.S. Marines.] We lost a lot of good men. I was platoon sergeant. We finally got ashore. After landing, there were 12 men remaining out of our original 48. We finally found the command post on the southeast end of the island. Two or three more of our group were killed. We tunneled underground to get to Japanese soldiers and a wounded admiral. I got to the admiral first. I wanted his sword, hara-kiri knife, and flag. I got them and took them off myself.' You know, with this dream, I get a vivid sense that I'm right there and all this is happening just the way it was in the battle."

In later sessions, he returned to this nightmare and related battle experiences, giving descriptions of the role of his attitude of invulnerability in his battle experiences. He made these statements: "When we landed on the Tarawa beaches, it was wall-to-wall people, both dead and living. The first night, we slept behind piled-up bodies for shelter. Talking about that now, it feels like a dream. You learn to black it out. That kind of thing almost got to me. You get to thinking, was it worth it, and who was to blame? Could I have done something? I just have the sure sense that my believing that I would survive and come home helped me get through a lot of that."

Alan's demeanor and tone, when first describing this dream, conveyed quiet intensity in a controlled effort to fully report his nightmare and experience. Next emerged a tone of caring and then some wavering in his voice as he said he had not described this dream or related war experiences and feelings to anyone. Alan's commonly understated expression of feeling, if contrasted with Jim's, demonstrates the great variations in the degree of the invulnerable's central trait of detachment.

Unforgettable was the experience a few weeks after the Tarawa nightmare report, when Alan, after speaking of his recent career loss, returned to talk of his young Marine buddies who died on Tarawa. He paused, and his eyes filled with tears as he said, "Many good men died that day"—there was an eloquent silence and a struggle for words—"I sometimes wonder why." It is hard to describe Alan's expression of quiet courage and discovery as he ventured into this feeling of loss he had so long kept to himself. Alan's many years of not sharing his mixed feelings of loss clearly indicate some detachment. Nevertheless, unlike Jim, Alan expressed, tolerated, and grasped the appropriateness of his hurt, anger, and sadness with his losses after just a few weeks of treatment.

These and related clinical observations indicate to me that the great variations in detachment shown by invulnerables, such as the differences between Alan and Jim, correlate with what are probably varied degrees of splitting. For example, Alan's memory of the horror of sleeping behind stacked Marine bodies on Tarawa was brought up with related feelings reported as deeply split off, unreal, and dream-like. By contrast, his memory of lost buddies was brought up with related grieving feelings of sadness and anger, only very slightly split apart. What little splitting operated here was at a surface, preconscious level. Conscious control of feelings seemed to contribute as much or more to Alan's detachment here. By contrast, Jim's sadness and anger related to loss and divergent personality segments were deeply split off and unexpressed for 3 years of psychoanalysis. In Jim's first 2 treatment years, strong feeling in the transference was rigidly denied, giving the impression of the existence of more primitive, deeply split-off feelings and personality segments.

Alan's unique detachment is, in some ways, best articulated by his own reflective comments. He noted, "I'm a very private person. I've told you things about the war and myself that I've not told my wife, children, or anyone. This talk is helping me." He went on to say, "You know, one thing I think's going on with those dreams is that I lost a couple of friends over there in the Pacific." (Battle histories document that Alan was in the 6th Regiment of the bloody 2nd Marine Division described in Leon Uris's famous novel, Battle Cry. Most of the original members were killed or seriously wounded in the war. Only a handful survive today. Out of the 242 men in his platoon who landed on Tarawa, only 42 survived. Alan was in charge of the survivors.) "You know, it's been my later-life salvation that I've not let myself get too close to males because I lost such friends. When I'm socializing, I prefer talking to women. Now, how is it I'm saying so much to you? Oh, well, it does seem to help."

As impressive as Alan's battle experiences and conflicts has been his capacity for effective insight. He has been able to acknowledge and work with interpretations of his furious and aggressive feelings and thoughts toward hostile new company management; his controlled fury (temper) in World War II battles; and, to a lesser extent, his irritation with his wife and her relatives at their more disruptive moments. Unlike Jim, Alan has acknowledged and dealt with anger in the transference from the start of treatment. Here, it is relevant to note that, because he has only been in treatment for 2 years at this writing, the data concerning Alan's traumas and related conflicts during the first 6 years of his life are more limited than in the case of Jim. Nevertheless, there are still important data on Alan that serve to document and extend some main themes of Jim's case.

Graphically addressing the crucial issue of the invulnerable's detachment in interpersonal relationships, Alan described his own such trait thus: "You could say I've been a loner all my life. While I got along well in school with socializing and sports, still I had a temper. I guess that helped make for a certain distance. It was we loners that survived the battles. I learned not to get close to anybody. When we were fighting on Bloody Ridge, I had to take from our group of Marines a couple of guys to go on patrols. I knew we'd do best on the patrols when I picked loners, like myself, and those were the ones I picked." Alan further said, "We were the unit called Huxley's Harlots, the one in Battle Cry. I was runner for the old man. On Saipan, the old man was killed when I was just 5 feet away. That was the first Japanese use of rockets. I was scared. We lost Golding and Peter Lake there." When asked about his feelings during and after these battle experiences, Alan responded, "That drove home the Marine training to not get close to anybody." Most eloquent at this point were the slight waver in his voice and then his silence as he recalled the lost leader/surrogate father.

IMMEDIATE CONTEXT OF LIFE EXPERIENCES

Having presented some essentials of Alan's life, his related invulnerable mental state, and some of his mastery of high risk, I now turn to the data of his main objects and some dynamic themes involved in his family background, which his associations partly revealed.

First, let us consider the context of his life experiences occurring in the months just before the re-emergence of this nightmare. About 2 years before the nightmare, Alan had two major encounters with loss and disruption. His father, with whom he had retained strong feeling and closeness throughout his life, had suffered a stroke and was generally deteriorating. His company, which had earlier undergone a hostile takeover, now had directors who were radically disagreeing with Alan's policies and practices and were moving to undercut his position in any way possible. This corporate war had very much preoccupied him and was an important matter he wished to discuss in his upcoming initial consultation with me. Prior to the consultation, he had dealt with this massive career disruption by using stoic denial. Considering his intuitive intelligence, he would have anticipated being confronted with this denial during his initial psychoanalytic consultations.

While his marriage had a high degree of stability and emotional and sexual compatibility, his wife nevertheless periodically manifested an overzealous dedication to various relatives (who were nuns) and their religious orders that sometimes interfered with their marital life, even though Alan addressed this issue with denial. They also disagreed over which part of the country in which to retire.

It was actually with first associations to his Tarawa nightmare that Alan revealed important clues to the complex, dynamic web of his relationship with his mother and siblings, the correlated world of his struggle with internal objects, and his intense conflicted feelings (at this stage, especially intense aggressive feelings).

With Alan's presenting nightmare, he provided these intial associations: "The saber, hara-kiri knife, and flags were returned to me by the Navy after the war, and I sent them home. When I got home, I could not find the stuff; that was in the early 1950s and just before. My mother had those war mementos and would not release them. Just 3 months ago, my brothers and sisters and I were together at the family reunion. My older brother presented me with the box that contained the flags and knives. I was flabbergasted. I did not understand. He was a colonel in the Air Force and has all his mementos. Well, anyhow, I was very happy to get my things back."

Alan went on to describe a unique aspect of his nightmare, as follows: "At first, I'd keep the box with the knife and saber under my bed. With this last nightmare, I awoke from the dream (grabbing the sword.) I had to move the box out from under the bed and put it in the closet." Describing his feelings during and after the dream, Alan said, "I wake up from that one all tense and sweaty. Once I'm awake, it's a sense of relief to get away from it."

First, Alan's physical move toward the sword was another example of a critical re-enactment phenomenon, very similar to Jim's graphic, literal beating nightmare and associations to the stepfather beating him, which he connected to his successful pattern of defensive fighting. Alan's deeply ingrained reflexes of hunting and successful use of weapons had been pushed to their most terrible limits when he succeeded in surviving the Tarawa assaults, as few men had. Given the horrors of Tarawa as described by Alan, official war histories, and Battle Cry, the wonder in this case is that Alan did not have more frequent and more disabling nightmares.

Some obvious dynamic developmental themes of anger with control, and anger at invasion by the mother and siblings during crucial steps of individuation, seem pointed to by the material. However, in such cases of unique massive trauma, one must be alert for devastating environmental experiences encountered by the patient and family. Such experiences tend to be as deeply repressed and as hard to face as childhood fantasies and conflicts. For instance, a few weeks after the nightmare and more associations, Tarawa came up again. At this time, Alan reported the devastation inflicted on his mother and family when, in the disastrous chaos of the battles, with thousands of marchers killed and thousands more wounded, a traded and misplaced dog tag and the frenzy of battle carnage led officers to tell his family that Alan had been killed on Tarawa. This experience seemed to significantly mold the family's control and suppression of reminders of Tarawa. At the same time, Alan's mother had been a controlling matriarch who probably had earlier elicited her son's repressed urge toward angry rebellion.

ALAN'S FAMILIAL BACKGROUND WITH ITS MASTERED ADVERSITIES

Although early treatment repressions probably still block the most painful early memories in Alan's case, consistently cross-checked family information and transference data, as well as the patient's history of mood and characterological function, indicate that there were not as

many or prolonged severe early childhood traumas in Alan's development as there were in Jim's. Concomitantly, Alan and his siblings all
have impressive histories of successful marriages (lasting more than 20
years), successful child rearing, and outstanding career accomplishments. The first-year transference phenomena of the two cases can be
compared as follows: Alan articulated feelings of a need for, and posses-
sion of, my image, which he has maintained during vacation breaks; Jim
was unable to accomplish these tasks until he had had more than 3
years of analysis. Hence, while I expect further details and effects
involved with Alan's early childhood traumas to emerge with further
treatment, I hypothesize that these will be substantially less in degree
than those of Jim.

Alan was the third son in a family where the three oldest siblings
were brothers and the three youngest were sisters. Giving him a
modified sort of only-child experience were the facts that when he was
growing up, his older brothers were away in the Air Force, and his
sisters were between 4 and 8 years his junior. The aforementioned
setting of Alan's childhood experiences has the feel of that portrayed in
Marjorie Kinnan Rawlings's novel *The Yearling*.

The following summarizes the clinically pertinent disruptions in
hard, though adaptive, rural life. The family lived in farm country
where considerable hard work and hunting were required simply to
survive. Alan recalls that he walked a long way to school, and in the
winter, this had to be done in freezing weather with minimal protection. Starting in latency years and continuing thereafter, hard farm
work was required in the early morning hours, and again after school
for 4 to 6 hours, as well as on weekends. There was a period of family
change during Alan's latency years, when his two older brothers moved
away from home to become full-time Air Force pilots. Work demands
were increased as the family suffered financial setbacks with the Depression. At about this time, his younger sisters were born. Added to
these experiences were occasional beating episodes, the loss of a unique
and beloved coon dog, and the father's twice-yearly absences when he
left the farm to work in the saw mills.

As the first 9 months of Alan's treatment progressed, along with
the partial symptomatic relief and widening self-awareness, there occurred an extensive series of traumatic memories. These memories
were of his humiliating experiences when he was removed from his
corporate post, and a long list of exceptional battle experiences encountered during the Pacific campaign.

Many details of the patient's childhood memories document impressive examples of how childhood learning experiences and identifications specifically contributed to the patient's remarkably successful
wartime and peacetime mastery of extreme risk situations. Elucidation

of this material in more detail than has been given in my introductory statements regarding Alan's childhood cultural setting is beyond this chapter's scope and will require a separate complete report.

A final example illustrates therapeutic work with Alan's Tarawa nightmare and related dynamic issues. At the 8-month point in treatment, after a week's break, Alan returned to war scenes, saying, "On Tarawa, after we rested and regrouped among the bodies and shell holes, on the third day, I still had the sense it was not my time to go. I spotted a Japanese flag 100 yards in front of our lines. I stripped to my shorts, tied down my helmet, and with a tommy gun and knife, ran to the flagpole and got it down. I was good at hitting the ground. The old man was pissed at me when I got back, but I did get back." I made the transference observation that with the break in treatment, he could have had painful feelings like those he had had when amidst the bodies. He made the connection that he did feel lost and upset about the missed sessions. This material provides an instructive example of the coexistence of Alan's personality trait of invulnerability with his need to maintain distance in interpersonal relationships; at the same time, unlike Jim's, Alan's defensive distance was (and is) notably less marked, and he has had access to feelings, including that of loss, relatively early in treatment. This situation has also come across in his descriptions of current family life. This access to painful loss and related feelings seems to indicate a form of evidence of Alan's relatively stable and responsive first 6 years of life, which stand in marked contrast to the same years in Jim's life.

Conclusion

The story of Jim's childhood and analysis demonstrates that, beginning when he was 1 year old and continuing throughout his childhood, there were imprinted upon him traumatic images of and identifications with parenting adults in situations where they mastered great risk and stress to combat destruction. The identifications were seen to take on a preoedipal, oedipal, or later tenor, according to the epoch in which they were made. Comparing this chapter's cases, we can see evidence of later, more flexible identifications with Alan, and earlier, more rigid identifications with Jim. In these and related cases, there are some overriding similarities in the particular process of forming traumatic images of and identifications with the adults mastering great risk, regardless of the developmental phase of occurrence. Concomitantly with the forming of traumatic imagery, the invulnerable state of mind develops in its most set form. Jim, and the others like him, show that this unique mental state consists of the child's confidence of achieving grand tasks, which he associates with the acceptance of work, pain, punishment, and loss. This contrasts with the sense of omnipotent grandiosity, in which the analysand is confident of achieving great things with little to no work, pain, punishment, or loss.

It is noteworthy how many such boyhood identifications were with mothers, or surrogate mothers, who were mastering adversity. While this is an important trend, these cases demonstrate a complex web of traumatic images and related identifications with either sex at different epochs, which is woven into the fabric of the true invulnerable's drive to master risk realistically and successfully.

Jim's repeated successes in mastering risks in all developmental epochs strongly imply that the existence of such inherited ego skills as high intelligence, rapid reflexes, and other physical skills contributed to his success and survival. Alan and Sam manifest evidence of similar inherited traits. At the same time, the well-documented and repeated pattern of confronting and mastering risks is clearly not solely a matter of such inherited skills, which we often see in children who do not manifest these patients' particular mastering patterns.

The story of Jim's life and his analysis, in addition to his comments about his terrifying identity loss when first out of detective work, indicate that in his inner world to exist is to test one's strength in mastering risk; concomitantly, ceasing to take on and master risk threatens to shatter and disillusion one's personal identity. The imprinting of such a mental state brings to mind the studies by Terr (1981, 1983) of the children involved in the school bus kidnapping in Chowchilla, California, all of whom experienced massive psychic trauma at varying developmental epochs. Such characteristic responses as re-enactment phenomena and nightmare experiences were found in these children, regardless of their age. The traumatic imaging and identifying processes contributing to the invulnerable's state of mind can similarly have their effect during varying developmental epochs. Jim's case gives some indication of this, although since there was substantial trauma in all of the epochs, it is impossible to say exactly how much each experience contributed to his invulnerable state of mind. The overall impression is that this state of mind, with its images and identifications, was developed in an additive fashion from his first year into his late teens and beyond. This chapter's partial reports on Alan and Sam begin to delineate the emergence of true invulnerable traits in different developmental phases than occurred with Jim. Alan's extended adolescent experience of years in the most trying battle conditions stands out as an example.

In sum, while the mechanisms of this axis of traumatic imagery and re-enactment remain constant, the patient's full characterological and affective structure is enormously influenced by the developmental epoch in which the major trauma occurs. This chapter, I hope, demonstrates that it is only through psychoanalytic case studies that we can fully elucidate the existence and functions of a mastery re-enactment pattern such as Jim's. His driven pursuit of and attachment to seriously damaged, deteriorating women was molded by the images derived from his traumatic experience at age 2½ of sharing a bed and embraces with his great-aunt, who was dying of cancer. Such reflections also illuminate Jim's suffering with memories of battered bodies of homicide victims, which was abated by gradually working with free associations back through the long trail of deteriorating and otherwise out-of-control bodies in Jim's life.

This is obviously an area where further case studies should add clarification. It would also seem that further research with direct observation of children and families will be helpful in substantiating, refining, or refuting these clinical observations and my opening thesis.

Anthony (1974) graphically makes the point of the central role of mastery of risk in the mental processes and life histories of true invulnerables by summing up the ancient myth of Hercules, who might be called the first true invulnerable. With this report of Jim's analysis and of his childhood and adult development, we have the advantage in that we can glimpse this main process of mastering risks throughout his childhood and adult life. Comparing the life history of Hercules with that of Jim reveals some startling similarities.

The principal mastering achievements of Hercules, very briefly, are as follows: (1) As an infant, he slew snakes. (2) He developed great physical prowess and strength. (3) He slew a killer lion. (4) He was driven insane, in which state he killed a family, but he proceeded to survive and take his punishment. (5) He strangled another lion, using his cloak as a wrapping of invulnerability. (6) He took on and completed the grimy task of cleaning huge stables. (7) He conquered a mad bull. (8) He recovered golden apples. (9) He successfully struggled with death.

Jim's corresponding achievements were as follows: (1) He subdued pet rattlesnakes. (2) He repeatedly developed exceptional physical prowess. (3) He made a career of tracking and subduing killers (the murderer being the most threatening creature in the urban jungle). (4) He developed serious levels of anxiety and depression, and survived. (5) His successful grappling with dangerous criminals gave him a career reputation that was a kind of coat of invulnerability. (6) He had a childhood job of cleaning chicken coops and stables. (7) He subdued the belt beatings of a stepfather. (8) He recovered the treasures of robbery victims. (9) As in the struggle with the out-of-control race car, Jim repeatedly struggled with death and survived. While we are not generally looking for literal correlations between the mastering achievements of modern invulnerables and those of Hercules, the range of Jim's mastery experiences nevertheless documents a fairly unique world experience, with startling resemblance to that of the mythical Hercules.

My three cases, I think, document important developmental roles (via identifications with parents or surrogate parents) of the patients' (1) dealing with madness in family members or their surrogates (e.g., the madness of war in Alan's case); (2) successfully persisting at dirty, physical work; and (3) developing substantial physical skills, such as strength and speed. Subsequently, in adult life, they have manifested unusual capacities for handling such experiences, and even an attraction to them.

Again, while invulnerables like Jim are aided by unique positive identifications, they are concomitantly tortured by a series of traumatic images that can also be seen as negative identifications with some terrifying objects they have encountered at varying stages in their developmental sagas. For example, Jim's identification with his great-aunt in her struggle against cancer contributed to his underlying fantasies of having a penis oozing worms and a woman with a garbage disposal vagina. Alan's identification with warriors engaged in killing, in addition to the role of actually killing enemies in his adolescence, greatly intensified his conflict over expressing aggression when the corporate takeover cornered, provoked, and undermined him in later adult life. I believe that such traumatic images or threatening identifications, with their concomitant affect storms, generate another unique quality of the invulnerable, which is an exquisite need to retain control of emotions and objects.

Finally, let us sum up what this chapter has enabled us to give in the way of responses to Anthony's research questions, posed in the introduction.

As to whether there is a point in life when natural selection begins to operate, or whether invulnerability gradually builds up, I have the impression that both factors are operative. I think the case data indicate that in Jim's first year, some factors of natural selection (high intelligence, physical resilience, and capacity for rapid and effective physical learning) were operative, permitting Jim to survive. In addition, his pattern of repeatedly taking on high risks and mastering them give me the impression of a coat of invulnerability gradually building up. I think the case gives evidence that what is a large part of the invulnerable's protective coating turns out periodically to function as his Achilles heel. In other words, the rigid drive toward mastery served periodically to bring Jim into overwhelming amounts of contact with high risk that he was intermittantly unable to master, thereby bringing on conditions of overwhelming anxiety or depression.

Anthony has also asked whether the wear and tear of everyday existence reduces the efficacy of immunity. In the case of Jim, I think it was not the wear and tear of everyday existence, but rather an excessive and rigid application of the drive to mastery, that reduced the efficacy of his immunity.

Let us now consider the question that is so crucial to both clinical practice and the design of preventive programs. Is the immunity paid for by the concomitant related development of insensitivity, detachment, and self-absorption? In the cases of Jim, Sam, and Alan, and in related studies, I find consistent evidence that detachment in intimate relationships is a price paid in varying degrees for immunity. This distancing derives, in large part, from the invulnerable's exquisite control needs discussed earlier. By contrast, I do not find evidence that insensitivity and self-absorption are any more present in invulnerables I have treated than in other patient populations.

Both the transference data and the developmental history data in these cases document that Jim, Sam, and Alan repeatedly mastered hostile fates and were not treated benignly by the world. Responding to Anthony's last question as to the possibility of distinguishing between early and late, and true and false, invulnerables, it seems clear that a single in-depth study does not give us the data with which to make these distinctions. Nevertheless, my treatment experience with other invulnerables shows me that careful reporting of psychoanalytic cases does help us to make these distinctions.

Transference data, like those in the cases described here, add greatly to developmental data in distinguishing between early and late invulnerables. Although my data on Alan are not yet complete, his capacity in early analysis to express hurt and anger over separations indicates that he was not pushed toward early, rigid invulnerable identifications, as was Jim. Furthermore, psychoanalytic research into early and late invulnerability promises rich dividends in improved preventive and screening programs. I hope these case reports have made the general point that attention to the presence of traits and mechanisms involved in the invulnerable state of mind and in the characterological drive to mastery makes positive contributions to the psychoanalytic understanding and treatment of individuals such as Jim. Granting this point, I think there is a need for much more in-depth case reporting in this area. There seem to be noteworthy modifications of the invulnerable's mind set and character, depending upon the developmental stage or stages in which his drive to mastery and related personal and developmental events have emerged. It may be productive, in the future, to make subclassifications of the invulnerable character typology.

Other future research, in my opinion, suggested by these reflections would include comparative studies of characterological subgroups conducted along with clinics oriented toward diagnosis and brief treatment. It would seem worthwhile to do a prospective study designed to have interviewers separate true invulnerables, false invulnerables, and noninvulnerables with narcissistic personality disorders, during intake and brief follow-up interviews. Having made these separations, we would then be in a position to test our prediction that repetitive mastering behavior, with its concomitant advantages and deficits, would mainly appear in the group of true invulnerables.

It is likely that such clinical research studies may productively set a course for the establishment of an independent characterological diagnostic group of the invulnerable personality. There is some likelihood that the use of such a category could make positive contributions to improving our work with individuals heretofore classified in the diagnostic groups of generalized anxiety disorder, narcissistic personality, posttraumatic stress disorder, and some masochistic disorders.

In the area of preventive psychiatry, it seems to me that this chapter and related case reports give additional evidence of the need to further expand Anthony's work of providing at-risk children with interpersonal experiences that combine caring with a healthy respect for the young child's capacity to cope independently with risk situations. It appears that there is plenty of room for expansion of such programs to apply them to families of disaster victims while gathering further data.

Reflection on the present cases and on earlier pioneering research tells me there is a large need for additional related research in the area of disability and work-related injury and illness. I have preliminary data indicating that attention to thorough characterological diagnosis with sensitivity to the presence of invulnerable traits, in addition to carefully designed treatment interventions, can significantly reduce the duration and degree of disability in patients with primary psychiatric disabilities and with psychiatric disabilities secondary to injuries.

In conclusion, I hope that this report has communicated the value of the concepts of prior invulnerability studies and the ideas they stimulate for our work with patients and future research planning.

REFERENCES

Anthony, E. J. (1974). The syndrome of the psychologically invulnerable child. In E. J. Anthony & C. Koupernik (Eds.), *The child in his family: Children at psychiatric risk* (International yearbook, Vol. 3). New York: Wiley.
Anthony, E. J. (1978). From birth to breakdown: A prospective study of invulnerability. In E. J. Anthony, C. Koupernik, & C. Chiland (Eds.), *The child in his family: Vulnerable children* (International yearbook, Vol. 4). New York: Wiley.

Brett, E. A., & Ostroff, R. (1985). Imagery and post-traumatic stress disorder: An overview. *American Journal of Psychiatry, 142,* 417–424.

DeWind, E. (1984). Some implications of former massive traumatization upon the actual analytic process. *International Journal of Psycho-Analysis, 65,* 273–281.

Glover, E. (1929). Screening function of traumatic memories. *International Journal of Psycho-Analysis, 10,* 90–93.

Greenacre, P. (1949). A contribution to the study of screen memories. *Psychoanalytic Study of the Child, 3,* 75–84.

Terr, L. C. (1981). Psychic trauma in children: Observations following the Chowchilla school bus kidnapping. *American Journal of Psychiatry, 138,* 14–19.

Terr, L. C. (1983). Chowchilla revisited: The effects of psychic trauma four years after a school bus kidnapping. *American Journal of Psychiatry, 140,* 1543–1550.

Van Der Kolk, B. A. (1984). *Post-traumatic stress disorder: Psychological and biological sequelae.* Washington, DC: American Psychiatric Press.

Conclusion IV

13

Adversity, Resilience, and the Study of Lives

BERTRAM J. COHLER
University of Chicago

Risk research, if it does nothing else, should induce a degree of humility in its investigators confronted with the extraordinarily difficult task of separating causation from correlation. It will bring out of the shadows of neglect the *invulnerable* child who survives despite adversity, forcing us to look at processes of coping and adapting rather than solely at those that reflect failure and incompetence.—Garmezy (1972, p. 31)

While there has been much study of the determinants of personal adjustment, more is known about circumstances leading to psychopathology than about the ability to maintain psychological resilience when confronted with such adversity as unexpected tragedy, family conflict, or serious disappointments. Economic privation, social disorganization, and accumulation of unfortunate life changes are among the factors believed to be associated with impaired adjustment. The effect of misfortune may be heightened through increased constitutional vulnerability, such as that resulting from increased genetic loading for major psychopathology.

Even in the presence of both adverse life circumstances and some increased constitutional vulnerability, most persons are able to function effectively, finding ways of buffering the effects of unpleasant life experiences. The important questions in the study of mental health and the life course may have less to do with why the more vulnerable persons succumb to psychopathology than with the question of how persons remain invulnerable or resilient, able to cope with the effects of misfortune and adversity (Albee, 1980; Garmezy, 1972).

The study of factors associated with vulnerability and resilience raises important questions regarding the determinants of continuity and change across the course of life (Bloom, 1964; Clarke & Clarke, 1976; Emde, 1981; Kagan, 1980, 1984). These questions involve the complex interplay of temperament, social context, and life changes as factors entering into the capacity to withstand adversity and to remain resilient when confronted with such circumstances as economic privation, psychiatric illness within the family, and parental abuse and neglect. Little is known about factors associated with the capacity to remain resilient when confronted by adverse circumstances, particularly among persons who are already more vulnerable to psychopathology as a result of such innate characteristics as increased genetic loading for psychopathology.

Reviewing material from myth, legend, and ethnography, Anthony (1974b) notes that, among some persons, adversity represents a challenge to be overcome; an increased sense of personal competence results from successfully meeting these challenges to adjustment. As Anthony observes, invulnerability or resilience is too often viewed merely as the absence of psychopathology, rather than the result of coping with problems threatening present adjustment. Furthermore, too often it is assumed that circumstances such as poverty or family disorganization must inevitably lead to increased suffering and turmoil; there is insufficient understanding of the meaning of such events for persons experiencing them, or recognition that such events may also lead to renewed efforts to master this adversity.

For example, while parental psychiatric illness may be an adverse event for a child, there is little reason to assume that this misfortune necessarily leads to lowered levels of psychosocial functioning, or that children are necessarily unable to cope with problems presented for them as a consequence of parental psychopathology. Because they are most often confronted by persons showing personal distress, which may be accompanied by greatly increased vulnerability and difficulty in managing adversity, the mental health professions may have given too little recognition to adaptive capacity; they may have devoted too little attention to the study of persons who are able either to overcome adversity or, where there are few alternatives, to become reconciled to such misfortune. When a person is confronted by unanticipated diagnosis of a terminal illness, there may be few alternatives for the patient and significant others except to recognize feelings of sadness and fear, maintaining a sense of self-worth and personal integrity when confronted by adversity for which there is no real solution.

The study of determinants of resilience and coping, which is concerned with predicting response to adversity, requires consideration of the characteristics associated with particular life changes, as well as the timing of these changes in terms of the life course. These characteristics of events must be considered together with attributes of persons, including such innate characteristics as temperament, as well as constitutionally determined vulnerability for experiencing increased distress when confronted with particular kinds of adversity at particular points in the course of life. This predictive approach, based on information regarding the type of life change, the social context in which particular changes take place, and the attributes of persons, must be complemented by a narrative approach, which is concerned with the manner in which persons experience and interpret or "make sense" of these life changes.

Little is known of the manner in which persons create a narrative that renders adversity coherent in terms of experienced life history, or of the manner in which presently constructed meanings of life changes may be altered in order to maintain a sense of personal integration. For some persons, at particular points in the life course, the fact of such misfortunes as poverty or the untimely death of a parent during early childhood is used as an explanation for the failure to realize personal goals; for other persons, this misfortune becomes the impetus for increased effort in order to attain these goals.

The present chapter considers both predictive and narrative approaches to the study of resilience. In order to better predict response to life changes, it is first necessary to consider the nature of these changes that require coping responses in an effort to maintain continued resilience, and then to consider such factors as constitutional predisposition and the course of development from earliest childhood, which are believed to determine later coping responses when a person is confronted by subsequent adversity.

Life Changes and Mental Health

It is well known that life changes may be experienced as life stress, leading to the expression both of physical symptoms and of psychological distress (Thoits, 1983). Study of the association of stress and illness was given particular emphasis in W. B. Cannon's (1932) discussion of biological adaptation and maintenance of homeostasis, as well as in classic discussions by Adolf Meyer (1951), Selye (1956), and Dubos (1965). Barbara P. Dohrenwend's (1961) pioneering study of the relationship of stressful events and psychiatric symptoms has inspired much subsequent research on the properties of life events most important in contributing to impaired mental health.

Classification of Life Events

Research summarized by the Dohrenwends (1974) suggests that, regardless of their affective quality as either pleasant or unpleasant and adverse, life changes pose unique problems requiring increased efforts at adaptation; increased feelings of distress are the result of the failure to resolve problems posed by these changes. Findings reported by Holmes and Rahe (1967), Masuda and Holmes (1967, 1968), Paykel and Uhlenhuth (1972), and others have shown that some life changes are judged to be particularly adverse and are capable of evoking significant distress, even among persons generally able to adjust to life changes (Brown & Harris, 1978; Fontana, Hughes, Marcus, & Dowds, 1979; Pearlin & Lieberman, 1979; Pearlin, Lieberman, Menaghan, & Mullan, 1981; Thoits, 1983).

Intensive study across the past decade has suggested that not all life changes are experienced as a source of increased distress (Kessler, Price, & Wortman, 1985; Pearlin, et al., 1981; Thoits, 1983). Events most likely to adversely affect mental and physical health are those that persons feel they have little control over; that are undesirable, aversive, or hazardous to personal adjustment; that are unexpected and "accidental," including off-time in terms of a shared timetable for the life course (Hagestad & Neugarten, 1985; Neugarten & Hagestad, 1976; Neugarten, Moore, & Lowe, 1965; Roth, 1963; Sorokin & Merton, 1937); that are major in terms of their implications for maintaining present understanding of self and the meaning of life (Weber, 1906); and that are additive or interactive in their effect.

These research findings, which have generally been based on checklists of life changes, have also been the subject of considerable critical discussion. Even beyond such questions as the accuracy of recall of changes taking place many months or years prior to the time of the study, there is question regarding the psychological meaning of summated scores on these checklists (Brim, 1980; Brim & Ryff, 1980; Hultsch & Plemons, 1979; Pearlin, 1982, 1983; Reese & Smyer, 1983). In the first place, there is some question regarding the role of even the most adverse life changes as determinants of episodes of major psychiatric illness (Brown & Birley, 1968; Brown, Harris, & Petro, 1973).

Indeed, Beck and Worthen (1972) have shown that events attributed by schizophrenic adults as precipitants of disturbance were markedly idiosyncratic and would not have been regarded as particularly adverse in normative studies rating the adversity of particular life changes. Consistent with the perspective proposed by Murray and Associates (1938), Gergen (1977), and Hultsch and Plemons (1979), those events most troublesome for present adjustment may be markedly more idiosyncratic—not only among troubled persons, but also among those who are psychologically well—than has been suggested by research attempting to rate the upsetting qualities of a variety of life changes.

Hultsch and Plemons (1979) have criticized this checklist approach to the study of life changes not only for failing to take persons' own understandings of these events into account, but also as assuming a degree of stability and linear continuity in the relationship between life changes and adjustment in the life history that has not been supported by presently available findings (Emde & Harmon, 1984; Kagan, 1980, 1984). For example, findings reported by Maas and Kuypers (1974) suggest that persons maintaining greater continuity in personality and life style from middle to old age appear to be less well adjusted than persons reporting changes over time in interests and life styles.

Brim and Ryff (1980) have suggested that the study of life stress and adjustment should emphasize the process by which persons make particular attributions for life events, rather than being concerned with such general characteristics as the extent to which events are viewed as pleasant or unpleasant in a checklist of possible life changes. For example, persons generally rely upon most recent events in judging the salience of life changes for adjustment. Those events selected as attributed sources of change are also the most vivid and all-encompassing. Less dramatic events, or those that might be continuous or interrelated in affecting adjustment, may be overlooked.

An additional problem in the study of life changes, vulnerability, and adjustment concerns distinctions among types of life changes (Brim & Ryff, 1980; Reese & Smyer, 1983).[1] Much of the work in the area of life events and mental health has emphasized the extent of changes without considering the nature of these changes. Three major types of life changes may be identified: those related to normative transitions across the life course (Fiske, 1980a, 1980b; Lowenthal, Thurnher, Chiriboga, & Associates, 1975; Pearlin, 1975, 1980, 1982; Reese & Smyer, 1983); those due to unexpected and generally adverse accidents of fate (Bandura, 1982b; Gergen, 1977, 1982); and those encountered in the performance of such major life roles as those of parent, spouse, and worker (Goode, 1960; Minkler & Biller, 1979; Pearlin, 1983).

Many of what are considered life changes are those eruptive, unpredictable accidents of fate such as serious illness, which cannot be anticipated or predicted in advance. Eruptive changes must be differentiated from normative transitions, or changes that are expected as a result of shared understandings of the course of life. These expected transitions reflect agreement among persons within particular cohorts regarding expectable duration of life; major delineations within the life course, such as infancy or young and middle adulthood; and timing of transitions into and out of major life roles, such as marriage and work.

This social timetable (Durkheim, 1915; Hagestad & Neugarten, 1985; Neugarten, 1979; Neugarten & Hagestad, 1976; Roth, 1963; Sorokin & Merton, 1937) permits the comparative evaluation of present attainments in terms of socially recognized milestones across the course of life. The accomplishment of particular role transitions may be either "on time," in terms of that age expected for most persons of one's cohort, or may show a departure from this shared timetable of the course of life—either "off-time early," in the case of role transitions such as adolescent motherhood, or "off-time late," in the case of men who marry and become parents for the first time in middle age.

There is little evidence that on-time, recognized changes or transitions such as the "empty nest" or retirement have an adverse effect on morale and mental health when they occur at approximately the expected point in the course of life (Cohler & Boxer, 1984; Neugarten, 1979). Even otherwise eruptive adverse events appear to be less disruptive or adverse than has often been maintained when they occur at expected points in the life course. For example, although the death of a spouse has been rated as a source of marked and lasting personal distress, findings reported by Kessler and McLeod (1984) and Bankoff (1983) suggest that the extent to which this event has a lasting impact depends upon the point in the life course at which the loss of the spouse takes place. Consistent with the formulation of Neugarten (1979) Neugarten and Hagestad (1976), and Hagestad and Neugarten (1985), the effects of widowhood appear limited in both time and impact among older women, who have had an opportunity to rehearse the role of widow, for whom widowhood is an "on-time," expectable event, and for whom there is a role convoy of associates having experienced the same event.[2]

Off-time adverse events, such as off-time early widowhood or forced early retirement due to business reversal or failure, appear to have a particularly profound impact upon adjustment. This is true both because there is little chance for anticipatory socialization, and because there may be no convoy of consociates (Kahn & Antonucci, 1980; Plath, 1980) who have experienced similar events and who can facilitate adjustment to the new status. Lack of opportunity for role rehearsal and lack of relevant consociates may explain why role-connected life changes that are off-time early—including those, such as work or school promotions, that are more positive in tone—appear to adversely affect adjustment to a greater extent than role-connected life changes that are delayed or off-time late (Pearlin, 1975, 1980, 1983).

Strain and overload within roles, as well as conflict across roles, also affect mental health, although in ways somewhat different from eruptive events. Role strain appears primarily to affect morale or life satisfaction, rather than to lead to increase in the number or type of symptoms generally associated with impairment in mental health. The impact of role strain upon morale and adjustment may be quite different, depending upon other aspects of present life. What appears at some points in the life course as role overload may at other times appear as challenge. For example, young adults just beginning careers may accept difficult and time-consuming work assignments as opportunities for proving their merit and winning valued promotions. By contrast, if a person is married and with young children at home, time-consuming and demanding work may be resented by both that person and the spouse as interfering in family life.

Persons characteristically develop techniques for managing everyday hassles that are relatively consistent over time, although these techniques may also be role-specific (Lazarus & Folkman, 1984; Menaghan, 1983; Pearlin & Schooler, 1978). Unexpected, adverse life changes appear to be more directly related to the onset of significant personal distress (Pearlin et al., 1981; Pearlin & Schooler, 1978); they generally require adaptive response in emergency situations that are generally not a part of everyday life.

Life Changes and Mental Health in the Childhood Years

Much of what is known regarding life changes and mental health has been based on the study of adulthood through middle age. Findings such as those reported by Uhlenhuth, Lipman, Balter, and Stern (1974) suggest that the number of unexpected life changes, as well as the potential for disruption of adjustment, increases through midlife and then gradually declines in later life. Unexpected and adverse events, as well as role strain, diminish in both number and intensity as a consequence of such role exits and losses as retirement and widowhood. However, older women who are kinkeepers for a large number of interdependent lives (Cohler, 1983; Kessler & McLeod, 1984; McMiller & Ingham, 1985; Pruchno, Blow, & Smyer, 1984) may continue to experience a larger number of family-related adverse events than men.

Just as little is known about the significance of life changes earlier in adulthood for adjustment in later life, little is known about the impact of adverse life changes in childhood upon both present and subsequent adaptation (Rutter, 1981b).[3] Reviewing findings regarding the relationship between life changes and childhood adjustment, Rutter (1981b) has noted the paucity of research in this area. Events discussed by Rutter include primarily such expected role transitions as the birth of a brother or sister, where only the youngest children show particular signs of distress, or parental divorce, where responses among children of different ages are so variable that it is difficult to determine the impact of this life change upon adjustment (Wallerstein & Kelly, 1980).

The role of childhood experience as a determinant of adult capacity to withstand misfortune may be less salient than was formerly maintained. Indeed, the course of development across the childhood years appears to be more resilient to transitory adversity, and to be less resistant to spontaneous reversibility following such unfortunate experiences, than was previously assumed (Chess, 1979; Clarke & Clarke, 1976; Dennis, 1973; Emde, 1981; Emde & Harmon, 1984; Kagan, 1980, 1984; Kagan & Klein, 1973; Kagan, Klein, Finley, Rogoff, & Nolan, 1979; Kohlberg, Ricks, & Snarey, 1984; Skeels, 1966).

Consistent with the views of Waddington (1957, 1966), Emde (1981) suggests that the course of development may be like a river: Finding one channel blocked, development proceeds to take a parallel path in the same direction. For example, Goldin-Meadow and Mylander (1984) have shown that deaf infants develop the capacity to communicate wishes and goals in the same manner as hearing infants, using a complex sign language that shows dramatic linguistic competence. Following Ricoeur's (1977) discussion of the interpretive perspective in psychoanalysis, I (Cohler, 1982) have suggested that assumptions of irreversibility and directionality in human development may be more a reflection of socially shared assumptions regarding the organization of stories than a generalization from research findings showing any cause-and-effect relationship between earlier events and later development.

It has been assumed, stemming from a belief in the primacy of childhood experiences for adult adjustment, and based in large part upon the "critical-period" hypothesis, that particular eruptive events taking place in childhood might have particularly significant impact on adult adjustment. Furthermore, it has also been assumed that the earlier in life at which the adverse event occurs, the greater its subsequent impact upon adjustment will be. This assumption has received relatively little systematic examination. Findings from Brown and Harris's (1978) retrospective study do suggest that the death of a parent when a child is young has a particularly adverse impact upon adult mood. However, a review of prospective studies (Garmezy, 1983), including those with random selection of children for study (Clayton & Darvish, 1979), suggests that few long-term effects of the loss of a parent are evident, particularly among children who are younger at the time of the loss of the parent. Adolescent boys losing a father show more prolonged grief than either boys or girls at other ages.

There has been considerable debate regarding the capacity of young children to understand death and to participate in bereavement (Garber, 1981). Consistent with Kagan's (1979, 1980) argument regarding the psychological impact of the strange situation upon the actions of toddlers, it is possible that the particular impact of parental death, as well as other separations from parents in childhood (Bowlby, Robertson, & Rosenbluth, 1952; Robertson, 1970; no date)—for example, as reflected in expression of protest and despair—may in large part be attributed to the child's inability to understand finitude or to distinguish between more and less permanent separations.

If we rely primarily upon findings from study of life changes in the adult years, it appears that off-time early events may be more disruptive than off-time late ones. Off-time late events are less likely to be experienced by children than by adults because of the short span of life to date. Since there can be little preparation or anticipatory socialization prior to the event, and few consociates with whom to share the experience (Neugarten & Hagestad, 1976; Plath, 1980) and to depend upon for support, younger children who lose a parent through death or divorce, who develop a dibilitating illness, may have fewer coping resources than children not experiencing these potentially disruptive events or somewhat older children.

Consistent with this view of the particularly adverse impact of off-time early changes in life, Kagan (1979, 1983) and Kagan, Kearsley, and Zelazo (1978) have noted the impact of events perceived by the child as discordant with expectations. Reinterpreting findings regarding responses to separation from caretakers in the "Strange Situation" paradigm developed by Ainsworth and her associates (Ainsworth, 1982; Ainsworth, Blehar, Waters, & Wall, 1978), Kagan suggests that the primary reason for this adverse impact is its unexpected and unanticipated occurrence rather than the mother's absence as such. Again, if the child has not reached the point in cognitive development necessary in order to understand changes resulting from these adverse events, the extent of this adversity may be even greater.

Reconsideration of earlier findings regarding effects of temporary separation from the mother (Garmezy, 1983) suggests that these effects may not be as adverse as formerly supposed. Implicitly supporting Kagan's assumptions regarding discrepancy in expectations as the basis for the adverse quality of these separations, Garmezy notes that much can be done to help children anticipate separations, and that this would reduce their discrepant and unanticipated qualities. When young children are provided with supports buffering the effects of unanticipated occurrence, they appear not to react to these effects with the same degree of distress.

Defense, Coping, and Resilience

A consideration of response to adverse life changes underscores the variety of approaches that persons may adopt in order to integrate these changes into the course of their lives. Some persons prefer not to think about such events (Cohen & Lazarus, 1973; Lazarus, 1980)—a response that appears to work well in coping with such adverse events as imminent surgery (Janis, 1958)—while others may make great efforts to seek all available information. Too often, the mode of approach in solving these problems has been understood in terms of the notion of "defense," which has been borrowed, sometimes inappropriately, from psychoanalytic concepts of intrapsychic conflict and defense in ways that are not always appropriate.

Psychoanalytic Approaches to the Study of Defense and Coping

Discussing the psychoneuroses, Freud (1894, 1896) emphasized the value of adjustment as a result of freedom from the experience of disturbing and painful ideas or feelings, particularly the conflict between wishes and socially determined opposition to the expression of these wishes, through repression or refusal to admit these feelings into awareness.

Even in his very early papers, Freud emphasized the significance of "normal" defenses (characterized by avoiding the pain associated with re-enactment of previously remembered experiences and by successfully warding off feelings of unacceptable tension), as well as "distorted" defenses (in which there is both excitation or pleasure and pain, connected in such a manner that the pleasure is sought but the pain is experienced, leading to feelings of being overwhelmed) (Freud, 1915–1917). As a result, pleasure can become a source of pain, or the real world itself can be seen as dangerous, since it may provide opportunity for satisfaction of a wish that will only further increase the sense of conflict (Freud, 1926).

The initial concept of defense against sexual wishes, associated with the family romance in the case of hysteria, was later extended by Freud (1915–1917, 1926) to a variety of neurotic disturbances beyond hysteria itself. Work by Abraham (1924), Glover (1932a, 1932b), and Reich (1933) further extended the concept of defense to include a means of protection, through action, against recognition of unacceptable wishes and goals. While repression, or refusal to admit a wish into awareness, was recognized as the model of the process of defense, other defenses were described as well (Freud, 1926).

Each defense was thought to function in a similar manner, protecting against anxiety resulting from experience of unacceptable wishes, as well as from the significance of difficult or painful life circumstances (A. Freud, 1936, pp. 59–61). In each instance, defenses serve to protect against feelings of being overwhelmed, with the quality of life experiences responsible for the sophistication and appropriateness of defenses when expressed. Problems in the regulation of tensions can be so significant that means of protection, serving to protect present adaptation, may lead to distortion of relations with the external world.

Much of this discussion of defense and adjustment was systematized by A. Freud's (1936) volume, which portrays the relationship between intrapsychic conflict and means of protection from awareness of underlying wishes as disguised through neurotic symptoms or character structure, particularly as observed in the context of the psychoanalytic interview, rather than as reconstructed on the basis of a hypothetical formulation such as that earlier provided by Abraham (1924). Drawing upon Freud's (1905, 1915–1917) epigenetic formulation of personality development, as systematized and elaborated by Abraham (1924) and Erikson (1963), efforts have been made to order the defenses in a manner parallel to other lines of development (Engel, 1962; Menninger, Mayman, & Pruyser, 1963; Semrad, 1967; Semrad, Grinspoon, & Feinberg, 1973; Vaillant, 1971, 1976, 1977).

However, based on observational study of the therapeutic process, A. Freud has noted—both in her earlier (1936) discussion of the defenses and in her later (1965) volume on normality in development—that defenses may not be as readily ordered according to a chronology of personality development as had been supposed. In an otherwise sympathetic review of psychoanalytic approaches to the study of defenses, recognizing the significance of unacceptable and unrecognized wishes as determinants of actions, Swanson (1961) has also shown that there is very little support for assumptions that the several defense mechanisms may be ordered in an epigenetic manner.

Since epigenetic classifications of development, including the purported genetic ordering of defense mechanisms, appear to represent little more than an analogy between Freud's early laboratory study (Cohler, in press; Freud, 1895, 1925; Sulloway, 1979), then there is little reason to attempt such systematizations that are so experience-distant (Kohut, 1971; Klein, 1976). Consistent with A. Freud's (1936, p. 53) explicit warning against premature efforts at ordering the defenses, Swanson's discussion provides additional support for her view that persons characteristically use a variety of defenses in dealing with conflict inspired by wishes.

Vaillant's (1976, 1977) findings do suggest that three levels or grades of defense may be distinguished, characterized by the extent to which environmental contingencies are distorted in an effort to provide protection from encounters with conflict, and by the extent to which these particular defenses are used in an inflexible and extreme manner. D. Miller and Swanson's (1960) findings provide an alternative two-category ordering of defenses: those that provide comforting fantasies when confronted by an intolerable reality, and those that provide for displacement of one need by another that is socially more acceptable.

A. Freud has observed that the "healthy" person uses a variety of defenses from all presumed levels of personality development. However, there is little reason to believe that a hierarchy of defenses exists that fosters management of age-appropriate conflicts in the manner earlier portrayed by Abraham, Glover, and others, and most recently systematized by Erikson (1963). At the same time, as A. Freud (1936), D. Miller and Swanson (1960), and Vaillant (1971, 1976) suggest, some defenses are more complex and sophisticated than others, restricting or promoting satisfying relations with other persons and facilitating or interfering in resolution of salient life tasks.

Early discussion of conflict and defense assumed that all aspects of mentation are devoted to need satisfaction. Intense wishes, unacceptable to awareness, was thought to control thought and actions in such a manner that all activities ultimately represent compromises with efforts at the search for satisfaction of these unacknowledged needs. All energy was seen as harnessed in an effort at satisfaction of these unacceptable wishes, which were thought to originate in the family romance. However, publication of Nunberg's (1932) classic text, together with Hartmann's (1939) classic essay on ego psychology and R. W. White's (1960, 1963) discussion of effectance and independent ego energies, has led to a dramatic reformulation of psychoanalytic perspectives, in which the energy providing the basis for mentation is not necessarily linked to satisfaction of particular unconscious wishes. As Hartmann (1950a, 1950b, 1955) notes, ego functions (actually "cognitive competences," in contemporary terms) are partially rooted in constitution, partially in life experiences, and partially in the course of maturation itself, independent of needs and life experiences.

Some ego functions enjoy primary autonomy from needs or wishes, although they may later be drawn into such conflict. Perception, memory, and other basic cognitive functions develop with maturation and are further shaped by the transaction between intrinsic processes and the environment (Piaget, 1975). While these cognitive functions may later become involved in conflict, they are not inevitably and intrinsically created by satisfaction of needs.

Other cognitive competences—perhaps rooted in defenses against expression of intrapsychic conflict, such as transformation of feelings into ideation, and blocking off the expression of ideation—may later move outside the sphere of wishes, providing the basis of an intrinsic capacity of intellectuality. When used beyond satisfaction of needs, these cognitive competences acquire what Hartmann (1939, 1950a) has portrayed as "secondary autonomy." These cognitive competences are relatively outside needs and wishes, although, under certain circumstances, these cognitive competences may be reinvolved in the process of conflict, need, and defense. As Hartmann (1950a) observes:

> Through what one could call a "change of function," what started in a situation of conflict may secondarily become part of the non-conflictual sphere (Hartmann, 1939). Many aims, attitudes, interests, [and] structures

of the ego have originated in this way (see also G. Allport, 1937). What developed as a result of defense against an instinctual drive may grow into a more or less independent and more or less structured function. . . . [B]ecause we know that even the results of this development may be rather stable, or even irreversible in most normal conditions, we may call such functions autonomous, though in a secondary way (in contradistinction to primary autonomy of the ego . . .). (p. 123)

Recognition that cognitive functions are not necessarily developed in order to satisfy important needs led to increased study of the conditions under which these functions remain relatively independent of need satisfaction or in the service of repetitive and circumscribing efforts to replay and resolve earlier experienced deficits in development. Since the role of play and creativity in development could be understood apart from needs, focus of study shifted away from concern exclusively with drive and defense to concern with development of sense of mastery, self-esteem, and effectance in development over the first years of life.

Central in this new approach to the study of childhood personality development was R. W. White's (1963) monograph on independent ego energies. White extended and built upon Hartmann's dual concepts of primary and secondary autonomy, noting that energy is inherent in the body and propels all later actions in transactions with reality. While one or another cognitive function may at some times be drawn into conflict, ordinary effort and manipulation of objects lead the infant to an increased sense of effectance in the real world, propelling yet additional exploratory activities. As White has noted, "the living organism does not typically sit and learn. It learns through action, and what it learns is a design or readiness for future action" (1963, p. 34). Furthermore, "playful exploration and manipulation take place because one feels inclined toward such behavior and finds it naturally satisfying" (1963, p. 34).

Reviewing Piaget's observations on the development of his own children, White (1959, 1963) has suggested that the search for variety and novelty, and for active mastery of the environment, may be more intrinsic to human nature than the need to reduce tensions and control drives. As a result of this intrinsic striving for effectance, the child develops a sense of competence or subjective sense of the capacity to interact effectively with the environment, which arises from effectance activities as well as from those motivated by conflict. Each particular transaction with the external world provides an increased sense of efficacy; the overall sense of competence is a result of repeated successful transactions with the environment.

Although borrowing from metapsychology, particularly Rapaport and Gill's (1959) extension of metapsychology to include the adaptational point of view, White's formulation is based primarily upon findings from the observational study of development (R. W. White, 1960, 1963), rather than Freud's philosophy of science as contained in metapsychology (Cohler, in press; Gill, 1976; Klein, 1976). Study of the determinants of conflict and defense must continue to be founded upon clinical study and findings from systematic research (A. Freud, 1936; Gill, 1976; Kohut, 1971), rather than based on efforts to deduce personality processes from postulated concepts such as the epigenesis of defenses, which, as Freud (1925) notes in his autobiography, was based upon an effort to extend earlier laboratory findings in the discipline of developmental neurobiology to the study of human behavior as a kind of metaphor (Sulloway, 1979).

Defense, Coping, and Resilience

Earlier study of the interplay of defense with intrapsychic conflict and processes of development led to increased appreciation of the extent to which not all cognitive functions need necessarily be drawn into conflict. Acceptance of the processes of primary and secondary autonomy fostered detailed studies of coping and development across the childhood years, particularly the interplay between maturational processes and the widening world of the child's experience (Murphy, 1960a, 1960b, 1962, 1970; Murphy & Moriarty, 1976). More recently, attention has been focused on issues of coping across the adult years; these studies have been based on a set of quite different assumptions, often implicitly borrowing concepts from the psychoanalytic tradition. Subsequent application of this quite different tradition to the study of childhood adjustment has only further confused the study of coping and mental health.

The psychoanalytic tradition has focused on the representational world (Sandler & Rosenblatt, 1962); it has been concerned with the appearance of compromise formations or psychological enactments of conflict, through dreams, symptoms, and transferences, between unacceptable wishes based on early childhood sexuality and the time–space world. More recent, social-psychological inquiry has been concerned with the consequences for adjustment resulting from particular role strains and both normative and eruptive life changes.

While some investigators (Haan, 1977, 1982; Menninger, 1954; Menninger et al., 1963; Murphy, 1960b, 1970; Murphy & Moriarty, 1976; Vaillant, 1971, 1976, 1977) have attempted to relate these traditions, the quite different conceptual frameworks used in psychoanalysis and social psychology raise questions regarding the advantages of this approach. Murphy (1970) appears to recognize this dilemma when she notes that "since the term defense mechanism was appropriated for the intrapsychic maneuvers, transformations, and other operations dealing with affects and instincts, another term is needed to refer to the ego's dealing with the actual external or objective situation itself" (p. 69).

Consistent with the tradition of ego psychology, focusing upon concepts such as primary and secondary autonomy (Hartmann, 1939), independent ego energies (R. W. White, 1963), and the need to study mechanisms of adaptation and coping in the same detail as previously noted for the study of defenses (R. W. White, 1974), Murphy proposes the concept of "coping" as a means of representing these transactions. In using this term, Murphy maintains that even classical discussion of the defenses refers to relations with the time–space world (A. Freud, 1936; Novey, 1968). She suggests that, in contrast with defensive operations, which serve to protect the person from threat (of the awareness of unacceptable wishes), coping operations are in the service of mastery of conflict with the external world.

Murphy (1960b, 1962, 1970) views the relationship of defense and coping in terms similar to Hartmann's (1939) discussion of primary and secondary autonomy. Particular ego functions may at some points be in the service of defense, while at other points they may be in the service of coping (Murphy, 1960b, 1962, 1970). Murphy views the use of defensive processes as a part of coping efforts, called upon at times when the child is in danger of feeling overwhelmed, maintaining that it is only when defenses become too intense or paramount in the child's life, interfering with efforts at adjustment, that these defenses may lead to the appearance of psychopathology.

Janis (1958), D. Miller and Swanson (1960), Kroeber (1963), and Haan (1977, 1982) have adopted a position consistent with Murphy's formulation. Drawing largely on the study of adult lives, and using data from longitudinal studies conducted by the Institute of Human Development at Berkeley (Baylery, 1963; MacFarlane, 1963, 1964), Kroeber (1963) and Haan (1977, 1982) have posited a number of linear personality dimensions with defensive and coping alternatives. For example, intellectualization, or the use of ideas in protecting against the experience of feeling, is the defensive pole of a dimension that has intellectuality, or enjoyment in the study of ideas, at the coping pole. Haan (1977) has also posited a third outcome, more extreme than defense, which she terms "fragmentation."

Although Haan (1982) maintains that she does *not* view coping as related to defense, but rather as a separate process, her discussion of findings suggests that they may be linked in empirical study. She also insists that she sees these dimensions of personality as processes rather than as traits, although much of her empirical work uses self-report questionnaires and ratings in which items are phrased as traits. Definitions of other ego processes than defense and coping (Haan, 1977) are also phrased as personality traits.

Social Science Perspectives on Coping and Solving Problems

In contrast with this concern regarding conflict, defense, and autonomous or coping aspects of personality, which appears to be based on psychoanalytic perspectives on personality development, a second research tradition, largely informed by social psychology, has been concerned with the process by which persons seek to master feelings of distress evoked either by normative on-time, life changes or eruptive, off-time events, as well as the experience of strain engendered by performance of expectable roles (Goode, 1960; Lazarus, Averill, & Opton, 1974; Lazarus & Folkman, 1984; Pearlin & Schooler, 1978). This tradition makes few assumptions regarding the structure of personality, including distinctions between psychological conflicts and those involving person and environment. Rather, circumstances are perceived as having an impact upon personal adjustment as a whole, which is measured in terms of negative emotional states, lowered morale, and increased reports of such psychiatric symptoms as anxiety and depression (French, Rodgers, & Cobb, 1974).

Concepts of coping and mastery have quite different significance when understood in terms of this social-psychological tradition than when understood from the psychoanalytic/ego-psychological perspective. From the social-psychological perspective, coping responses represent strategies used by persons in an effort to deal with problems posed by life context; these strategies permit avoidance of feelings of distress and continued positive self-esteem (Menaghan, 1983). Lazarus and Folkman (1984) define coping as "constantly changing cognitive and behavioral efforts to manage specific external and/or internal demands that are appraised as taxing or exceeding the resources of the person" (p. 141). Distinctions between defense and coping are as irrelevant here as the distinction between intrapsychic conflict and conflict stemming from person–environment interactions (Lazarus, 1980; Lazarus & Folkman, 1984). Study of the process of appraisal of and response to specific threatening events is of particular significance for those working within this tradition (Antonovsky, 1979l; Billings & Moos, 1981; Lazarus, 1966; Lazarus & Folkman, 1984; Mechanic, 1962, 1974; Menaghan, 1983; Moos & Billings, 1982; Pearlin & Schooler, 1978).

Investigators working within the social-psychological tradition of coping research assume a continuing process in which the meaning of transactions with the real world are evaluated in terms of both possible disruptions of present adjustment, and the potential for ever-increased sense of efficacy or competence (Janis & Mann, 1977; Lazarus & Folkman, 1984; Mechanic, 1974, 1977; Meichenbaum, Butler, & Gruson, 1981). Lazarus has been most explicit in describing a feedback system similar to the Test-Operate–Test-Exit (TOTE) system portrayed by G. Miller, Galanter, and Pribram (1960), in which continuing, or primary, appraisal of the stream of experience is able to provide the first warning of possible disruptions of present adjustment, including immediate threats (characterized as eruptive events), anticipated life changes, and opportunities for increased realization of personal satisfaction (e.g., those presented by accepting new responsibilities at work). Secondary appraisal provides further evaluation of means for dealing with the threat or reality of disruption of adjustment, as well as for taking advantage of challenges or opportunity. Reappraisal of the success of these actions (planned or enacted) leads to further modifications in actions, designed either to deal with adversity or to take advantage of opportunity.

Lazarus and Folkman (1984) have suggested that coping serves two major functions: managing or changing the problem (problem-focused coping), and regulating one's own response to the problem (emotion-focused coping). While such emotion-focused techniques as "psyching" oneself to meet a challenge may be useful in some specific contexts, the problem with this approach is that it may also lead to distortion of reality, making solution of the problem even more difficult. In contrast, problem-focused coping requires cognitive reappraisal of the event that is posing a challenge to adjustment, and then acting on the basis of the problem as defined. Focusing on the experience of students taking doctoral examinations, Mechanic (1974) has proposed a three-step process of dealing with situational demands, creating the motivational state necessary to meet those demands, and maintaining the capacity required to deal with the event.

Menaghan (1983) and Lazarus and Folkman (1984) emphasize the significance of appreciating available resources, enduring styles of response to challenging events, and efforts directed at meeting those challenges in understanding the coping process. Csikszentmihalyi (1975) has proposed that challenge, or "flow," is characterized by the experience of a balance between circumstances and skills and talents. Increased anxiety is experienced when persons feel that their available skills are inadequate to deal with circumstances, while boredom results from the perception that skills and talents are much greater than those required to deal with circumstances.

Antonovsky (1979), Kobasa (1979, 1982), Kobasa, Maddi, and Kahn (1982), and Lazarus and Folkman (1984) all stress the significance of health and vitality in meeting these challenges, while Bandura (1977,

1982b), Block and Block (1980), Gurin and Brim (1984), and Lazarus and Folkman (1984) also emphasize the importance of maintaining a sense of self-efficacy or control, as well as of having social skills and being able to use available social supports. However, Pearlin and Schooler (1978) and Menaghan (1983) question the significance of generalized coping styles, including trait conceptions of coping; they note that, at least in study of response to role strain and overload, there is little consistency of techniques used across roles.

While generally accepting the concept of coping as a process of appraisal, action, and reappraisal, most clearly discussed in work by Pearlin and his associates and by the Lazarus research group, Billings and Moos (1981) and Moos and Billings (1982) have further extended the study of coping processes by focusing explicitly upon factors affecting the choice of a coping method. Distinguishing between cognitive or psychological strategies and action or behavioral strategies, these investigators have delineated three particular methods or strategies: active coping, or focusing upon personal appraisal of challenging events and the most effective responses to them; active behavioral coping, involving particular actions to overcome the challenge; and avoidance coping, the goal of which is to avoid confrontation with challenging events. Moos and Billings (1982) suggests that this tripartite distinction of method of coping, together with the locus of coping as either problem- or emotion-focused, will provide the most complete possible understanding of response to challenge. The problem with this approach is that it also makes assumptions that coping styles are invariant across situations, which have not been supported either in the investigators' own research or that of Pearlin and Schooler (1978).

Normative transitions, adverse events, and role strains appear to have particular associated coping responses, not responses generalizable across events or roles. Particular coping responses are always a function of complex interactions between persons and events, in the manner suggested by Stern, Stein, and Bloom (1954), Stern (1970), French et al. (1974) and Caplon (1980). All adversity is not alike, just as particular role strains have particular meaning for persons at particular points in the life course. Issues of resilience and mastery must be phrased in more specific terms than they have been in research to date, taking into account distinctions among the three major sources of challenge to adjustment (role strain, normative transitions, and adverse, eruptive life changes), as well as factors entering into appraisal of the meaning of these events (Brim & Ryff, 1980).

Social-psychological perspectives on the coping process emphasize continuing interaction between person and environment, involving a feedback evaluation process in which experience is assessed in terms of its potential for interference with or promotion of adjustment; this process increases levels of sense of personal integration and realization of valued goals. This perspective has been useful in the development of a research tradition for study of the relation of persons and events in determining adjustment—a tradition that does not rely upon assumptions of a psychoanalytic metapsychology focused more on the philosophy of science than on clinical findings (Cohler, in press; Gill, 1976; Klein, 1976). The conceptual framework employed by this social-psychological perspective, as well as research findings, question the need for a concept of a continuum of defense and coping as a means of understanding responses to life changes.

As used within psychoanalytic theory, the concept of defense refers to such processes as blocking off awareness of unacceptable wishes related to the nuclear complex (Freud, 1910) or the triadic family romance; these processes lead to the formation of particular symptoms, which serve as a compromise formation simultaneously providing partial satisfaction of these unacceptable wishes. It may be questioned whether this concept of defense has meaning when employed to portray styles of adjusting to life changes. Rather than extending this concept from the study of intrapsychic processes, particularly as revealed through the study of transference re-enactments in the psychoanalytic situation (Stone, 1954, 1961), discussion of the processes used in adjusting to life changes should refer to strategies used by persons in evaluating and responding to experienced threats and challenges, in order to provide solutions that foster present and subsequent adjustment (Bibring, 1959).

With the exception of continuing studies by Fiske (Lowenthal) and her colleagues (Fiske, 1980a, 1980b; Lowenthal et al., 1975) and by Pearlin, Lieberman, and their colleagues (Menaghan, 1983; Pearlin et al., 1981), there has been little continuing study of the impact of life changes over time and across cohorts. Little is known about continuity over time in coping styles when people are confronted with particular life changes. The selection of particular strategies for solving problems, and even the function of these strategies in resolving problems and dealing with adversity and challenge, are related not just to life changes, but also to one's place in the course of life.

For example, among younger persons, increased suspiciousness and preoccupation with the motives of others are not very effective means for dealing with adversity. However, among very old persons, a so-called "paranoid" stance is predictive of increased longevity after transition from independent living to residential care (Lieberman & Tobin, 1983). Some persons are able to overcome particular adversity or to deal with particular role strains at particular points in the course of life, but they may be unable to cope with stress and strains at either earlier or later points. Findings from studies of the onset of and recovery from schizophrenia suggest that older patients with episodic forms of this disturbance appear more resilient when confronted with personally salient adversity than they did at earlier ages (Cohler & Ferrono, in press). Once again, it becomes clear that the most interesting questions in the study of resilience and coping, as in the study of vulnerability, concern changes in the significance of particular strategies of solving problems associated with particular points in the course of life.

Furthermore, persons within one cohort, who are experiencing particular sociohistorical events in common may use particular means of coping with the impact of role strains, normative events, and unexpected adversity that may not be characteristic of other cohorts. Other than in Elder's continuing study of the Great Depression cohort (Edler, 1979, 1985; Elder, Liker, & Cross, 1984; Elder, Nguyen, & Caspi, 1985; Elder & Rockwell, 1978, 1979), there has been little concern with determining the effects of aging, phase of life course, and cohort as factors associated with the selection of particular coping styles when confronted with changes resulting from normative transition, unexpected adversity, and role strains.

Consideration of continuity and change over time must also include the study of issues of coherence and sense of self in responding to challenges posed by adversity and change. Appriasal of and response to life changes are closely related to a person's present conception of self, including perceived self-efficacy and control (Bandura, 1977, 1982b) and presently experienced coherence or narrative of the life history as a whole (Antonovsky, 1979; Cohler, 1982; Feinstein, 1979; Kris, 1956). This personal narrative, reflecting the coherence of a presently remembered past, experienced present, and anticipated future, is defined by factors as diverse as enduring temperamental influences, place in the course of life, and effects of sociohistorical events affecting a particular cohort. It governs the manner in which particular coping strategies are defined as relevant.

Developmental Study and the Origins of Coping Processes

Inspired in large part by the narrative commitment characteristic of this culture and clearly reflected in both psychoanalytic and social learning perspectives on development (Brim & Ryff, 1980; Cohler, 1982; Ricoeur, 1977), which assumes that lives, like texts, can be understood as organized stories with beginnings, middles, and ends, and that later outcomes may be traced back to origins determining these outcomes, much attention has been devoted to the origins of coping processes during earliest childhood. Since psychoanalysis is among the intellectual frameworks in which this narrative commitment has been most explicitly formulated, it is understandable that the developmental study of coping would be inspired by metapsychological perspectives, particularly the "genetic (epigenetic) point of view," and that derived from ego psychology, or the so-called "adaptive point of view" (Rapaport & Gill, 1959).

The development of stable individual differences in coping techniques are assumed to result from the interplay of relatively stable, constitutionally based cognitive styles or control principles (G. Klein, 1958; R. Gardner, Holzman, Klein, Linton, & Spence, 1959; Witkin, Dyk, Faterson, Goodenough, & Karp, 1962; Witkin, Lewis, Machover, Meissner, & Wapner, 1954) and variations in early experience, such as continuity and consistency of "good enough mothering" (Winnicott, 1960). Based on this formulation, much subsequent study has focused on the emergence of maturationally relevant competencies during infancy and early childhood (Escalona, 1968; MacFarlane, Allen, & Honzik, 1954; Murphy, 1962; O'Malley, 1977).

Additional study has been concerned with the development of the sense of the self as competent—able to bring internal states into harmony with the demands of reality—as a result of the child's experience of early caretaking (Kohut, 1971, 1977). For example, consistent with Sander's (1962, 1976, 1983) characterization of developmentally determined changes in the mother-child relationship during early childhood, Goldberg (1977) has noted the importance of temperamental factors as the basis of the infant's contribution, reflected in variations in the extent to which cues of need states are "readable" by caretakers and responsive to the care that is provided. Less well-organized infants, those more difficult to comfort, are more difficult to care for.

Variations in the quality of the caretaker-child relationship—influenced both by temperamental characteristics of child and caretaker, and by the subsequent complex interaction of stable individual differences of child and caretaker—do appear to be related to the child's subsequent capacity to cope with life changes and to remain resilient when confronted with misfortune (Chess & Thomas, 1984; E. Werner & Smith, 1982; see also Farber and Egeland, Chapter 10, this volume, and Musick, Stott, Spencer, Goldman, & Cohler, Chapter 9, this volume). However, developmental research has too often placed undue emphasis on continuity rather than discontinuity in the study of lives over time (Kagan, 1980, 1984); the basis for later competence traced in the years of earliest childhood has been shown in a number of studies not to yield linear predictors of development with much stability over time (Bayley, 1970; Kagan, 1980; Sameroff & Chandler, 1975; Sameroff, Seifer, & Zax, 1982).

Findings such as those reviewed by Emde (1981), and Emde and Harmon (1984), and reports of the adult outcome of a woman fistula-fed as an infant (Engel, 1967; Engel & Reichsman, 1956; Engel, Reichsman, Horway, & Hess, 1985; Reichsman, 1977; Viederman, 1979) suggest that the course of development may be more flexible and less linear or epigenetic than suggested by both psychoanalytic and cognitive epistemology. Across the course of childhood, as in adulthood, personality development remains open to a variety of influences, including social context; even the effects of relatively significant adversity appear to be reversible (Clarke & Clarke, 1976; Kagan et al., 1979).

As Felsman and Vaillant (Chapter 11, this volume) suggest, the nature of misfortune may be less important than its duration. Temporary disruptions of maternal care may be less adverse than continuing instability of the caretaker–child bond (Rutter, 1979a, 1981a). Emphasis upon issues of continuity, focusing on enduring, early-formed, stable coping styles, may lead to disregard of such other factors as family milieu, development, and even unpredictable life circumstances, which also influence both the nature of and changes in coping styles over time (Garmezy, 1983; Rutter, 1981b, 1984; B. L. White & Associates, 1978; B. L. White, Kaban, & Attanucci, 1979; B. L. White & Watts, 1973).

There has been much interest in the significance of the caretaker-child relationship in the origins of the capacity for resilience. On the one hand, findings from B. L. White's longitudinal study of the origins of competence have suggested that early social exchange between child and caretaker has relatively little lasting impact on the development of competence; much of the contact between mothers and children in this study centered on teaching the children to speak. On the other hand, as Bowlby (1973, 1977), Sroufe (1979; Sroufe, Fox, & Pancake, 1983), E. Werner and Smith (1982), and Musick et al. (Chapter 9, this volume) have all noted, the quality of the child's attachment bonds to the caretaker appears related both to increased sense of self-reliance during childhood and to later resilience when confronted by adversity.

Process studies of coping across the adult years, focusing on the complex interplay of person and situation, have suggested that there are relatively few consistent individual differences over time in preferred manners of resolving problems (Lazarus & Folkman, 1984; Menaghan, 1983; Pearlin & Schooler, 1978). To date, other than in the pioneering studies of Rutter (1975) and of Garmezy and his associates (Garmezy, 1981, 1983; Garmezy & Tellegen, 1984), there has been little effort to use this social-psychological approach in the study of coping across the childhood years.

There has also been little study of developmental factors related to the selection of coping strategies (Sroufe & Rutter, 1984; see also Earls, Beardslee, & Garrison, Chapter 3, this volume; Felsman & Vaillant, Chapter 11, this volume; Fisher, Kokes, Cole, Perkins, & Wynne, Chapter 8, this volume). Changes noted through middle childhood and adolescence in the choice of coping strategies are a function both of social context per se (Pearlin *et al.*, 1981; Rutter, 1984; see also Earls *et al.*, Chapter 3, this volume) and of the shift from maturational factors to those based on social context as the most significant factors in personality development and change (Cohler & Boxer, 1984; Rutter, 1981b; E. Werner & Smith, 1982).

Particularly during the early childhood years, limitations upon particular coping strategies are a function of such maturational factors as difficulty in conceiving of the future, which limits the child's capacity to engage in grief and mourning (Garber, 1981). Differences in the means by which children and adults evaluate and respond to adversity and opportunity are still not clearly understood. Rutter (1981b) has suggested that, as temperamental characteristics are modified by experience, there may be increased variability and differentiation in the manner in which children are able to perceive and respond to problems created by life circumstances.

Resilience, Vulnerability, and Coping with Adversity

Particularly in studies of the determinants of the major psychiatric disorders (schizophrenia and both the unipolar and bipolar affective disorders), there has been increased recognition that constitutional factors such as genetic loading or vulnerability, together with developmental delay in infancy and early childhood, increase vulnerability to later disorder, which occurs in the context of events experienced by such persons as adverse and a source of conflict in present adaptation. In an effort to understand issues of vulnerability and resilience in psychiatry, increased attention has been devoted to the interplay of temperament and life circumstances as factors entering into the origins and course of psychopathology (Escalona, 1968; Thomas & Chess, 1977; Wertheim, 1978). Findings reported by Thomas, Chess, Birch, and Korn (1963), Thomas and Chess (1977), and Chess and Thomas (1984), regarding the stability over time of individual differences in temperament, provide additional support for the importance of Freud's (1905) concept of the "complemental series," emphasizing the interplay of constitution and experience in determining personal adjustment. In fact, Freud viewed biological factors as primary determinants of development during the early infantile period, a perspective later endorsed by Piaget as well (Cohler, in press).[4]

Noting that many persons with major psychiatric disorders show periods of symptom-free functioning fluctuating with episodes of disturbance, Zubin and Spring (1977) and Zubin and Steinhauer (1981) maintain that vulnerability to disorder represents one of the most important aspects of constancy in human development over time; constitutionally based vulnerability appears to interact with particular, interrelated, unexpected adverse life events in producing episodes of disturbance. The work of Zubin and his colleagues provides additional support for the position advanced by Gottesman and his colleagues (Gottesman & Shields, 1982; Hanson, Gottesman, & Heston, 1976; Hanson et al., 1977) that extent of vulnerability varies among persons. Genetically determined vulnerability for major psychopathology may be present to some extent among all persons. Episodes of disturbance may be the result of a necessary set of adverse events that occur in a particular manner and are viewed by persons as particularly disturbing for them at particular points in the course of life (Gutmann, Griffin, & Grunes, 1982).

One possibility, suggested by Zubin and Steinhauer (1981), is that genetic factors may be responsible for the adequacy of learning from experience; persons who are more vulnerable may also be less able to profit from past experience in order to cope with problems in the present. The problem with this perspective is that all unknown factors are attributed to possible genetic determinants, which await discovery by more sophisticated research techniques than exist at present. It remains to be determined whether these markers are characteristic of psychotic states in general, or are specific to particular forms of disturbance. It also remains to be seen whether these markers of vulnerability are primary, or merely accompany other psychophysiological changes observed in particular disorders.

Clearly, there is variability within the population in the extent to which particular forms of disturbance are genetically determined, as well as in the relative saturation of or loading for a particular disturbance among persons in particular families. Findings reported by Gershon and his colleagues (Cytryn, Gershon, & McKnew, 1984; Gershon et al., 1982), based on a comparative study of unipolar and bipolar disturbance, suggest both that bipolar illness is determined by heritable characteristics to a greater extent than unipolar illness, and that genetic saturation within the family line is important in determining the extent of vulnerability to major psychiatric disorder. It is important to note that the interaction of external events and constitutional vulnerability in contributing to the onset of psychiatric episodes is more complex than has often been realized (Wender, 1979).

Consistent with findings reviewed by Hanson et al. (1977), Zubin and Spring (1977), and Zubin and Steinhauer (1981), it may be assumed that each person has some degree of vulnerability, posing particular limitations in coping with particular eruptive, adverse life changes. However, when confronted with misfortune, most persons show marked resilience following an initial period of crisis and strain; they are able to respond reasonably effectively to such challenges to adjust-ment. For example, the children studied by Coles (1964) were mostly able to respond to challenges posed by desegregation in the South in ways that fostered continued adjustment, although some few children were challenged to a degree to which they could not respond.

The children followed in the Coping Studies of Murphy (1962) and Murphy and Moriarty (1976), in a stable Midwestern community, were able to "dose" challenges for themselves, taking their next steps in development at points at which they were able to respond to challenge. Consistent with A. Freud's (1936) discussion of means used by adoles-cents to cope with the increased drive demands of adolescence, Mor-iarty and Toussieng (1976) demonstrated this same capacity for "dos-ing" experience in the response of Coping Studies subjects as adolescents to the social changes and alternative life styles appearing in the late 1960s. Some of these adolescents, particularly the boys, re-affirmed supposedly traditional values, while another group sought opportunities for new experiences. In most instances, as shown in detailed discussion of particular young people, the teenagers were able to regulate the extent of their immersion in the emerging youth culture in ways that felt comfortable for them.

Little is known about the capacity to dose experience in terms that permit efforts at mastery and maintenance of feelings of competence. It is clear that temperament, life circumstances, and cultural context must all be relevant (Ogbu, 1981). Tense infants who show diminished plea-sure in movement and are unable to modulate tensions may later find it difficult to modulate or dose experience in ways providing a positive sense of mastery (Cohler, 1980; Kohut, 1971, 1977; Winnicott, 1960). Among these persons, any amount of challenge may evoke inflexible coping strategies; as a result, they often fail to resolve a particular crisis, and this leads to increased feelings of personal distress. As Csikszentmihalyi (1975) has noted, feelings of personal integration are fostered by situations in which challenge and skills are matched, but anxiety may be increased in those situations in which persons feel inadequate to master challenge. It is important to maintain a dual focus on experienced sense of competence and on the demands posed by particular life circumstances (Menaghan, 1983; Pearlin & Schooler, 1978).

Adverse, off-time, unexpected events may have particular poten-tial for evoking episodes of disturbance among already constitutionally vulnerable persons. However, the agreement regarding the potential of these events for disturbance may be much less evident than might be expected on the basis of scaled ratings of adversity, such as those provided by Holmes and Rahe (1967), Masuda and Holmes (1967, 1968), or Paykel, Prusoff, and Uhlenhuth (1972), which do not differentiate among the three major kinds of life changes—role strain, eruptive or unexpected and adverse events, and normative transitions.

Parental midlife marital separation or divorce may be a particular source of distress for one already vulnerable young adult son or daughter, while other (often younger) brothers or sisters may be better able to cope with the consequences of such events. In the same manner, as Freud (1937) has noted in discussing determinants of the psychoneuroses, subsequent episodes may result from repeated experience to other subjectively experienced life changes, and may not necessarily be related to previous episodes.

Little is known about the adult life course of persons with particular vulnerability (Clausen, 1984; Cohler & Ferrono, in press; Gutmann et al., 1982). As difficult as it is to understand the origins of vulnerability, and the relationship of vulnerability and episodes of disturbance, it is even more difficult to understand the roots of psychological resilience. For example, Meissner (1970) has described a family seen jointly with me, in which the maternal grandmother, the mother, and both the youngest and the oldest of three daughters had been repeatedly hospitalized for schizophrenia. The question posed by study of this family was not only why two daughters experienced psychiatric illness when confronted with life changes not generally viewed as particularly adverse, but also why one daughter remained invulnerable to psychiatric illness. The mother had been hospitalized after the birth of each of her three daughters, while the oldest daughter, of college age, had been hospitalized whenever she attempted to leave the parental home to live in the college residence. The youngest daughter, then in high school, suffered schizophrenic episodes concurrent with those of the oldest daughter, while the middle daughter, a talented musician, received recognition for her attainments, lived apart from the family, and showed little evident vulnerability. She visited each of her sisters in the hospital, was empathic with their problems and those of the family as a whole, and yet managed to avoid becoming enmeshed in the family crisis.

Notable in the hospitalization of other women in the family was the fact that while hospitalization had been associated with life changes, these changes would ordinarily not have been viewed as sufficiently adverse to lead to psychotic episodes. The oldest daughter had attended a nearby junior college, and the transition from home to independent living had been made gradually, without parental pressure, and without alteration of long-standing patterns of interdependence across generations (Boszormenyi-Nagy & Spark, 1973; Coelho, Hamburg, & Murphey, 1967; Silber et al., 1961). Even this most gradual life change, however, was stressful for the already vulnerable oldest daughter; in turn, her distress affected the equally vulnerable youngest daughter. Clearly, psychiatric hospitalization of a sibling is a stressful event within any family (Howard, 1978). Even where there are problems of differentiation of self and others, this event is not one characteristically assumed to be of such magnitude as to lead to psychiatric episodes among siblings, except among already vulnerable persons.

Developmental Perspectives on Resilience

All persons are potentially vulnerable to personal distress at different times and for different reasons; they may react in an inflexible and stereotyped manner when confronting adverse events that are particularly salient and painful because of individual differences in life experiences. In a similar manner, the concept of invulnerability, stress resistance, or resilience is also relative, referring to the capacity to maintain feelings of personal integration and sense of competence when confronted by particular adversity.[5]

Another way of understanding this issue is to assume that basic energy is available for the task of modulating both external stimuli and the experience of bodily states and thoughts. Otherwise well-functioning persons, with no unusual vulnerability or sensitivity, will generally meet on-time or normative developmental tasks with a sense of competence, using available tasks and skills in the service of mastery. Challenges to development based on such normative transitions as graduation from grade school or high school are, by definition, dosed as long as they are on time and expectable; this permits preparation, in addition to the support of consociates experiencing similar events (Neugarten & Hagestad, 1976; Plath, 1980).

For example, among preschoolers already vulnerable to any disruption in development, even expectable events represent a threat to present adjustment. Under these circumstances—and depending upon such innate characteristics as tempo, and other aspects of prenatal and neonatal life likely to predispose to lessened resilience (Heider, 1966; Mednick, 1978; Thomas & Chess, 1984; Thomas, Chess, Birch, & Korn, 1963; E. Werner, Bierman, & French, 1971; E. Werner & Smith, 1977, 1982), as well as the emotional climate of the family—the more vulnerable child may react to an expectable event by withdrawing from parents, denying problems in having to share parental concern with another, or a variety of other responses.

After a period of difficulty, perhaps resulting in temporary loss of toilet training or other evidence of returning to less developmentally appropriate solutions to socialization issues, the child "recovers" from the disruption and becomes willing to take the next developmentally appropriate step, such as entrance into nursery school. Again, this depends upon the balance of resilience and vulnerability, as well as the nature of the adversity. From this perspective, "coping strategies" refers primarily to appraisal and response to challenges stemming from the world outside the child as these interact with the child's needs and concerns. Increased reliance on less flexible (defensive) coping approaches, which are also less amenable to change over time, may make adjustment more difficult in situations where complex and flexible solutions are required.

Resilience and Adversity: Coping Strategies among Children within Socially Disorganized Families

FAMILIES IN POVERTY

Over the past decade, Garmezy and his students have been involved in a series of related studies designed to isolate factors associated with increased resistance to stress in childhood. Findings based on the study of disadvantaged inner-city children suggested that maintenance of the capacity to relate positively to peers, and, to a limited extent, adequate intelligence, differentiated the better-adapted from the more poorly adapted children in this high-stress group.

The first research with the inner-city group used economic privation as a measure of adverse outcomes. There are a number of problems with this concept of stress, including problems in determining precisely those aspects of economic privation that are stressful (Elder, 1974, 1985). Study of generations of families living in poverty requires focus upon those aspects of poverty that are most significant for children as factors interfering with adjustment and the maintenance of resilience. Furthermore, differentiations need to be made between families living in recent or temporary poverty and the multigeneration welfare families portrayed by Stack (1974). Indeed, Garmezy (1981) notes that the large majority of children living in poverty are well able to adjust to this life circumstance. According to an earlier literature review (Garmezy & Nuechterlein, 1972), these children do not appear to differ from their more advantaged counterparts. Economic privation and advantage become socially constructed understandings that these children have of themselves and their development (Brim & Ryff, 1980; Hultsch & Plemons, 1979).

While children of the slums may show some degree of invulnerability, it is also true that children of the suburbs may not necessarily be invulnerable; they may only not yet have been forced to deal with life circumstances that would test areas of vulnerability (Coles, 1975). It is not uncommon for children of the suburbs to establish impressive secondary school records, characterized by impressive intellectual attainments and social success, only to experience personal distress at college that sometimes leads to the development of psychiatric symptoms. Removed from an environment in which they have felt safe and admired, these gifted young people feel threatened by adversity that interacts with areas of vulnerability never before tested.

Subsequent research by Garmezy's research group, using a stress score based on Coddington's (1972a, 1972b) measure of life event stress in the lives of children, together with a detailed parental interview of life circumstances, led to the following conclusions. First, consistent with the inner-city studies, those children who were more stress-resistant in terms of achievement and behavior at school and adjustment at home, and who showed at least average intellectual ability, were better able to maintain a socially decentered perspective (Pellegrini, 1980). Second, more stress-resistant children were better able to remain engaged in and attend to school and showed good cognitive control, particularly when there was adequate intellectual functioning (Ferrarese, 1981). Divergent thinking (Guilford, 1950; Wallach & Kogan, 1965), together with adequate intellectual resources and a sense of humor, was also associated with increased adequacy of school performance, including social involvement with peers (Masten, 1982). Reflecting Allport's (1937) observations regarding sense of humor as essential in positive mental health, children with a good sense of humor were flexible, creative children who could think of alternative solutions for problems created by life changes. Viewed in terms of the literature on coping in adulthood, these children were effective in appraising alternatives for solving problems with which they were presented (Lazarus & Folkman, 1984).

While it is difficult to determine the impact of particular adverse events (apart from normative transitions and role strain) as factors associated with variations in resilience among these children, findings of Garmezy's research group have been consistent with those of other investigators whose work Garmezy (1981) has reviewed, as well as with that of Murphy (1974; see also Chapter 4, this volume), Felsman (1981), and Felsman and Vaillant (Chapter 11, this volume). Together, these investigators suggest that children who remain resilient are able to use flexible coping strategies in overcoming adversity, rather than reacting in a brittle and rigid manner.

More resilient children appear to have increased levels of sensory-neural integration, which help them to resist the effects of adversity; they show reflective rather than impulsive cognitive styles (Kagan, 1966), using extended trial action or thought (Rapaport, 1951). In addition, these more resilient children demonstrate higher intelligence; more divergent or creative thinking in approaching problems; increased capacity to select out the particular aspects of adversity required to be overcome; and use of goal-oriented strategies in order to plan means for taking these steps without becoming lost in the hopelessness of the situation. They also maintain good control over feelings, with capacity to plan ahead and to think rather than to act. They show increased persistence and a greater sense of mastery over their own lives. Of particular significance, and found also among children living with other forms of social disorganization, these more resilient children show increased capacity for finding comfort and satisfaction in their own efforts at soothing and solace, rather than depending upon others for such comfort.

PARENTAL PSYCHOPATHOLOGY

Findings similar to those regarding children subjected to adversity of poverty have been reported by investigators studying children with a parent hospitalized for psychiatric illness. Children in these families have often experienced unstable caretaking over periods of many years; multiple caretakers during times when parents (typically mothers) were hospitalized; and continuing problems as a result of living with caretakers whose actions and moods are often unpredictable, and who may have idiosyncratic understandings of the real world (Cohler, Gallant, Grunebaum, & Kaufman, 1983; Grunebaum, Gamer, & Cohler, 1983; Grunebaum, Weiss, Cohler, Hartman, & Gallant, 1982).

   Much of our present understanding of the means by which children of psychiatrically ill parents maintain resilience comes from detailed studies by Garmezy and his colleagues (Garmezy, 1981; Garmezy, Masten, Nordstrom, & Ferrarese, 1979), and from Anthony's (1974b, 1976) initial studies of "invulnerability." Anthony (1976) has noted that the children he studied resisted becoming engulfed in the parental psychopathology; showed curiosity in understanding what it was that troubled the ill parent; maintained a compassionate but detached approach to the troubled parent; were not overwhelmed by a series of interconnected troublesome life events; and were able to receive some emotional support from the well parent. Similar findings emerged in Garmezy's (1971, 1974, 1981) study of resilient offspring of psychologically troubled parents, as well as in Rutter's (1979b, 1981b) reports on the study of invulnerable offspring of psychotic parents. Indeed, about 10% showed genuine creativity—a figure that compares with observations regarding similar children observed by Heston (1966), Heston and Denny (1968), and Kaufman, Grunebaum, Cohler, and Gamer (1979).

   In each of these independent studies, a group of children of schizophrenic parents was identified who appeared to be even more effective, creative, and competent than counterparts from families in which there was no history of parental psychiatric illness. Based on a study of persons in a self-contained and geographically isolated Scandinavian community, Karlsson (1968) has reported that a higher proportion of creative adults and first-degree relatives diagnosed with schizophrenia than less creative counterparts. These findings would suggest that the same genetic determinants are involved in the unusual perceptions characteristic of distinctive creative attainment and of schizophrenic illness.

Outcomes favoring invulnerability or vulnerability depend on the degree of genetic loading or saturation, as well as on the often accidental contact with particular life changes likely to lead to the onset of psychiatric symptoms (Rutter & Garmezy, 1983). Much attention has been focused on the small number of vulnerable children of parents with major psychopathology who show psychiatric distress. It is equally important to consider the large number of offspring who remain invulnerable—able to adjust favorably to life circumstances that include such disruptions as continued parental discord, family preoccupation with the mental health of the troubled parent, and increased expectations for the offspring themselves to assume a degree of personal maturity and responsibility not expected among their age-mates.

Often, children of troubled parents are expected to monitor parental mental health, to watch for signs of increased parental depression or personal disorganization, and to assume some degree of parental care for their own troubled parents. At the same time, as Anthony (1971, 1974b), Garmezy (1983), and Fisher *et al.* (Chapter 8, this volume) all have noted, these children may cope with problems presented by parental psychiatric illness, such as *folie à deux* and parentification, through maintaining curiosity about the origins and course of the ill parent's disturbance, developing an objective yet compassionate approach, and assuming caretaking roles only after a lengthy period of exposure and development of psychological immunity.[6]

One 12-year-old son of a schizophrenic mother complains that he can't bring his friends over to the house after school because he can never be sure what state his mother will be in: "Sometimes she acts so crazy that it scares my friends. They think she's some sort of monster like Frankenstein." Significant in this boy's comment is the fact that he has a number of close friends and that he has a number of other interests outside the house, including participation in the school band and a morning paper route. His multiply rehospitalized mother has successfully resisted the effects of antipsychotic medication in ways similar to those described by Van Putten, Crumpton, and Yale (1976) and Van Putten, May, Marder, and Wittmann (1981) for a small number of cases. Complaining that he never expected to be married to a "crazy" woman, this boy's father has long since succeeded in obtaining a divorce and moving to another community, where he has remarried and started another family.

This boy, full of life, is able to reach out to other adults. His mother's brother, who has a son of about the same age, has provided a second home and is regarded as like a father. This boy has also been able to interest his teachers in various projects such as a class newspaper, and spends much of his time out of school working on the newspaper, playing in the band, or involved with other projects. As both Anthony (1974b) and Kaufman *et al.* (1979) have noted, the capacity of offspring to use other adults as substitutes for emotionally unavailable parents is an important characteristic differentiating more from less resilient offspring of psychiatrically ill parents. As a result of his ability to avoid spending time at home, particularly at times when his mother is disturbed, this presently resilient boy is able to avoid becoming enmeshed in his mother's disturbance.[7] To date, we know little regarding means for increasing competence among those young people "at risk" for psychiatric illness (Marlowe & Weinberg, 1985; Ricks, 1980; Shure, 1981; Tyler & Gatz, 1977; Wine, 1981; Wrubel, Brenner, & Lazarus, 1981).

While it does not necessarily result in the appearance of symptoms, the strain for children that is engendered by living with a psychiatrically ill parent and the accompanying adverse family changes (Grunebaum *et al.*, 1983; Rutter, 1981b) may lead to other signs of personal distress. This distress appears to be more significant among the children of parents (primarily mothers) with an affective disorder than among children of parents with a schizophrenic disorder. Much of the discussion to date has concerned social competence (Kent & Rolf, 1979; Lewine, Watt, & Fryer, 1978), particularly the capacity to make friends and to use adults in positive ways (Garmezy, 1983; Kaufman *et al.*, 1979; Rolf, 1976; see also Musick *et al.*, Chapter 9, this volume).

As Rutter (1981b), Garmezy (1983), and Worland, Weeks, and Janes (Chapter 7, this volume) have all noted, intellectual ability is also important. Children who are better able to understand events in their lives are also better able to figure out strategies for coping with these events.[8] Reviewing the basis of Piaget's lifelong interest in the study of adaptation to reality, Anthony (1971; see also Chapter 6, this volume) notes that Piaget had a mother who was recurrently psychiatrically ill. Anthony suggests that Piaget's reluctance to consider emotional life beyond shared moral sentiments, as in his interruption of a just-begun personal analysis, was motivated by concern that he might lose his own precious ties to reality. However, this insistence upon adherence to reality facilitated mastery and increased resilience.

While there is little evidence that higher intelligence alone promotes more effective coping, several studies of the young children of schizophrenic mothers suggest that intelligence is positively associated with resilience (Worland *et al.*, Chapter 7, this volume), as is the capacity to organize free play and to actively reach out to others for help in observed sessions of mother–child interaction (Earls *et al.*, Chapter 3, this volume; Musick *et al.*, Chapter 9, this volume). Consistent with findings reported by Kaufman *et al.* (1979), more competent offspring of both schizophrenic and depressed mothers are better able to use other adults as resources in time of distress. Similar findings have been reported among offspring of psychiatrically ill parents by Fisher *et al.* (Chapter 8, this volume). Furthermore, consistent with earlier findings reported by Rodnick and Goldstein (1974), these more competent children also tend to have parents hospitalized later in the child's development, with some parental capacity for positive responding still available to the child (Fisher *et al.*, Chapter 8, this volume). This latter finding is also consistent with Anthony's (1974b) report that resilience is enhanced by having at least one parent able to effectively respond to the child's needs.

In sum, the children of psychiatrically ill parents who are better able to cope with the adversity of unreliable and often emotionally inaccessible caretakers have innate ego strength, creative abilities, and increased personal and physical attractiveness; these traits enable these children to continue to reach out to others for support. To the extent that their parents are able to provide care and assistance, these more resilient children appear to be successful in engaging the parents. When a disturbed parent is not accessible, these children do not give up in their efforts to obtain adult care, turning instead to such other available adults as relatives, teachers, and family friends. Finally, these children often have greater intelligence and come from families higher in social status; in turn, these qualities foster increased instrumental mastery and greater social skills.

The social skills and early socialization into self-reliance characteristic of middle-class families (Kohn, 1969; Winterbottom, 1958) facilitate efforts at increased personal autonomy and responsibility. These children also develop hobbies, take jobs outside the home, and find other activities that prevent them from becoming enmeshed in parental psychopathology (Anthony, 1971, 1974b). Finally, on the basis of clinical study, it may be suggested that these more resilient children use the adversity of their earlier years as a challenge to be overcome. The very fact of their troubled childhood becomes used as an element of a developing narrative of a life devoted to disproving the "odds" of developing psychiatric illness; the children may work even harder to avoid the same affliction as their parents.

At the same time that these better-coping children develop techniques for avoiding involvement in parental psychopathology, their very success in this endeavor may be achieved at considerable personal cost. Many of these children develop interests in science and technology (Grunebaum et al., 1982) without parallel sustained concern with intimate relationships. Successful in their studies, they may be less able to sustain the kind of close relationships that are important in coping with such important role transitions of adulthood as marriage and parenthood.

Often, these successfully coping children rely effectively upon denial as a "defense," are reluctant to explore their own feelings, and maintain rigid concern with the mechanical world. Similar concerns about the cost of maintaining resilience have been noted by Rutter (1981b, p. 24) in reviewing studies of response to life changes among adults. Rutter observes that those persons who were more resilient also appeared to have less caring relations with others and were unduly concerned with their own needs and interests.

There has also been little study of changes in coping techniques across early and middle childhood and the adolescent years, or among boys and girls of either schizophrenic or affectively disordered parents. For example, findings reported by Mednick and colleagues (Mednick, Schulsinger, Teasdale, Schulsinger, Venables, & Rock, 1978) suggest that maternal psychopathology may be more directly linked to later psychiatric illness among women than among men supporting earlier clinical observations of G. Gardner (1967) who suggests that maternal psychopathology may be more directly associated with later psychiatric illness among girls than among boys, while my colleagues and I (Cohler, Gallant, Grunebaum, Weiss, & Gamer, 1976) and Rutter (1970) suggest that boys may find it more difficult than girls to cope with the impact of parental psychiatric illness. These findings are consistent with those reported by Elder and Rockwell (1979) that the effects of the Great Depression were more adverse for those who were preschool boys than those who were preschool girls at the time of economic privation. Underemployment and unemployment often cause men to lose morale and to leave their families; this is particularly difficult for sons, who may be in the midst of resolving complex, ambivalent feelings and who lose an important source of identification, rather than daughters, who continue to enjoy both maternal care and the opportunity to resolve issues of mother–daughter rivalry.

Finally, it should be noted that little progress has been made in the development of standardized instruments for evaluating coping and resilience. Dibble and Cohen (1974) have reported on an instrument to be used by mothers in evaluating coping behavior of young children, and used by researchers in larger-scale epidemiological study. Based on Murphy and Moriarty's (1976) report on coping and resilience, Zeitlin (1980) has developed a profile of coping behaviors, which are rated on the basis of direct observation of children. While adequate interobserver reliability is reported, Zeitlin notes the problems inherent in developmental study, where changing social context interacts with maturational factors, leading to little stability in rating over time.

Caution regarding the evaluation of resilience in longitudinal study has been recommended by Rutter (1984), Farber and Egeland (Chapter 10, this volume), and Fisher *et al.* (Chapter 8, this volume), all of whom note the problems of evaluating stability in resilience over time. As a consequence of regression to the mean, the child who appears most resilient at one point in time may occupy a less extreme position upon subsequent evaluation. A partial solution for this problem is to provide multiple measurement points, rather than measurement only at two points.

Resilience and Experienced Life History

The predictive approach to the study of characteristic means for appraising and resolving problems associated with adversity has been important in delineating the various means used. At the same time, this approach provides little information regarding the manner in which persons understand or interpret misfortune. For some persons at some points in the course of life, particular forms of adversity are experienced as insurmountable obstacles; others are able to use these misfortunes as the basis for renewed efforts at coping, leading to continued resilience. As both Hultsch and Plemons (1979) and Brim and Ryff (1980) have noted, more detailed study is required of the dimensions that are salient for particular persons in interpreting and responding to problems associated with particular life changes. There are still relatively few studies of the manner in which persons reflect upon their own past experiences as a resource promoting later resilience and coping. Murphy (1982) has published a case study detailing her earlier work with a girl who showed multiple learning problems, leading to developmental disability. With years of patient work, this girl was able to gain increased self-confidence; her school attainments increased, and she ultimately became a self-supporting adult able to cope with adversity and turmoil. Murphy shows that the child's experience of a supposed limitation in coping ability, and her determination to overcome this limitation, served to motivate her achievement in ways that never would have been thought possible. Colona (1981) has noted similar determination to overcome the limitations of a physical handicap in her continuing study of blind children observed from early childhood through adulthood.

In his book describing the adversity imposed by the extraordinary disorganization of his family, which led him to delinquency during childhood, W. Brown (1983) has recounted his effort to use this earlier difficulty as a resource in realizing later professional success—first as a youth officer helping other troubled youths, and later as a scholar in the area of delinquency and culture. In a similar manner, Elder (1974) and Elder and Rockwell (1979) show that one effect of having grown up in the poverty inspired by the Great Depression was increased determination to do better in life. Among the Great Depression cohort, experience of early adversity was used as a force propelling persons toward success in later life, albeit more as a consequence of the fear of failure than of confidence in the certainty of success. Anthony's account of Piaget's biography suggests that his career was influenced by a determination to overcome obstacles, particularly those imposed by having an episodically psychiatrically ill mother. Piaget's search for the rules according to which children order reality was fostered by concern that without such determined adherence to reality, he would suffer a fate similar to that of his mother.

Common to each of these accounts in which past adversity has become the basis for later resilience is the use of the personal narrative, or presently experienced life history, in an effort to cope effectively with earlier adversity. At the same time, at least in Elder's (1974) study of the Great Depression cohort, this use of the personal past as a resource in maintaining resilience also leads to some problems; these include limitations of flexibility in solving problems and increased concern about taking risks, both of which appear to constrain the ability to evaluate alternatives in the search for the most effective problem-solving strategies (Lazarus & Folkman, 1984). However, little is known about the manner in which persons create particular narratives and become committed to particular strategies for resolving problems that are most consistent with their sense of self and the totality of their life histories.

The value of an interpretive approach as a complement to the predictive approach becomes even greater as a result of findings emerging from longitudinal studies (Emde, 1981; Jones, Bayley, MacFarlane, & Honzik, 1971; Kagan & Moss, 1963; Livson & Peskin, 1980; Moss & Susman, 1980; Rutter, 1984; see also Felsman & Vaillant, Chapter 11, this volume), showing that lives are not as ordered and predictable over time as had previously been assumed. To the extent that lives show predictability, this order may be more a function of shared understanding regarding the linear organization of the expectable course of life in this culture than of continuity reflected by data collected at multiple observation points.

In an effort to account for apparent discontinuity observed in lives over time, Kagan and Moss (1963), Clarke and Clarke (1981), and Peskin and Livson (1982) have all described "sleeper effects" in development, in which particular developmental attributes are associated with outcomes later in life, but not necessarily at more intermediate points. Although, at least to some extent, these reported relationships may reflect the unreliability of the underlying measures, they may also reflect the discontinuous nature of lives over time when viewed from the relatively experience-distant perspective of the predictive approach.

Focus on demonstration of stability and order, rather than on discontinuity across the course of life, may have led investigators to miss the most interesting questions about lives. The important issue is not how lives stay the same over time, or even how the means used for solving problems associated with misfortune show continuity across different ages; rather, it is how to account for factors leading to change in coping strategies across the course of life (Emde & Harmon, 1984; Neugarten, 1969, 1979). Rather than viewing human development in a linear, epigenetic, or orthogenetic perspective, which has characterized earlier discussion (Abraham, 1924; Erikson, 1963; Freud, 1905, 1915–1917; H. Werner, 1940), it may be more relevant to adopt a perspective stressing dramatic, often discontinuous transformations of personality over time, often as a result of chance encounters fashioned by an individual into a life story that is experienced as having continuity (Bandura, 1982a; Cohler, 1982; Cohler & Carney, in press; Emmerich, 1968; Gergen, 1977, 1982; Rutter, 1984).

As a consequence of changing approaches to the study of lives over time, there has been increased awareness of the importance of studying persons' own accounts of their lives (Hultsch & Plemons, 1979). Persons differ both in the extent and the means according to which reconstructed experience of the past is used to turn present adversity into challenge or opportunity (Cohler, 1980). These accounts are based on a story or personal narrative (Antonovsky, 1979; Cohler, 1982; Feinstein, 1979; Kris, 1956); of the presently experienced past and present and the anticipated future, including adverse, eruptive events as these events are perceived to have affected the course of life (Cohler, 1982; Freeman, 1984; Kris, 1956).

Retrospective study of lives necessarily involves a linear narrative commitment because of the culturally shared template within our own society of the story as a creative act having a beginning, a middle, and an end, with the elements of the story organized in a coherent manner (Ricoeur, 1977). Even when works of art set out to violate these shared assumptions, with a presentation purposively denying these assumptions, the shared view is the normative account forming the structure for understanding the artist's departure from this accepted account.

As a result of the commitment to a linear narrative, both for stories and for lives, that is shared by all persons in our own society, it is always possible to reorganize these experiences so that they *appear* to fit into an ordered narrative. Indeed, the failure to be able to maintain a coherent life history is characteristic of psychopathology of the self (Kohut, 1977). At the same time, it should be noted that persons differ in the extent to which they are explicitly concerned with maintenance of this linear narrative commitment; this concern, as a coping tehnique for preserving resilience, may also vary across the life course.

The "life review," as portrayed by Butler (1963), is one example of the reliance upon a strict linear order as a coping technique in dealing with the crisis of finitude. Butler has noted that older persons differ in the extent to which they engage in a life review, or integration of the remembered past in an effort to find meaning in life, which in turn is an effort to resolve the crisis of finitude of life represented by increased realization of the finality of death (Marshall, 1981; Munnichs, 1966). Findings reported by Lieberman and Falk (1972) suggest that middle-aged persons are more likely to use reminiscence, or present recon-structions of the past, in the service of active solution of problems, while older persons are more likely to use reminiscence as a life review, providing solace and comfort when confronted with the finality of death.

In an effort to maintain a coherent personal narrative, or interpre-tation of the significance of the experienced past for the present, an individual relies upon presently imagined past experiences, including those that have become a part of family legend, and accidents of fate or aleotoric events (Bandura, 1982a; Gergen, 1977, 1982; Rutter, 1984), regardless of their actual occurrence. The narrative that is constructed from these elements represents the most complete possible account that a person is able to provide, at any particular time, of the interrela-tionship among events taking place over a lifetime, including their significance for present intents and actions.

For example, Piaget (Bringuier, 1980) relates an event from his own childhood in which, while he and his nanny were out for a walk, a kidnapper was supposed to have attempted to take him from his car-riage. Piaget notes that he could remember the event as if it were yesterday, including the policeman summoned by the nanny, the length of the policeman's cape, and the place of the abduction. Years later, the nursemaid had to tell the grateful parents that the whole scene was untrue, and that it had been fabricated to obtain a monetary reward.

Piaget narrates this story in the process of questioning the empha-sis placed by psychoanalysis upon past experiences as direct, linear determinants of later wishes and intents. It is clear that psychoanalysis has long struggled to resolve problems regarding the relationship of early experience to later outcomes. As early as the *Project for a Scientific Psychology* (Freud, 1895), never destroyed yet never published, Freud described events from early childhood that were associatively con-nected by analysands with present conflicts. As already noted in the discussion of psychoanalytic formulations of a genetic ordering of the defenses, much of the previous concern within psychoanalysis with the genetic point of view was based on Freud's determination to find a means for the study of experience that would be in accord with the philosophy of science during the late 19th century (Klein, 1976; Sulloway, 1979). This metapsychological study, reflecting cultural commitment to history as ordered in a linear manner, must be differentiated from the clinical method, which is devoted to understanding the analysand's particular construction of experience.

The capacity to continually rewrite the story of one's own life is shared by those who study lives (Freeman, 1984), and may be one of the reasons why it has been so difficult for developmental psychology to understand the complex determinants of the life history or personal narrative (Emde, 1981; Emde & Harmon, 1984). As Kagan (1980, 1984), Emde (1981), and Emde and Harmon (1984) have noted, predictive developmental study is overly concerned with demonstration of a linear or epigenetic ordering of the course of development, and has been unable to account for the discontinuity so often reported in studies of lives over time.

The clinical theory in psychoanalysis (Klein, 1976), which is concerned with the process by which the personal narrative changes over time, may be one method that may be used as a means for increased understanding of the dynamics determining changing uses of the personal past across the course of life. As Winnicott (1951), Green (1975, 1978), and Schafer (1981, 1983) have emphasized, one of the major accomplishments of clinical psychoanalytic interventions—and, to a lesser extent, all psychotherapy—is the joint construction by analyst and analysand of a mutually shared, jointly acceptable life story. Furthermore, the clinical psychoanalytic method demands that both participants become aware of their own assumptions about self and the course of experience, including the predisposition to a linear or epigenetic ordering of the past when such a linear commitment may not fit the analysand's own experience of the past.

The jointly constructed narrative or account of the analysand's life history replaces the one that the analysand has presented at the outset, and that has made it so difficult to overcome the compulsion to repeat the past (Cohler, 1981, 1982; Cohler & Freeman, in press); the reconstruction relies upon the analyst's empathic skills for apprehending the manner in which others experience their own lives. The consequence of this experience-near effort is an explicit focus on the process of creating a life history or personal narrative, particularly through observation of the variety of enactments of the past brought into the analytic setting by the analysand, together with changing perspectives on these enactments as a result of making them explicit in terms of present wishes and intents.

This explicit concern with the process of creating a life story that is experienced as coherent, and that fosters increased capacity to deal with adversity, provides a unique opportunity for studying the manner in which persons use the experienced past in an effort to resolve present dilemmas. It should be recognized that analyst and analysand, characteristically sharing a concern with history as linear and ordered, may come to recognize that some past adversity that has been attributed by the analysand and others to a particular life change over which there may have been some control could actually have been an accident of fate or a chance event.

A coherent life history that serves as a template for determining future actions may include explicit recognition of such chance events, and may also reflect an effort to make particular meaning or reason out of prior adversity. The joint creation of a revised personal narrative through the psychoanalytic process includes explicit consideration of the problems imposed by the commitment to a linear, connected view of history among persons in this society, including analyst and analysand. It is this explicit attention to the reasons for stories that are told and events that are recounted in the analysis of transference and other enactments, as experienced and understood by both participants, that provides a unique opportunity for studying the determinants of the personal narrative, including the effect of shared commitment to a view of lives as organized in a linear manner.

The problem with the predictive approach to the study of lives, as contrasted with the interpretive approach (such as is represented by study of the psychoanalytic process), is that the predictive approach makes it difficult to differentiate the particular narrative commitment that forms the basis of data collection and analysis from the one that is experienced by those persons whose lives are being studied. This commitment on the part of investigators to either a linear or an orthogenetic ordering of lives over time makes it difficult to study the impact of chance events on the course of life; to study the changing context in which the past is interpreted across the course of life; or to study the manner in which persons presently understand the relationship between past and present experience, so critical in understanding the meaning of earlier adversity for present adjustment.

For example, while variations that are experienced in the quality of maternal care are believed to have some impact upon the nature of both present and subsequent adjustment, the nature of this impact is still not clearly understood (Rutter, 1979a, 1981a). In the first place, as Piaget's charming anecdote suggests, it is the memory of the event and not the event itself that is important in later life. The important motivating factor is the presently remembered event, and not the event as it actually happened in the past.

In the second place, there is little reason to assume that the event remembered at a particular point in the course of life will be remembered in the same way at some later point. Vaillant and McArthur (1972) report that memories of their adolescence provided by middle-aged men differed in systematic ways from the memories provided by these men during their college years. Elder (1985) reports that even memories of life in military service in World War II differed markedly over a period of two decades—a period that was also characterized by movement from young adulthood to the "stable adult years" (Cohler & Boxer, 1984).

Future research on the use of the experienced personal history as a resource in resolving misfortune must include the present point in the life course, as socially defined within particular cohorts, as an essential determinant of the manner in which the past is reconstructed in resolving misfortune. Within a particular cohort, defined in terms of shared sociohistorical events, life changes—the building blocks of the personal narrative—are differently remembered, and they change their function at successive points in life as a result of socially defined changes in the meaning of age and aging from earliest childhood to oldest age (Cohler & Corney, in press).

Nowhere is this changing perspective on the past across the course of life better shown than in Elder's continuing study of the impact of the Great Depression upon the subsequent course of life (Elder, Liker, & Cross, 1984). Comparing persons from families showing at least a one-third decrease in income with those not showing this income loss, Elder has found that the experience of privation led to conservatism and sense of concern, particularly among the men in the study; this pattern has continued in this cohort as long as these men have been followed, through late middle age (Elder & Rockwell, 1979).

Predictive and interpretive approaches may each make an important contribution to the study of resilience in lives over time. It is necessary to combine these two perspectives if we are to understand the origin and later transformations of the capacity to resolve misfortune. The predictive approach suffers from the limitations imposed by socially constructed concepts of lives and stories: These are necessarily understood in a linear manner, but this commitment cannot be included as a factor in the study of persons' reconstruction of their lives over time. The predictive approach also suffers from the failure to include shifting meanings attributed to past experiences across the course of life as determinants of present efforts at resolving problems for continued morale and adjustment.

Predictive studies of coping and resilience have the virtue, at least in theory, of being verifiable in terms of external criteria beyond the coherence of the narrative itself. At the same time, this verifiability requires some sacrifice of understanding of wishes and intents, including the sacrifice induced by the need to maintain a coherent autobiography that permits persons to deal with adverse events (e.g., early childhood poverty or disruptions in caretaking, which might otherwise be assumed to be a source of increased later vulnerability). At least to some extent, in the effort to provide verifiable findings, predictive studies are unable to account for precisely those aspects of the life history that may be most important in understanding resilience over time, in response to particular forms of adversity.

Conclusion

Resilience to adversity—the ability to cope with unexpected, eruptive events, pressures imposed by strains of everyday life, and lack of available social supports in dealing with expected life transitions—appears to be relative, determined by constitutionally imposed limitations upon the range of available strategies for solving problems, as well as by the constraints imposed by particular life changes. At least to some extent, variations in resilience during childhood, resulting from temperament and the experience of particular events (e.g., significant losses and extreme poverty), have an impact upon later choice of coping strategies. At the same time, across the adult years, maturational constraints yield to those determined by shared understandings of the course of life, and to expectable life transitions, as important determinants of coping strategies.

Over the past several years, there have been important changes in understanding the means by which persons deal with personal misfortune and problems imposed by role strain and overload. Findings from these studies have raised important questions regarding the generalizability of strategies for resolving problems across particular events and roles. Other findings have clarified the process by which persons cope with adversity and role strain.

This advance in understanding the means used by adults in coping with problems arising in their lives has raised serious questions regarding the adequacy of prior formulations of coping processes derived from the study of intrapsychic conflict. Based on metapsychology, or the philosophy of science within psychoanalytic theory, rather than upon clinical theory, which emerges from the detailed study of lives, earlier discussions of defenses relied too greatly upon Freud's metaphor of epigenesis in psychic life derived from his earlier study in developmental neurobiology. Even though critics of an epigenetic ordering of defenses, from Anna Freud to Guy Swanson, have questioned the value of this ordering, efforts have continued to employ an approach that seems to have little value in understanding the dynamics of adjustment to life changes.

Clinical psychoanalytic perspectives are particularly concerned with the constructions that persons make of their lives. To date, the relationship of this intrapsychic experience and adjustment to life changes has not been clarified; little correspondence has been shown between wishes or thoughts and actions. Indeed, much effort is devoted in the clinical psychoanalytic process to clarifying this correspondence for particular persons. Much more must be learned about determinants of wishes and intents before it will be possible to specify the conditions according to which these wishes and thoughts influence particular coping strategies.

Efforts at understanding this relationship between wishes and actions may be best pursued according to a narrative rather than a survey approach to the study of lives. Survey perspectives can provide important information regarding characteristics of coping strategies that are useful in resolving personal misfortune. However, detailed narrative study may provide important information regarding the manner in which the past is used as a means of resolving present problems. This study must include recognition that conceptions of past, present, and future change over time, not only for persons, but also across cohorts. The dialectic approach, pioneered by Riegel (1978), would be of great value in understanding the continuing transaction between personal and collective history, at different ages and across groups of persons with shared experience of particular events.

Much of the discussion of resilience has focused on positive aspects of the capacity to resist the otherwise adverse effects of events as dramatically different as early childhood economic privation, physical and psychiatric illness, and discontinuities in child care. Findings from studies of persons otherwise vulnerable as a consequence of increased genetic risk for major psychopathology, or of growing up in extreme poverty or social disorganization, all report on unexpected resilience characterized by positive life attainments.

It should be noted that these studies have not yet focused on the particular coping strategies associated with differences in resilience. It is possible that persons continue to show resilience only because they have not yet encountered that adversity, unique to their own life experience, that interacts with constitutionally derived vulnerability in order to produce episodes of major psychiatric disorder. From this perspective, continued resilience may simply be good fortune on the part of otherwise vulnerable persons.

Even assuming that resilience represents a positive response to adversity, it is likely that morale may be adversely affected by the continued effort at coping with misfortune, or that resilience in one set of circumstances may not be related to later resilience. For example, adults in the cohort of the Great Depression, who were distinguished by being able to rise out of economic privation, may not be sensitive to the misfortunes of others. These men and women express continuing concern regarding the ever-present danger of sliding back into poverty, and tend to be somewhat careful and tentative in their appraisal of and response to life experiences.

Personal success may be attained at the cost of spontaneous enjoyment of life. Resilient offspring of parents with episodic psychiatric disorder often show strong interests in science and other pursuits in which predictability and "thing-oriented" perspectives may be more important than the attainment of satisfying relationships. Often, these offspring feel pressured to maintain maturity and responsibility for themselves and others, which may have later costs in terms of continuing adjustment. However, there have been few studies following persons identified as resilient over longer periods of time. Studies such as that of Monica, a housewife and mother who had been a fistula-fed baby (Engel & Reichsman, 1956; Engel et al., 1985; Viedermann, 1979), support the assumption that resilience, as marked by later life success, may be attained at the cost of some degree of spontaneity and flexibility.

Just as vulnerability is relative, depending upon complex interactions between constitutional factors and life circumstances, resilience appears to be governed by a similar interaction. Much previous longitudinal study has been concerned with tracing continuity over time, rather than with studying possible discontinuities and transformations across the course of life. Resilience appears to be less an enduring characteristic than a process determined by the impact of particular life experiences among persons with particular conceptions of their own life history or personal narrative.

Determinants of the stories that persons presently maintain of past adversity, together with factors leading them to overcome their misfortunes, are still not well understood. Particular talents and skills, and attractiveness to adults willing to assist these children of misfortune, play some part in overcoming adversity. However, there are many persons with similar talents who use the fact of adversity as justification for their own continued distress. Interpretive approaches complement systematic predictive approaches in understanding the determinants and course of vulnerability and resilience in the study of lives.

ACKNOWLEDGMENTS

Suggestions provided by Frances M. Stott and Andrew Boxer were of great help in completing this chapter. The support of the Center for Developmental Studies, University of Chicago, is acknowledged. Grant Nos. AG-0010 from the National Institute on Aging and MH-14668 from the National Institute of Mental Health facilitated completion of this chapter.

NOTES

1. Since the Dohrenwends' (1974, 1981) pioneering research, there have been many efforts at understanding the dimensions of life changes that are important in determining the extent to which persons can respond in ways that positively affect adjustment. Brim and Ryff (1980) propose vividness or dramatic quality, recency of occurrence, size or magnitude, power or degree of adversity implied, and complexity or extent of linkage with other events as determinants. Danish, Smyer, and Nowak (1980) propose on- versus off-timing of an event, duration or length of time an event lasts, the orderliness of an event in terms of the sequence of expected life events, the interrelation of an event with other events, and the generality of an event, among many others.

Following Lowenthal and Chiriboga (1973), Hultsch and Plemons (1979) suggest including the age at which an event takes place, the extent to which changes imply gains or benefits versus losses, and the timing and sequence of events across the course of life. Reese and Smyer (1983) suggest a new conceptualization of changes either as processes with some duration and with antecedents, contexts, and outcomes; as transitions or briefer processes that are in the process of taking place; or as markers that a change has taken place. These changes may be considered in terms of 10 separate criteria: focus on self versus others; extent of impact on adjustment; extent to which persons can exercise control over existence and course of changes; desirability of an event; extent to which an event is expected; frequency of an event among consociates; reversibility of change; and point in the course of life at which an event is likely to take place.

2. It may well be that the reason why the loss of a spouse is so much more difficult for men losing their wives than for women losing their husbands is because there are so few surviving older men that it is difficult for these men either to rehearse their role or to find other widowed men to be of assistance during this time of transition. It is more commonly expected that wives will outlive husbands than that husbands will outlive wives. Furthermore, definitions of gender identity, which led many men in earlier cohorts to be unable to care for the household or to do daily chores, may have made it more difficult for these men to manage their lives in the absence of their spouses. It remains true that occurrence of psychiatric symptoms and frequency of relocation to institutional settings are more frequent among men losing their wives through death than among older women losing their husbands through death.

3. Coddington (1972a, 1972b) created a measure of stressful life events for children similar to the original measure developed by Holmes and Rahe (1967) for adults. Findings obtained using that scale have been reviewed by Garmezy and Tellegen (1984), who have attempted a revision of the initial Coddington instrument; the revision includes positive as well as negative events, and the past year is used as the period inquired about. Attempts to obtain a normative group were complicated by an increased refusal to participate in the study among families including children with higher stress scores. Interviews with mothers of these children elicited additional sources of stress not included in the paper-and-pencil measure. Little detailed information is available regarding the ecology of stress for these children. Since the approach followed by Garmezy and his colleagues does not differentiate among adverse off-time changes, role transitions, and role strain (it includes both life changes and life event stress as a part of a single index),

and since few findings have been reported to date, it is difficult to evaluate the promise of this approach.

4. The timing of the appearance of psychiatric symptoms is not necessarily related to the concept of critical periods as previously used in the study of personality development and mental health. Based on findings from ethological studies (Freedman, 1974; Hinde, 1963, 1983) regarding determinants of the infant's first attachment to its mother, it had been assumed that all of development could be viewed as a series of "moving windows" that were open only for very limited periods of time. Failure to realize particular developmental attainments within these developmental points of particular sensitivity was believed to be a source of problems in subsequent development (Bowlby, 1969, 1977, 1983). This perspective was introduced into the study of developmental psychopathology as a result of Bowlby's (1951) initial formulation regarding emotional development and factors interfering in the formation of the mother–child bond, and Harlow's studies of monkey children separated from their mothers (Harlow & Harlow, 1966).

While some limited support has been reported for particular aspects of the critical-period hypothesis over relatively short intervals in development, and in regard to particular functions (Colombo, 1982), there has been little support for the assumption that particular psychopathology results from the failure of developmental events within particular critical periods in early development. Connolly (1972) questions whether the critical-period or sensitive-period hypothesis is viable in the study of human infancy to the extent that has been reported for nonhuman species. Reviewing classic studies regarding longer-term effects of disrupted caretaking in infancy, Rutter (1981a) has questioned whether maternal deprivation necessarily has the adverse effects initially attributed to it. Reconsidering their own findings regarding critical periods and social isolation in monkeys, Novak and Harlow (1975) have suggested that supposed nonreversible effects may be reversed or corrected at later points in development.

5. The problem with the term "stress-resistant," as used by Garmezy and his associates, is that it implies absolute rather than relative invulnerability or resilience. Consistent with the position discussed in this chapter, "resilience" is always a probabilistic concept. There is a point at which all persons confronted with particular adversity find themselves unable to provide effective responses, leading to feelings of fragmentation (Kohut, 1977). Developmental study can add much to understanding of the conditions under which a particular means of coping with adversity is no longer effective in resolving a sense of personal crisis.

6. While this lengthy period of "exposure" to parental psychopathology, particularly disturbances of thinking and of reality processing, might lead to the transmission of irrationality across generations (Lidz, 1963; Lidz, Fleck, & Cornelison, 1965; Mishler & Waxler, 1968; Wynne, 1981; Wynne, Singer, Bartko, & Toohey, 1977), there is little evidence that the offspring of schizophrenic parents evidence greater transactional thought disorder than counterparts from psychologically well families. Influences implicated in the origins of thought disorder among persons becoming schizophrenic are not the same as influences upon the children of schizophrenic parents. Indeed we (Cook & Cohler, 1986) have reviewed findings suggesting that the increased thought disorder found among parents of young adult schizophrenics, as contrasted with parents of psychologically well young adult offspring, may be the consequence of (1) anxiety induced by discovery of the offspring's disturbance; (2) factors associated with hospitalization and adopting the role identity (McCall & Simmons, 1978) of parents of psychiatric patients; and (3) having lived for a long time with offspring who process reality in unusual ways. Socialization is reciprocal, involving not just "forward" transmission from parent to offspring, but "backward" transmission from child to parent at the same time. At least to some extent, it is possible that schizophrenic offspring teach their caretakers to think in ways characteristic of deviance in communicating clearly with others.

7. There is little reason to believe that the intervention between genetic diathesis and adverse life changes likely to precipitate illness is greater in the first years of life than at other points in the course of life (Hanson, Gottesman, & Meehl, 1977). Indeed, consistent with findings regarding the onset of such major psychopathology as schizophrenia (Kramer, 1978; Neugebauer, Dohrenwend, & Dohrenwend, 1980), prevalence rates increase across the period from age 15 to age 25 in present cohorts—a point in the life course corresponding to an expanding role portfolio, when already vulnerable persons are unable to adjust to multiple demands and expectations (Cohler & Boxer, 1984). It should be noted that additional cases of schizophrenia have been reported across the adult years, even into later life (Cohler & Ferrono, in press). Since the genetics of affective disorders, particularly the bipolar disorders, appear similar in most respects to the genetics of schizophrenia (Rosenthal, 1970), there is little reason to believe that appearance of a depressive illness would occur more frequently in early childhood than later in life.

8. There has been little systematic study of the manner in which children cope with parental psychosis, and virtually no study of differences in coping techniques among children of schizophrenic and depressed parents. Some research (Rosen, Klein, Levenstein, & Shahinian, 1969) has suggested that coping strategies useful for schizophrenic patients may not be those most beneficial for depressed patients. It is possible that offspring of parents with schizophrenia and affective illness will have different means for coping with the effects of parental illness, and that coping effects will also vary according to both age and sex of offspring.

REFERENCES

Abraham, K. (1924). A short study of the libido viewed in the light of mental disorders. In *Selected papers on psychoanalysis*. New York: Basic Books, 1953.

Ainsworth, M. (1982). Attachment: Retrospect and prospect. In C. M. Parkes & J. Stevenson-Hinde (Eds.), *The place of attachment in human behavior*. New York: Basic Books.

Ainsworth, M., Blehar, M., Waters, E., & Wall, S. (1978). *Patterns of attachment: A psychological study of the strange situation*. Hillsdale, NJ: Erlbaum.

Albee, G. (1980). A competency model must replace the defect model. In L. A. Bond & J. C. Rosen (Eds.), *Competence and coping during adulthood*. Hanover, NH: University of Vermont Press/University Press of New England.

Allport, G. (1937). *Personality*. New York: Henry Holt.

Allport, G. (1964). Mental health: A generic attitude. In *The person in psychology*. Boston: Beacon Press, 1968.

Antonovsky, A. (1979). *Health, stress, and coping*. San Francisco: Jossey-Bass.

Anthony, E. J. (1976). How children cope in families with a psychotic parent. In E. Rexford, L. Sander, & T. Shapiro (Eds.), *Infant psychiatry: A new synthesis*. New Haven, CT: Yale University Press, 1976.

Anthony, E. J. (1974a). A risk–vulnerability intervention model for children of psychotic parents. In E. J. Anthony & C. Koupernik (Eds.), *The child in his family: Children at psychiatric risk* (International yearbook, Vol. 3). New York: Wiley.

Anthony, E. J. (1974b). The syndrome of the psychologically invulnerable child. In E. J. Anthony & C. Koupernik (Eds.), *The child in his family: Children at psychiatric risk* (International yearbook, Vol. 3). New York: Wiley.

Bandura, A. (1977). Self-efficacy: Toward a unifying theory of behavioral change. *Psychological Review, 84*, 191–215.

Bandura, A. (1982a). The psychology of chance encounters and life paths. *American Psychologist, 37,* 747–755.

Bandura, A. (1982b). Self-efficacy mechanism in human agency, *American Psychologist, 37,* 122–147.

Bankoff, L. (1983). Social support and adaptation to widowhood. *Journal of Marriage and the Family, 45,* 827–839.

Bayley, N. (1963). The life-span as a frame of reference in psychological research. *Vita Humana (Human Development), 6,* 125–139.

Bayley, N. (1970). Development of mental abilities. In P. H. Mussen (Ed.), *Carmichael's manual of child psychology.* New York: Wiley.

Beck, J., & Worthen, K. (1972). Precipitating stress, crisis theory, and hospitalization in schizophrenia and depression. *Archives of General Psychiatry, 26,* 123–129.

Bibring, G. (1959). Some considerations of the psychological process in pregnancy. *Psychoanalytic Study of the Child, 14,* 113–121.

Billings, A., & Moos, R. (1981). The role of coping responses and social resources in attenuating the stress of life events. *Journal of Behavioral Medicine, 4,* 139–157.

Block, J., & Block, J. (1980). The role of ego-control and ego-resiliency in the organization of behavior. In W. A. Collins (Ed.), *Development of cognition, affect, and social relations: The Minnesota Symposium on Child Psychology* (Vol. 13). Minneapolis: University of Minnesota Press.

Bloom, B. (1964). *Stability and change in human characteristics.* New York: Wiley.

Boszormenyi-Nagy, I., & Spark, G. (1973). *Invisible loyalties: Reciprocity in intergenerational family therapy.* New York: Harper & Row.

Bowlby, J. (1951). *Maternal care and mental health.* Geneva: World Health Organization.

Bowlby, J. (1969). *Attachment and loss: Vol. 1. Attachment.* New York: Basic Books.

Bowlby, J. (1973). Self-reliance and some conditions that promote it. In R. Gosling (Ed.), *Support, innovation and autonomy.* London: Tavistock.

Bowlby, J. (1977). The making and breaking of affectional bonds. *British Journal of Psychiatry, 30,* 201–210.

Bowlby, J. (1983). Attachment and loss: Retrospect and prospect. *American Journal of Orthopsychiatry, 52,* 664–678.

Bowlby, J., Robertson, J., & Rosenbluth, D. (1952). A two-year old goes to the hospital. *Psychoanalytic Study of the Child, 7,* 90–94.

Brim, O. G., Jr. (1980). Types of life events. *Journal of Social Issues, 36,* 148–157.

Brim, O. G., Jr., & Ryff, C. (1980). On the properties of life-events. In P. B. Baltes & O. G. Brim, Jr. (Eds.), *Life-span development and behavior* (Vol. 3). New York: Academic Press.

Bringuier, J. C. (1980). *Conversations with Jean Piaget* (B. M. Gulati, Trans.). Chicago: University of Chicago Press.

Brown, G., & Birley, J. (1968). Crises and life changes and the onset of schizophrenia. *Journal of Health and Social Behavior, 9,* 203–214.

Brown, G., & Harris, T. (1978). *Social origins of depression: A study of psychiatric disorder in women.* New York: Free Press.

Brown, G., Harris, T. O., & Petro, J. (1973). Life events and psychiatric disorders: Part 2. Nature of causal link. *Psychological Medicine, 3,* 159–176.

Brown, W. (1983). *The other side of delinquency.* New Brunswick, NJ: Rutgers University Press.

Butler, R. (1963). The life-review: An interpretation of reminiscence in the aged. *Psychiatry, 26,* 65–76.

Cannon, W. B. (1932). *The wisdom of the body.* New York: Norton.

Caplan, G. (1981). Mastery of stress: Psychosocial aspects. *American Journal of Psychiatry, 138,* 413–420.

Chess, S. (1979). Developmental theory revisited: Findings of a longitudinal study. *Canadian Journal of Psychiatry, 24*, 101–112.

Chess, S., & Thomas, A. (1984). *Origins and evolution of behavior disorders: From infancy to early adult life*. New York: Brunner/Mazel.

Clausen, J. (1984). Mental illness and the life course. In P. Baltes & O. G. Brim, Jr. (Eds.), *Life-span development and behavior* (Vol. 6). New York: Academic Press.

Clarke, S. D. B., & Clarke, A. M. (Eds.). (1976). *Early experience: Myth and evidence*. New York: Free Press.

Clarke, S. D. B., & Clarke, A. M. (1981). "Sleeper effects" in development: Fact or artifact? *Developmental Review, 1*, 344–360.

Clayton, P., & Darvish, H. (1979). Course of depressive symptoms following the stress of bereavement. In J. E. Barrett (Ed.), *Stress and mental disorder*. New York: Raven Press.

Coddington, R. D. (1972a). The significance of life events as etiologic factors in the diseases of children: I. A survey of professional workers. *Journal of Psychosomatic Research, 16*, 7–18.

Coddington, R. D. (1972b). The significance of life events as etiologic factors in the diseases of children: II. A study of a normal population. *Journal of Psychosomatic Research, 16*, 205–213.

Coelho, G., Hamburg, D., & Murphey, E. (1963). Coping strategies in a new learning environment. *Archives of General Psychiatry, 9*, 433–443.

Cohler, B. (1980). Developmental perspectives on the psychology of the self. In A. Goldberg (Ed.), *Advances in self psychology*. New York: International Universities Press.

Cohler, B. (1981). Adult developmental psychology and reconstruction in psychoanalysis. In S. Greenspan & G. Pollock (Eds.), *The course of life: Vol. 3. Adulthood and aging*. Washington, DC: U. S. Government Printing Office.

Cohler, B. (1982). Personal narrative and life course. In P. B. Baltes & O. G. Brim, Jr. (Eds.), *Life-span development and behavior* (Vol. 4). New York: Academic Press.

Cohler, B. (1983). Autonomy and interdependence in the family of adulthood: A psychological perspective. *The Gerontologist, 23*, 33–39.

Cohler, B. (in press). Approaches to the study of development in psychiatric education. In S. Weissman & R. Thurnblad (Eds.), *The place of psychoanalysis in psychiatric education*. New York: International Universities Press.

Cohler, B., & Boxer, A. (1984). Middle adulthood: Settling into the world—person, time and context. In D. Offer & M. Sabshin (Eds.), *Normality and the life course: A critical integration*. New York: Basic Books.

Cohler, B., & Carney, J. (in press). Developmental continuity and adjustment in adulthood. In N. Miller (Ed.), *The psychodynamics of aging*. New York: International Universities Press.

Cohler, B., & Ferrono, C. (in press). Schizophrenia and the life course. In N. Miller (Ed.), *Schizophrenia and aging*. New York: Guilford Press.

Cohler, B., & Freeman, M. (in press). Psychoanalysis and the developmental narrative. In S. Greenspan & G. H. Pollock (Eds.), *The course of life* (Revised). New York: International Universities Press.

Cohler, B., Gallant, D., Grunebaum, H., & Kaufman, C. (1983). Social adjustment among schizophrenic, depressed and well mothers and their school aged children. In H. Morrison (Ed.), *Children of depressed parents: Risk, identification, and intervention*. New York: Grune & Stratton.

Cohler, B., Gallant, D., Grunebaum, H., Weiss, J., & Gamer, E. (1976). Pregnancy and birth complications among mentally ill and well mothers and their children. *Social Biology, 22*, 269–278.

Cohen, F., & Lazarus, R. (1973). Active coping processes, coping dispositions, and recovery from surgery. *Psychosomatic Medicine, 35*, 375–389.

Coles, R. (1964). *Children of crisis* (Vol. 1). New York: Atlantic/Little, Brown.

Coles, R. (1975). *Children of crisis: Vol. 5. Privileged ones.* New York: Atlantic/Little, Brown.

Colombo, J. (1982). The critical period concept: Research, methodology, and theoretical issues. *Psychological Bulletin, 91*, 260–275.

Colona, A. (1981). Success through their own efforts. *Psychoanalytic Study of the Child, 36*, 33–44.

Connolly, K. (1972). Learning and the concept of critical periods in infancy. *Developmental Medicine and Child Neurology, 14*, 705–714.

Cook, J., & Cohler, B. (1986). Reciprocal socialization and the care of offspring with cancer and with schizophrenia. In N. Datan, A. Greene, & H. Reese (Eds.), *Intergenerational networks: Families in context*. Hillsdale, NJ: Erlbaum.

Csikszentmihalyi, M. (1975). *Beyond boredom and anxiety*. San Francisco: Jossey-Bass.

Cytryn, L., Gershon, E., & McKnew, D. (1984). Childhood depression: Genetic or environmental influences. *Integrative Psychiatry, 2*, 17–23.

Danish, S., Smyer, M., & Nowak, C. (1980). Developmental intervention: Enhancing life-event processes. In P. B. Baltes & O. G. Brim, Jr. (Eds.), *Life-span development and behavior* (Vol. 3). New York: Academic Press.

Dennis, W. (1973). *Children of the creche*. New York: Appleton-Century-Crofts.

Dibble, E., & Cohen, D. (1974). Companion instruments for measuring children's competence and parental style. *Archives of General Psychiatry, 30*, 805–815.

Dohrenwend, B. P. (1961). The social psychological nature of stress: A framework for causal inquiry. *Journal of Abnormal and Social Psychology, 62*, 294–302.

Dohrenwend, B. S., & Dohrenwend, B. P. (1974). *Stressful life-events: Their nature and effects*. New York: Wiley-Interscience.

Dohrenwend, B. S., & Dohrenwend, B. P. (1981). Life stress and illness: Formulation of the issues. In B. S. Dohrenwend and B. P. Dohrenwend (Eds.), *Stressful life events and their contexts*. New York: Prodist/Neale Watson.

Dubos, R. (1965). *Man adapting*. New Haven, CT: Yale University Press.

Durkheim, E. (1915). *The elementary forms of the religious life*. New York: Macmillan/Free Press, 1955.

Elder, G. H., Jr. (1974). *Children of the Great Depression*. Chicago: University of Chicago Press.

Elder, G. H., Jr. (1979). Historical change in life patterns and personality. In P. B. Baltes & O. G. Brim, Jr. (Eds.), *Life-span development and behavior* (Vol. 2). New York: Academic Press.

Elder, G. H., Jr. (1985). *Military times and turning points in men's lives*. Unpublished manuscript, Center for Population Studies, University of North Carolina at Chapel Hill.

Elder, G. H., Jr., Caspi, A., & Nguyen, T. V. (in press). Resourceful and vulnerable children: Family influences in hard times. In R. K. Silbereisen & K. Eyferth (Eds.), *Development in context: Integrative perspectives on youth development*. New York: Springer.

Elder, G. H., Jr., Liker, J., & Cross, C. (1984). Parent–child behavior in the Great Depression. In P. B. Baltes & O. G. Brim, Jr. (Eds.), *Life-span development and behavior* (Vol. 6). New York: Academic Press.

Elder, G. H., Jr., Nguyen, T. V., & Caspi, A. (1985). Linking family hardships to children's lives. *Child Development, 56*, 361–375.

Elder, G. H., Jr., & Rockwell, R. (1978). Economic depression and post-war opportunity: A study of life-patterns and health. In R. Simmons (Ed.), *Research in community and mental health*. Greenwich, CT: JAI Press.

Elder, G. H., Jr., & Rockwell, R. (1979). The life-course and human development: An ecological perspective. *International Journal of Behavioral Development, 2*, 1–21.

Emde, R. (1981). Changing models of infancy and the nature of early development: Remodeling the foundation. *Journal of the American Psychoanalytic Association, 29*, 179–219.

Emde, R., & Harmon, R. (1984). Entering a new era in the search for developmental continuities. In R. Emde & R. Harmon (Eds.), *Continuities and discontinuities in development*. New York: Plenum Press.

Emmerich, W. (1968). Personality development and concepts of structure, *Child Development, 39*, 671–690.

Engel, G. (1962). *Psychological development in health and disease*. Philadelphia: W. B. Saunders.

Engel, G. (1967). Ego development following severe trauma in infancy. *Bulletin of the Association of Psychoanalytic Medicine, 6*, 57–61.

Engel, G., & Reichsman, F. (1956). Spontaneous and experimentally induced depressions in an infant with a gastric fistula. *Journal of the American Psychoanalytic Association, 4*, 428–452.

Engel, G., Reichsman, F., Harway, V., & Hess, D. W. (1985). Monica: Infant-feeding behavior of a mother gastric fistula-fed as an infant: A 3-year longitudinal study of enduring effects. In G. Pollock & E. J. Anthony (Eds.), *Parental influences in health and disease*. Boston: Little, Brown.

Erikson, E. H. (1963). *Childhood and society* (rev. ed.) New York: Norton.

Escalona, S. (1968). *The roots of individuality*. New York: Aldine/Atherton.

Feinstein, A. D. (1979). Personal mythology as a paradigm for a holistic public psychology. *American Journal of Orthopsychiatry, 49*, 198–217.

Felsman, J. K. (1981). *Street urchins of Cali: On risk, resiliency and adaptation in childhood*. Unpublished doctoral dissertation, Harvard Graduate School of Education.

Ferrarese, D. (1981). Reflectiveness–impulsivity and competence in children under stress (Doctoral dissertation, University of Minnesota), *Dissertation Abstracts International, 42*, 4928B.

Fiske, M. (1980a). Changing hierarchies of commitment in adulthood. In E. Erikson & N. Smelser (Eds.), *Themes of work and love in adulthood*. Cambridge, MA: Harvard University Press.

Fiske, M. (1980b). Tasks and crises of the second half of life: The interrelationship of commitment, coping and adaptation. In J. Birren & R. B. Sloan (Eds.), *Handbook of mental health and aging*. Englewood Cliffs, NJ: Prentice-Hall.

Fontana, A., Hughes, L., Marcus, L., & Dowds, B. (1979). Subjective evaluation of life events. *Journal of Consulting and Clinical Psychology, 47*, 906–911.

Freeman, M. (1984). History, narrative, and life-span developmental psychology. *Human Development, 27*, 1–19.

Freedman, D. (1974). *Human infancy: An evolutionary approach*. Hillsdale, NJ: Erlbaum.

French, J. R. P., Jr., Rodgers, W., & Cobb, S. (1974). Adjustment as a person–environment fit. In G. C. Coelho, D. Hamburg, & J. Adams (Eds.), *Coping and adaptation*. New York: Basic Books.

Freud, A. (1936). *The writings of Anna Freud: Vol. 2. The ego and the mechanisms of defense*. New York: International Universities Press, 1966.

Freud, A. (1965). *The writings of Anna Freud: Vol. 6. Normality and psychopathology in childhood: Assessments of development*. New York: International Universities Press.

Freud, S. (1894). The neuro-psychoses of defense. *Standard Edition, 3*, 43–61. London: Hogarth Press, 1962.

Freud, S. (1895). Project for a scientific psychology. *Standard Edition, 1*, 281–387. London: Hogarth Press, 1966.

Freud, S. (1896). Further remarks on the neuro-psychoses of defense. *Standard Edition, 3*, 157–186. London: Hogarth Press, 1962.

Freud, S. (1905). Three essays on the theory of sexuality. *Standard Edition, 7*, 1–246. London: Hogarth Press, 1953.

Freud, S. (1910). Five lectures on psychoanalysis. *Standard Edition, 11*, 1–55. London: Hogarth Press, 1957.

Freud, S. (1915–1917). Introductory lectures on psychoanalysis. *Standard Edition, 15–16*. London: Hogarth Press, 1961–1963.

Freud, S. (1925). An autobiographical study. *Standard Edition, 20*, 1–70. London: Hogarth Press, 1959.

Freud, S. (1926). Inhibitions, symptoms and anxiety. *Standard Edition, 20*, 75–172. London: Hogarth Press, 1959.

Freud, S. (1937). Analysis terminable and interminable. *Standard Edition, 23*, 209–254. London: Hogarth Press, 1964.

Garber, B. (1981). Mourning in children: Toward a theoretical synthesis. *Annual for Psychoanalysis, 9*, 9–19.

Gardner, G. (1967). Role of maternal psychopathology in male and female schizophrenics. *Journal of Consulting Psychology, 31*, 411–413.

Gardner, R. (1962). Cognitive controls and adaptation: Research and adaptation. In S. J. Messick & J. Ross (Eds.), *Measurement in personality and cognition*. New York: Wiley.

Gardner, R., Holzman, P., Klein, G., Linton, H., & Spence, D. (1959). *Cognitive control: A study of individual consistencies in cognitive behavior.* (Psychological Issues Monograph No. 4) New York: International Universities Press.

Garmezy, N. (1971). Vulnerability research and the issue of primary prevention. *American Journal of Orthopsychiatry, 41*, 101–116.

Garmezy, N. (1972). Models of etiology for the study of children at risk for schizophrenia. In M. Roff, L. Robins, & M. Pollack (Eds.), *Life history research in psychopathology* (Vol. 2). Minneapolis: University of Minnesota Press.

Garmezy, N. (1974). The study of competence in children at risk for severe psychopathology. In E. J. Anthony & C. Koupernik (Eds.), *The child in his family: Children at psychiatric risk.* (International yearbook, Vol. 3) New York: Wiley.

Garmezy, N. (1981) Children under stress: Perspectives on antecedents and correlates of vulnerability and resistance to psychopathology. In A. I. Rabin, J. Aronoff, A. M. Barclay, & R. Zucker (Eds.), *Further explorations in personality*. New York: Wiley-Interscience.

Garmezy, N. (1983). Stressors of childhood. In N. Garmezy & M. Rutter (Eds.), *Stress, coping and development in children*. New York: McGraw-Hill.

Garmezy, N., & Devine, V. (1984). Project Competence: The Minnesota studies of children vulnerable to psychopathology. In N. F. Watt, E. J. Anthony, L. C. Wynne, & J. E. Rolf (Eds.) *Children at risk for schizophrenia: A longitudinal perspective.* Cambridge, England: Cambridge University Press.

Garmezy, N., Masten, A., Nordstrom, L., & Ferrarese, M. (1979). The nature of competence in normal and deviant children. In M. W. Kent & J. E. Rolf (Eds.), *Primary prevention of psychopathology: Vol. 3. Social competence in children*. Hanover, NH: University of Vermont Press/University Press of New England.

Garmezy, N., & Nuechterlein, K. H. (1972). Invulnerable children: The fact and fiction of competence and disadvantage. *American Journal of Orthopsychiatry, 42*, 328–329. (Abstract)

Garmezy, N., & Tellegen, A. (1984). Studies of stress-resistant children: Methods, variables, and preliminary findings. In F. L. Morrison, C. Lord, & D. P. Keating (Eds.), *Applied developmental psychology* (Vol. 1). New York: Academic Press.

Gergen, K. (1977). Stability, change and chance in understanding human development. In N. Datan & H. Reese (Eds.), *Life-span developmental psychology: Dialectical perspectives on experimental research*. New York: Academic Press.

Gergen, K. (1982). *Toward transformation in social knowledge*. New York: Springer-Verlag.

Gershon, E., Hamovit, J., Guroff, J., Dibble, E., Leckman, J., Sceery, W., Targum, J., Nurnberger, J., Goldin, L., & Bunney, W. (1982). A family study of schizoaffective bipolar I, bipolar II, unipolar, and normal control probands. *Archives of General Psychiatry, 39,* 1157–1167.

Gill, M. M. (1976). Metapsychology is not psychology. In M. M. Gill & P. Holzman (Eds.), *Psychology versus metapsychology: Psychoanalytic essays in memory of George S. Klein,* (Psychological Issues Monograph No. 36). New York: International Universities Press.

Glover, E. (1930). Grades of ego differentiation. In *On the early development of the mind.* New York: International Universities Press, 1956.

Glover, E. (1932a). On the etiology of drug addiction. In *On the early development of the mind.* New York: International Universities Press, 1956.

Glover, E. (1932b). A psychoanalytic approach to the classification of mental disorders. In *On the early development of the mind.* New York: International Universities Press, 1956.

Goldberg, S. (1977). Social competence in infancy: A model of parent–infant interaction. *Merrill–Palmer Quarterly, 23,* 163–177.

Goldin-Meadow, S., & Mylander, C. (1984). Gestural communication in deaf children: The effects and noneffects of parental input on early language development. *Monographs of the Society for Research in Child Development, 49*(3–4, Serial No. 207).

Goode, W. (1960). A theory of role strain. *American Sociological Review, 25,* 483–496.

Gottesman, I., & Shields, J. (1982). *Schizophrenia: The epigenetic puzzle.* New York: Cambridge University Press.

Green, A. (1975). The analyst, symbolization, and absence in the analytic setting. *International Journal of Psycho-Analysis, 56,* 1–22.

Green, A. (1978). Potential space in psychoanalysis: The object in the setting. In S. Grolnick, L. Barkin, & W. Muensterberger (Eds.), *Between reality and fantasy: Transitional objects and phenomena.* New York: Jason Aronson.

Grunebaum, H., Gamer, E., & Cohler, B. (1983). The spouse in depressed families. In H. Morrison (Ed.), *Children of depressed parents: Risk, identification, and intervention.* New York: Grune & Stratton.

Grunebaum, H., Weiss, J., Cohler, B., Hartman, C., & Gallant, D. (1982). *Mentally ill mothers and their children* (rev. ed.) Chicago: University of Chicago Press.

Guilford, J. P. (1950). Creativity. *American Psychologist, 14,* 469–479.

Gurin, P., Brim, O. G. Jr. (1984). Change in self in adulthood: The example of sense of control. In P. B. Baltes & O. G. Brim, Jr. (Eds.), *Life-span development and behavior* (Volume 6). New York: Academic Press.

Gutmann, D., Griffin, B., & Grunes, J. (1982). Developmental contributions to late-onset affective disorders. In P. B. Baltes & O. G. Brim, Jr. (Eds.), *Life-span development and behavior* (Vol. 4). New York: Academic Press.

Haan, N. (1977). *Coping and defending: Processes of self-environment organization.* New York: Academic Press.

Haan, N. (1982). The assessment of coping, defense, and stress. In L. Goldberg & S. Breznitz (Eds.), *Handbook of stress.* New York: Free Press/Macmillan.

Hagstad, G., & Neugarten, B. (1985). Age and the life-course. In R. Binstock & E. Shanas (Eds.), *Handbook of aging and the social sciences.* New York: Van Nostrand Reinhold.

Hanson, D., Gottesman, I. I., & Heston, L. (1976). Some possible childhood indicators of adult schizophrenia inferred from children of schizophrenics. *British Journal of Psychiatry, 129,* 142–154.

Hanson, D., Gottesman, I. I., & Meehl, P. E. (1977). Genetic theories and the validation of psychiatric diagnosis: Implications for the study of children of schizophrenics. *Journal of Abnormal Psychology, 6,* 575–588.

Harlow, H., & Harlow, M. (1966). Learning to love. *American Scientist, 54,* 244–272.

Hartmann, H. (1939). *Ego psychology and the problem of adaptation* (D. Rapaport, Trans.). New York: International Universities Press, 1958.

Hartmann, H. (1950a). Comments on the psychoanalytic theory of the ego. In *Essays on ego psychology: Selected problems in psychoanalytic theory*. New York: International Universities Press, 1964.

Hartmann, H. (1950b). Psychoanalysis and developmental psychology. In *Essays on ego psychology: Selected problems in psychoanalytic theory*. New York: International Universities Press, 1964.

Hartmann, H. (1955). Notes on the theory of sublimation. In *Essays on ego psychology: Selected problems in psychoanalytic theory*. New York: International Universities Press, 1964.

Heider, G. (1966). Vulnerability in infants and young children: A pilot study. *Genetic Psychology Monographs, 73*, 1–216.

Heston, L. (1966). Psychiatric disorders in foster home reared children of schizophrenic mothers. *British Journal of Psychiatry, 112*, 819–825.

Heston, L., & Denny, D. (1968). Interactions between early life experience and biological factors in schizophrenia. In D. Rosenthal & S. Kety (Eds.), *The transmission of schizophrenia*. New York: Pergamon Press.

Hinde, R. (1963). The nature of imprinting. In B. Foss (Ed.), *The determinants of infant behavior* (Vol. 2). New York: Wiley.

Hinde, R. (1983). Ethology and child development. In M. M. Haith & J. J. Compos (Eds.), *Handbook of child psychology: Vol. 2. Infancy and developmental psychobiology*. New York: Wiley.

Holmes, T., & Rahe, R. R. (1967). The Social Readjustment Rating Scale. *Journal of Psychosomatic Research, 11*, 213–218.

Howard, J. (1978). The influence of the children's developmental dysfunctions on marital quality and family interaction. In R. Lerner & G. Spanier (Eds.), *Child influences on marital and family interaction: A life-span perspective*. New York: Academic Press.

Hultsch, D., & Plemons, J. (1979). Life events and life-span development. In P. B. Baltes & O. G. Brim, Jr. (Eds.), *Life-span development and behavior* (Vol. 2). New York: Academic Press.

Janis, I. L. (1958). *Psychosocial stress: Psychoanalytic and behavioral studies of surgical patients*. New York: Wiley.

Janis, I. L., & Mann, L. (1977). *Decision making*. New York: Free Press/Macmillan.

Jones, M. C., Bayley, N., MacFarlane, J. W., & Honzik, M. (Eds.). (1971). *The course of human development: Selected papers from the longitudinal studies, Institute of Human Development, University of California at Berkeley*. Waltham, MA: Xerox College Publishing.

Kagan, J. (1966). Reflection and impulsivity: The geneality and dynamics of conceptual tempo. *Journal of Abnormal Psychology, 71*, 17–24.

Kagan, J. (1979). The form of early development: Continuity and discontinuity in emergent competences. *Archives of General Psychiatry, 36*, 1047–1054.

Kagan, J. (1980). Perspectives on continuity. In O. G. Brim, Jr., & J. Kagan (Eds.), *Continuity and change in human development*. Cambridge, MA: Harvard University Press.

Kagan, J. (1983). Stress and coping in early development. In N. Garmezy & M. Rutter (Eds.), *Stress, coping, and development in children*. New York: McGraw-Hill.

Kagan, J. (1984). Continuity and change in the opening years of life. In R. Emde & R. Harmon (Eds.), *Continuities and discontinuities in development*. New York: Plenum Press.

Kagan, J., Kearsley, R., & Zelazo, P. (1978). *Infancy: Its place in human development*. Cambridge, MA: Harvard University Press.

Kagan, J., & Klein, R. (1973). Cross-cultural perspectives on early development. *American Psychologist, 28*, 947–961.

Kagan, J., Klein, R., Finley, G., Rogoff, B., Nolan, E. (1979). A cross-cultural study of cognitive development. *Monographs of the Society for Research in Child Development, 44*, (Serial No. 180).

Kagan, J., & Moss, H. (1963). *From birth to maturity*. New York: Wiley.

Kahn, R., & Antonucci, T. (1980). Convoys over the life course: Attachment, roles, and social support. In P. B. Baltes & O. G. Brim, Jr. (Eds.), *Life-span development and behavior* (Vol. 3). New York: Academic Press.

Karlsson, J. L. (1968). Genealogic studies of schizophenia. In D. Rosenthal & S. Kety (Eds.), *The transmission of schizophrenia*. New York: Pergamon Press.

Kaufman, C., Grunebaum, H., Cohler, B., & Gamer, E. (1979). Superkids: Competent children of schizophrenic mothers. *American Journal of Psychiatry, 136*, 1398-1402.

Kent, M. W., & Rolf, J. (Eds.). (1979). *Primary prevention of psychopathology: Vol. 3. Social competence in children*. Hanover, NH: University of Vermont Press/University Press of New England.

Kessler, R. C., & McLeod, J. (1984). Sex differences in vulnerability to undesirable life events. *American Sociological Review, 49*, 620-631.

Kessler, R. C., Price, R., & Wortman, C. (1985). Social factors in psychopathology: Stress, social support, and coping processes. *Annual Review of Psychology, 36*, 531-572.

Klein, G. (1958). Cognitive control and motivation. In *Perception, motives and personality*. New York: Knopf, 1970.

Klein, G. (1976). *Psychoanalytic theory: An exploration of essentials*. New York: International Universities Press.

Kobasa, S. (1979). Stressful life events, personality, and health: An inquiry into hardiness. *Journal of Personality and Social Psychology, 37*, 1-11.

Kobasa, S. (1982). The hardy personality: Toward a social psychology of stress and health. In J. Sauls & S. Sanders (Eds.), *The social psychology of health and illness*. Hillsdale NJ: Erlbaum.

Kobasa, S., Maddi, S., & Kahn, S. (1982). Hardiness and health: A prospective study. *Journal of Personality and Social Psychology, 42*, 168-177.

Kohlberg, L., Ricks, D., & Snarey, J. (1984). Childhood development as a predictor of adaptation in adulthood. *Genetic Psychology Monographs, 110*, 91-173.

Kohn, M. (1969). *Class and conformity: A study in values*. Homewood, IL: Dorsey Press.

Kohn, M. (1977). *Social competence, symptoms, and underachievement in childhood: A longitudinal perspective*. Washington, DC: V. H. Winston.

Kohut, H. (1971). *The analysis of the self*. New York: International Universities Press.

Kohut, H. (1977). *The restoration of the self*. New York: International Universities Press.

Kramer, M. (1978). Population changes and schizophrenia, 1970-1985. In L. Wynne, R. Cromwell, & S. Matthysse (Eds.), *The nature of schizophrenia: New approaches to research and treatment*. New York: Wiley.

Kris, E. (1956). The personal myth: A problem in psychoanalytic technique. *Journal of the American Psychoanalytic Association, 4*, 653-681.

Kroeber, T. (1963). The coping functions of the ego mechanisms. In R. W. White (Ed.), *The study of lives*. New York: Aldine/Atherton.

Lazarus, R. (1966). *Psychological stress and the coping process*. New York: McGraw-Hill.

Lazarus, R. (1980a). The costs and benefits of denial. In B. P. Dohrenwend & B. S. Dohrenwend (Eds.), *Stressful life events and their contexts*. New York: Neale Watson/Prodist, 1981.

Lazarus, R. (1980b). The stress and coping paradigm. In L. A. Bond & J. C. Rosen (Eds.), *Competence and coping during adulthood*. Hanover, NH: University of Vermont Press/University Press of New England.

Lazarus, R., Averill, J., & Opton, E. M., Jr. (1974). The psychology of coping: Issues of research and assessment. In G. Coelho, D. Hamburg, & J. Adams (Eds.), *Coping and adaptation*. New York: Basic Books.

Lazarus, R., & Folkman, S. (1984). *Stress, appraisal and coping*. New York: Springer.

Lewine, R., Watt, N., & Fryer, J. (1978). A study of childhood social competence, adult premorbid competence, and psychiatric outcome in three schizophrenic subtypes. *Journal of Abnormal Psychology, 87*, 294-302.

Lidz, T. (1963). *The family and human adaptation: Three lectures.* New York: International Universities Press.

Lidz, T., Fleck, S., & Cornelison, A. (1965). *Schizophrenia and the family.* New York: International Universities Press.

Lieberman, M., & Falk, J. (1971). The remembered past as a source of data for research on the life cycle. *Human Development, 14,* 132–141.

Lieberman, M., & Tobin, S. (1983). *The experience of old age: Stress, coping and survival.* New York: Basic Books.

Livson, N., & Peskin, H. (1980). Perspectives on adolescence from longitudinal research. In J. Adelson (Ed.), *Handbook on adolescence.* New York: Wiley.

Lowenthal, M. F., & Chiriboga, D. (1973). Social stress and adaptation: Toward a life-course orientation. In C. Eisdorfer & M. P. Lawton (Eds.), *The psychology of adult development and aging.* Washington, DC: American Psychological Association.

Lowenthal, M. F., Thurnher, M., Chiriboga, D., & Associates. (1975). *Four states of life: A comparative study of men and women facing transitions.* San Francisco: Jossey-Bass.

Maas, H., & Kuypers, J. (1974). *From thirty to seventy: A forty year longitudinal study of adult life-styles and personality.* San Francisco: Jossey-Bass.

Marlowe, H., & Weinberg, R. (1985). Competence development theory and practice in special populations. Springfield, IL: Charles C Thomas.

MacFarlane, J. (1963). From infancy to adulthood. *Childhood Education, 39,* 336–342.

MacFarlane, J. (1964). Perspectives on personality consistency and change from the guidance study. *Vita Humana (Human Development), 7,* 115–126.

MacFarlane, J., Allen, L., & Honzik, M. (1954). *A developmental study of the behavior problems of normal children between 21 months and 14 years.* Berkeley: University of California Press.

Marshall, V. (1981). *Last chapters: A sociology of death and dying.* Belmont, CA: Wadsworth.

Masten, A. (1982). Humor and creative thinking in stress-resistant children (Doctoral dissertation, University of Minnesota). *Dissertation Abstracts International, 42,* 3737B.

Masuda, M., & Holmes, T. (1967). Magnitude estimations of social readjustments. *Journal of Psychosomatic Research, 11,* 219–225.

Masuda, M., & Holmes, T. (1968). Life events, perceptions, and frequencies. *Psychosomatic Medicine, 40,* 236–261.

McCall, G. J., & Simmons, J. J. (1978). *Identities and interactions: An examination of human associations in everyday life* (2nd ed.). New York: Free Press/Macmillan.

McMiller, P., Ingham, J. G. (1985). Are life events which cause each other additive in their effects? *Social Psychiatry, 20,* 31–41.

Mechanic, D. (1962). *Students under stress: A study in the social psychology of adaptation.* New York: Free Press/Macmillan.

Mechanic, D. (1974). Social structure and personal adaptation: Some neglected dimensions. In G. Coelho, D. Hamburg, & J. Adams (Eds.), *Coping and adaptation.* New York: Basic Books.

Mechanic, D. (1977). Illness, behavior, social adaptation, and the management of illness: A comparison of educational and medical models. *Journal of Nervous and Mental Disease, 165,* 79–87.

Mednick, S. (1978). Bergson's fallacy and high risk research. In L. Wynne, R. Cromwell, & S. Matthysse (Eds.), *The nature of schizophrenia: New approaches to research and treatment.* New York: Wiley.

Mednick, S., Schulsinger, F., Teasdale, T., Schulsinger, H., Venables, P., & Rock, D. (1978). Schizophrenia in high-risk children: Sex differences in predisposing factors. In G. Serban (Ed.), *Cognitive defects in the development of mental illness.* New York: Brunner/Mazel.

Meichenbaum, D., Butler, L., & Gruson, L. (1981). Toward a conceptual model of social competence. In J. D. Wine & M. D. Syme (Eds.), *Social competence*. New York: Guilford Press.

Meissner, W. (1970). Sibling relations in the schizophrenic family. *Family Process, 9*, 1–26.

Menaghan, E. (1983). Individual coping efforts: Moderators of the relationship between life stress and mental health outcomes. In H. Kaplan (Ed.), *Psychosocial stress: Trends in theory and research*. New York: Academic Press.

Menninger, K. (1954). Psychological characteristics of the organism under stress. *Journal of the American Psychoanalytic Association, 2*, 67–106.

Menninger, K., Mayman, M., & Pruyser, P. (1963). *The vital balance*. New York: Viking Press.

Meyer, A. (1951). The life-chart and the obligation of specifying positive data in psychopathological diagnosis. In E. E. Winters (Ed.), *The collected papers of Adolf Meyer: Volume 3. Medical teaching*. Baltimore: Johns Hopkins University Press.

Miller, D., & Swanson, G. (1960). *Inner Conflict and Defense*. New York: Henry Holt/Dryden.

Miller, G., Galanter, E., & Pribram, K. (1960). *Plans and the structure of behavior*. New York: Henry Holt/Dryden.

Minkler, M., & Biller, R. (1979). Role shock: A tool for conceptualizing stresses accompanying disruptive role transitions. *Human Relations, 32*, 125–140.

Mishler, E., & Waxler, N. (1965). Family interaction patterns and schizophrenia: A review of current theories. *Merrill–Palmer Quarterly, 11*, 269–315.

Mishler, E., & Waxler, N. (1968). *Interaction in families: An experimental study of family processes and schizophrenia*. New York: Wiley.

Moos, R., & Billings, A. (1982). Conceptualizing and measuring coping resources and processes. In L. Goldberger & S. Breznitz (Eds.), *Handbook of stress*. New York: Free Press/Macmillan.

Moos, H., & Susman, E. (1980). Longitudinal study of personality development. In O. G. Brim, Jr., & J. Kagan (Eds.), *Constancy and change in human development*. Cambridge, MA: Harvard University Press.

Munnichs, J. (1966). *Old age and finitude: A contribution to psychogerontology*. New York: Karger.

Moriarty, A., & Toussieng, P. (1976). *Adolescent coping*. New York: Grune & Stratton.

Murphy, L. B. (1960a). The child's way of coping: A longitudinal study of normal children. *Bulletin of the Menninger Clinic, 24*, 136–143.

Murphy, L. B. (1960b). Coping devices and defense mechanisms in relation to autonomous ego functions. *Bulletin of the Menninger Clinic, 24*, 144–153.

Murphy, L. B. (1962). *The widening world of childhood*. New York: Basic Books.

Murphy, L. B. (1970). The problem of defense and the concept of coping. In E. J. Anthony & C. Koupernik (Eds.), *The child in his family: The impact of disease and death* (International yearbook, Vol. 2). New York: Wiley.

Murphy, L. B. (1974). Coping, vulnerability, and resilience in childhood. In G. V. Coelho, D. Hamburg, & J. Adams (Eds.), *Coping and adaptation*. New York: Basic Books.

Murphy, L. B. (1982). *Robin: Comprehensive treatment of a vulnerable adolescent*. New York: Basic Books.

Murphy, L. B., & Moriarty, A. (1976). *Vulnerability, coping and growth: From infancy to adolescence*. New Haven, CT: Yale University Press.

Murray, H., & Associates (1938). *Explorations in personality*. New York: Oxford University Press.

Neugarten, B. (1969). Continuities and discontinuities of psychological issues into adult life. *Human Development, 12*, 121–130.

Neugarten, B. (1979). Time, age and the life-cycle. *American Journal of Psychiatry, 136*, 887–894.

Neugarten, B., & Hagestad, G. (1976). Aging and the life-course. In R. Binstock & E. Shanas (Eds.), *Handbook of aging and the social sciences*. New York: Van Nostrand Reinhold.

Neugarten, B., & Hagestad, G. (1985). In E. Shanas (Ed.), *Handbook of aging and the social sciences* (rev. ed.). New York: Van Nostrand Reinhold.

Neugarten, B., Moore, J., & Lowe, J. (1965). Age norms, age constraints, and adult socialization. *American Journal of Sociology, 70*, 710–717.

Neugebauer, B. (1981). The reliability of life-event reports. In B. S. Dohrenwend & B. P. Dohrenwend (Eds.), *Stressful life events and their contexts.* New York: Neale Watson/Prodist.

Neugebauer, B., Dohrenwend, B. P., & Dohrenwend, B. S. (1980). Formulation of hypotheses about the true prevalence of functional psychiatric disorders among adults in the United States. In B. P. Dohrenwend, B. S. Dohrenwend, M. S. Gould, B. Link, R. Neugebauer, & R. Wunsch-Hitzig (Eds.), *Mental disorders in the United States: Epidemiological estimates.* New York: Praeger.

Novak, M., & Harlow, H. (1975). Social recovery of monkeys isolated for the first year: I. Rehabilitation and therapy. *Developmental Psychology, 11*, 453–465.

Novey, S. (1968). *The second look: The reconstruction of personal history in psychiatry and psychoanalysis.* Baltimore: Johns Hopkins University Press.

Nunberg, H. (1932). *Principles of psychoanalysis: Their application to the neuroses* (M. Kahr & S. Kahr, Trans.) New York: International Universities Press, 1965.

Ogbu, J. (1981). Origins of human competence: A cultural–ecological perspective. *Child Development, 52*, 413–429.

O'Malley, J. M. (1977). Research perspective on social competence. *Merrill–Palmer Quarterly, 23*, 29–44.

Paykel, E., Prusoff, B., & Uhlenhuth, E. (1972). Scaling of life events. *Archives of General Psychiatry, 25*, 340–347.

Paykel, E., & Uhlenhuth, E. (1972). Rating the magnitude of life stress. *Canadian Psychiatric Association Journal, 17*, SS93–SS100.

Pearlin, L. (1975). Sex roles and depression. In N. Datan & L. Ginsberg (Eds.), *Life-span developmental psychology: Normative life crises.* New York: Academic Press.

Pearlin, L. (1980). The life-cycle and life strains. In H. Blalock, Jr. (Ed.), *Sociological theory and research.* New York: Free Press/Macmillan.

Pearlin, L. (1982). The social contexts of stress. In L. Goldberger & S. Breznitz (Eds.), *Handbook of stress.* New York: Free Press/Macmillan.

Pearlin, L. (1983). Role strains and personal stress. In H. B. Kaplan (Ed.), *Psychosocial stress: Trends in theory and research.* New York: Academic Press.

Pearlin, L., & Lieberman, M. (1979). Social sources of emotional distress. In R. Simmons (Ed.), *Research in community and mental health* (Vol. 1). Greenwich, CT: JAI Press.

Pearlin, L., Lieberman, M., Menaghan, E., & Mullan, J. (1981). The stress process. *Journal of Health and Social Behavior, 22*, 337–356.

Pearlin, L., & Schooler, C. (1978). The structure of coping. *Journal of Health and Social Behavior, 19*, 2–21.

Pellegrini, D. (1980). The social cognitive qualities of stress-resistant children (Doctoral dissertation, University of Minnesota). *Dissertation Abstracts International, 41*, 1925B.

Peskin, H., & Livson, N. (1982). Uses of the past in adult psychological health. In D. Eichorn, J. Clausen, N. Haan, M. Honzik, & P. Mussen (Eds.), *Present and past in middle life.* New York: Academic Press.

Piaget, J. (1975). *The equilibration of cognitive structures: The central problem of cognitive development* (T. Brown & K. J. Thampy, Trans.). Chicago: University of Chicago Press.

Plath, D. (1980). Contours of consociation: Lessons from a Japanese narrative. In P. B. Baltes & O. G. Brim, Jr. (Eds.), *Life-span development and behavior* (Vol. 3). New York: Academic Press.

Pruchno, R., Blow, F., & Smyer, M. (1984). Life events and interdependent lives: Implications for research and intervention. *Human Development, 27*, 31–41.

Rapaport, D. (1951). *Organization and pathology of thought: Selected sources.* New York: Columbia University Press.

Rapaport, D., & Gill, M. (1959). The points of view and assumptions of metapsychology. In M. M. Gill (Ed.), *The collected papers of David Rapaport.* New York: Basic Books, 1967.

Reese, H., & Smyer, M. (1983). The dimensionalization of life events. In N. Datan (Ed.), *Life span developmental psychology: Nonnormative life events.* New York: Academic Press.

Reich, W. (1933). *Character analysis* (T. P. Wolfe, Trans.). New York: Farrar, Strauss & Cudahy, 1945.

Reichsmann, F. (1977). An example of psychophysiologic research. In R. Simons & H. Parades (Eds.), *Understanding human behavior in health and disease.* Baltimore: Williams & Wilkins.

Ricks, D. (1980). A model for promoting competence and coping in adolescents and young adults. In L. A. Bond & J. C. Rosen (Eds.), *Competence and coping during adulthood.* Hanover, NH: University of Vermont Press/University Press of New England.

Ricoeur, P. (1977). The question of proof in Freud's psychoanalytic writings. *Journal of the American Psychoanalytic Association, 25,* 835–872.

Riegel, (1979). *Foundations or Dialectical Psychiatry.* New York: Academic Press.

Robertson, J. (1970). *Young children in the hospital* (2nd ed. with postscript). London: Tavistock.

Robertson, J. (no date). *The impact of temporary separation upon a two year old.* Chicago: Gittelson Film Library, The Institute for Psychoanalysis.

Rodnick, E., & Goldstein, M. (1974). Premorbid adjustment and the recovery of mothering function in acute schizophrenic women. *Journal of Abnormal Psychology, 83,* 623–628.

Rolf, J. (1976). Peer status and the directionality of symptomatic behavior: Prime social competence predictors of outcome for vulnerable children. *American Journal of Orthopsychiatry, 46,* 74–88.

Rosen, B., Klein, D., Levenstein, S., & Shahinian, S. (1969). Social competence and post-hospital outcome among schizophrenic and non-schizophrenic psychiatric patients. *Journal of Abnormal Psychology, 74,* 401–404.

Rosenthal, D. (1970). *Genetics of psychopathology.* New York: McGraw-Hill.

Roth, J. (1963). *Timetables: Structuring the passage of time in hospital treatment and other careers.* Indianapolis, IN: Bobbs-Merrill.

Rutter, M. (1970). Sex differences in children's responses to family stress. In E. J. Anthony & C. Koupernik (Eds.), *The child in his family: The impact of disease and death* (International yearbook, Vol. 2). New York: Wiley.

Rutter, M. (1979a). Maternal deprivation, 1972–1978: New findings, new concepts, new approaches. *Child Development, 50,* 283–305.

Rutter, M. (1979b). Protective factors in children's responses to stress and disadvantage. In M. W. Kent & J. E. Rolf (Eds.), *Primary prevention of psychopathology: Vol. 3. Social competence in children.* Hanover, NH: University of Vermont Press/University Press of New England, 49–74.

Rutter, M. (1981a). *Maternal deprivation reassessed* (2nd ed.). Harmondsworth, England: Penguin Books.

Rutter, M. (1981b). Stress, coping and development: Some issues and some questions. In N. Garmezy & M. Rutter (Eds.), *Stress, coping and development in children.* New York: McGraw-Hill, 1983.

Rutter, M. (1984). Continuities and discontinuities in socioemotional development: Empirical and conceptual perspectives. In R. Emde & R. Harmon (Eds.), *Continuities and discontinuities in development.* New York: Plenum Press.

Rutter, M., & Garmezy, N. (1983). Developmental psychopathology. In E. M. Hethering-
    ton (Ed.), *Handbook of child psychology* (4th ed). New York: Wiley.
Sameroff, A., & Chandler, M. (1975). Reproductive risk and the continuum of caretaking
    casualty. In F. D. Horowitz, M. Hetherington, S. Scarr-Salapetek, & G. Siegel
    (Eds.), *Review of child development research* (Vol. 4). Chicago: University of Chicago
    Press.
Sameroff, A., Seifer, R., & Zax, M. (1982). Early development of children at risk for
    emotional disorder. *Monographs of the Society for Research in Child Development, 47*(7,
    Serial No. 199).
Sander, L. (1962). Issues in early mother–child interaction. *Journal of the American Academy of
    Child Psychiatry, 1*, 141–166.
Sander, L. (1976). Infant and caretaking environment: Investigation and conceptualiza-
    tion of adaptive behavior in a system of increasing complexity. In E. J. Anthony
    (Ed.), *Explorations in child psychiatry*. New York: Plenum.
Sander, L. (1983). To begin with: Reflections on ontogeny. In J. Lichtenberg & S. Kaplan
    (Eds.), *Reflections on self psychology*. Hillsdale, NJ: The Analytic Press/Erlbaum.
Sandler, J., & Rosenblatt, B. (1962). The concept of the representational world. *Psychoana-
    lytic Study of the Child, 17*, 128–145.
Schafer, R. (1981). *Narrative actions in psychoanalysis*. Worcester, MA: Clark University Press.
Schafer, R. (1983). *The analytic attitude*. New York: Basic Books.
Selye, H. (1956). *The stress of life*. New York: McGraw-Hill.
Semrad, E. (1967). The organization of ego defenses and object loss. In D. M. Moriarity
    (Ed.), *The loss of loved ones*. Springfield, IL: Charles C Thomas.
Semrad, E., Grinspoon, L., & Feinberg, S. (1973). Development of an ego profile scale.
    Archives of General Psychiatry, 28, 70–77.
Shure, M. (1981). Social competence as a problem solving skill. In J. D. Wine & M. D.
    Syme (Eds.), *Social competence*. New York: Guilford Press.
Silber, E., Hamburg, D., Coelho, G., Murphey, E., Rosenberg, M., & Pearlin L. (1961).
    Adaptive behavior in competent adolescents: Coping with the anticipation of
    college. *Archives of General Psychiatry, 5*, 354–365.
Skeels, H. M. (1966). Adult status of children from contrasting early life experiences: A
    follow-up study. *Monographs of the Society for Research in Child Development* (31, Serial
    No. 105).
Sorokin, P., & Merton, R. (1937). Social time: A methodological and functional analysis.
    American Sociological Review, 42, 615–629.
Sroufe, L. A. (1979). The coherence of individual development. *American Psychologist, 34*,
    834–841.
Sroufe, L. A., Fox, N., & Pancake, V. (1983). Attachment and dependency in developmen-
    tal perspective. *Child Development, 54*, 1615–1627.
Sroufe, L., & Rutter, M. (1984). The domain of developmental psychopathology. *Child
    Development, 55*, 17–29.
Stack, C. (1974). *All our kin: Strategies for survival in a black community*. New York: Harper
    Torchbooks.
Stern, G. (1970). *People in context: Measuring person–event congruence in education and industry*. New
    York: Wiley.
Stern, G., Stein, M., & Bloom, B. (1954). *Methods in personality assessment*. New York: Wiley.
Stone, L. (1954). The widening scope of indications for psychoanalysis. *Journal of the
    American Psychoanalytic Association, 2*, 567–594.
Stone, L. (1961). *The psychoanalytic situation: An examination of its development and essential nature*.
    New York: International Universities Press.
Sulloway, F. (1979). *Freud, biologist of the mind: Beyond the psychoanalytic legend*. New York: Basic
    Books.

ADVERSITY, RESILIENCE, AND THE STUDY OF LIVES   423

Swanson, G. (1961). Determinants of the individual's defenses against inner conflict: Review and reformulation. In J. G. Glidewell (Ed.), *Parental attitudes and child behavior*. Springfield, IL: Charles C Thomas.

Thoits, P. (1983). Dimensions of life events that influence psychological distress: An evaluation and synthesis of the literature. In H. B. Kaplan (Ed.), *Psychosocial stress: Trends in theory and research*. New York: Academic Press.

Thomas, A., & Chess, S. (1977). *Temperament and development*. New York: Brunner/Mazel.

Thomas, A., & Chess, S. (1984). Genesis and evolution of behavioral disorders from infancy to early adult life. *American Journal of Psychiatry, 141*, 1-9.

Thomas, A., Chess, S., Birch, H., & Korn, S. (1963). *Behavioral individuality in early childhood*. New York: New York University Press.

Tyler, F., & Gatz, M. (1977). Development of individual psychosocial competence in a high school setting. *Journal of Consulting and Clinical Psychology, 45*, 441-449.

Uhlenhuth, E., Lipman, R., Balter, M., & Stern, M. (1974). Symptom intensity and life stress in the city. *Archives of General Psychiatry, 31*, 759-764.

Vaillant, G. (1971). Theoretical hierarchy of adaptive ego mechanisms: A thirty year follow-up of 30 men selected for psychological health. *Archives of General Psychiatry, 24*, 107-118.

Vaillant, G. (1976). Natural history of male mental health: V. The relation of choice of ego mechanisms of defense to adult adjustment. *Archives of General Psychiatry, 33*, 535-545.

Vaillant, G. (1977). *Adaptation to life*. Boston: Little, Brown.

Vaillant, G., & McArthur, C. (1972). Natural history of male psychologic health: I. The adult life cycle from 18-50. *Seminars in Psychiatry, 4*, 415-427.

Van Putten, T., Crumpton, E., & Yale, C. (1976). Drug refusal in schizophrenia and the wish to be crazy. *Archives of General Psychiatry, 33*, 1443-1446.

Van Putten, T., May, P., Marder, S., & Wittman, L. (1981). Subjective response to antipsychotic drugs. *Archives of General Psychiatry, 38*, 187-190.

Viederman, M. (Reporter). (1979). Monica: A 25 year longitudinal study of the consequences of trauma in infancy. *Journal of the American Psychoanalytic Association, 27*, 107-126.

Waddington, C. (1957). *The strategy of the genes*. London: Allen & Unwin.

Waddington, C. (1966). *Principles of development and differentiation*. New York: Macmillan.

Wallach, M., Kogan, N. (1965). *Modes of thinking in young children: A study of the creativity-intelligence distinction*. New York: Holt, Rinehart & Winston.

Wallerstein, J., & Kelly, J. (1980). *Surviving the breakup: How children and parents cope with divorce*. New York: Basic Books.

Watt, N., Anthony, E. J., Wynne, L. C., & Rolf, J. (Eds.). (1984). *Children at risk for schizophrenia: A longitudinal perspective*. Cambridge, England: Cambridge University Press.

Watt, N., & Lubensky, A. (1976). Childhood roots of schizophrenia. *Journal of Consulting and Clinical Psychology, 44*, 363-375.

Watt, N., Stolorow, R., Lubensky, A., & McClelland, D. C. (1970). School adjustment and behavior of children hospitalized for schizophrenia as adults. *American Journal of Orthopsychiatry, 40*, 637-657.

Weber, M. (1906). *The Protestant ethic and the spirit of capitalism*. New York: Scribner's, 1955.

Wender, P. (1979). Nurture and psychopathology: Evidence from adoption studies. In J. Barett (Ed.), *Stress and mental disorder*. New York: Raven Press.

Werner, E., Bierman, J., & French, F. (1971). *The children of Kauai: A longitudinal study from the prenatal period to age ten*. Honolulu: University Press of Hawaii.

Werner, E., & Smith, R. (1977). *Kauai's children come of age*. Honolulu: University Press of Hawaii.

Werner, E., & Smith, R. (1982). *Vulnerable but invincible: A study of resilient children.* New York: McGraw-Hill.

Werner, H. (1940). *The comparative psychology of mental development* (2nd ed.). New York: Harper & Row.

Wertheim, E. (1978). Developmental genesis of human vulnerability: Conceptual re-evaluation. In E. J. Anthony, C. Koupernik, & C. Chiland (Eds.), *The child in his family: Vulnerable children* (International yearbook, Vol. 4). New York: Wiley.

White, B. L., & Watts, J. C. (1973). *Experience and environment* (Vol. 1). Englewood Cliffs, NJ: Prentice-Hall.

White, B. L., & Associates (1978). *Experience and environment* (Vol. 2). Englewood Cliffs, NJ: Prentice-Hall.

White, B. L., Kaban, B., & Attanucci, J. (1979). *The origins of human competence: The final report of the Harvard Preschool Project.* Lexington, MA: Lexington Books/D. C. Heath.

White, R. W. (1959). Motivation reconsidered: The concept of competence. *Psychological Review, 66,* 297–333.

White, R. W. (1960). Competence and the psychosexual stages. In M. Jones (Ed.), *Nebraska Symposium on Motivation.* Lincoln: University of Nebraska Press.

White, R. W. (1963). *Ego and reality in psychoanalytic theory: A proposal regarding independent ego energies* (Psychological Issues Monograph No. 11). New York: International Universities Press.

White, R. W. (1974). Strategies of adaptation: An attempt at systematic description. In G. V. Coelho, D. A. Hamburg, & J. E. Adams (Eds.), *Coping and adaptation.* New York: Basic Books.

Wine, J. D. (1981). From defect to competence models. In J. D. Wine and M. D. Syme (Eds.), *Social competence.* New York: Guilford Press.

Winnicott, D. W. (1951). Transitional objects and transitional phenomena. In *Collected papers.* New York: Basic Books, 1958.

Winnicott, D. W. (1960). The theory of the parent–infant relationship. *International Journal of Psycho-Analysis, 41,* 585–595.

Winterbottom, M. (1958). The relation of need for achievement to learning experiences in independence and mastery. In J. W. Atkinson (Ed.), *Motives in fantasy, action, and society.* New York: Van Nostrand Reinhold.

Witkin, H. A., Dyk, R. B., Faterson, H. F., Goodenough, D. R., & Karp, S. (1962). *Psychological differentiation.* New York: Wiley.

Witkin, H. A., Lewis, H. B., Machover, K., Meissner, P. B., & Wapner, S. (1954). *Personality through perception: An experimental and clinical study.* New York: Harper & Row.

Wrubel, J., Benner, P., & Lazarus, R. (1981). Social competence from the perspective of stress and coping. In J. D. Wine & M. D. Syme (Eds.), *Social competence.* New York: Guilford Press.

Wynne, L. (1981). Current concepts about schizophrenia and family relationships. *Journal of Nervous and Mental Disease, 169,* 82–89.

Wynne, L., Singer, M., Bartko, J., & Toohey, M. (1977). Schizophrenics and their families: Recent research on parental communication. In J. M. Tanner (Ed.), *Developments in psychiatric research.* London: Hodder & Stoughton.

Zeitlin, S. (1980). Assessing coping behavior. *American Journal of Orthopsychiatry, 50,* 139–146.

Zubin, J., & Spring, B. (1977). Vulnerability—a new view of schizophrenia. *Journal of Abnormal Psychology, 86,* 103–126.

Zubin, J., & Steinhauer, S. (1981). How to break the logjam in schizophrenia: A look beyond genetics. *Journal of Nervous and Mental Disease, 169,* 447–492.

Index

425